# VOLUME ONE
# KNOWLEDGE & COMPREHENSION OF SCIENCE

**James L. Flowers, M.D., M.P.H.**

# A COMPLETE PREPARATION FOR THE MCAT*

## *MEDICAL COLLEGE ADMISSION TEST

## *Fourth Edition*

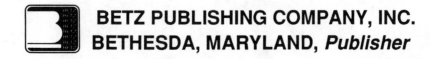

**BETZ PUBLISHING COMPANY, INC.**
**BETHESDA, MARYLAND,** *Publisher*

*A COMPLETE PREPARATION FOR THE MCAT* was originally published in 1978 as a one-volume work. The two-volume edition was published in 1981 and a revised two-volume edition was published in 1985.


Published since 1983 by:   BETZ Publishing Company, Inc.
P. O. Box 34631
Bethesda, Maryland 20817


FOURTH EDITION
*second printing*


Manufactured in the United States of America.


ISBN 0-941406-16-4 (volume 1)
ISBN 0-941406-15-6 (two-volume set)

# CONTENTS

**Chapter 3:    Review of General Chemistry**

**Chapter 4:    Review of Organic Chemistry**

# LIST OF FIGURES

## Chapter 3:    Review of General Chemistry

## Chapter 4:    Review of Organic Chemistry

**Chapter 5:    Review of Physics**

This book is dedicated to my parents,

especially my mother, Ozie,

and to other parents like them whose ambitions, dreams, and potentials may never be realized, but whose lives have been dedicated to seeing that their childrens' are.

It is also my privilege to acknowledge the special contributions of William C. Wallace, University of Illinois College of Medicine, formerly Director of the Harvard Health Careers Summer Program, Harvard School of Medicine, whose constant encouragement and support greatly enhanced this work, and also to acknowledge the Office of Health Resources Opportunity, Department of Health and Human Services, whose support gave incentive to this effort and helped assure its completion as a service to students who aspire to a career in medicine.

James L. Flowers, M.D., M.P.H

# PREFACE

Welcome to the fourth edition of *A Complete Preparation for the MCAT* by James L. Flowers, MD, MPH.

Now entering its tenth year of publication, the Flowers' Guide™ or Flowers' Manual™ as it is sometimes called was recognized early in its publication as a comprehensive preparation for the science knowledge subtest of the Medical College Admission Test. In 1981, reading and quantitative analysis sections were added in a second volume, and an essay writing module was added in 1985. The 1988 edition now includes material on *all* the MCAT subtests.

> **•*Volume 1--Knowledge and Comprehension of Science*:**
> Biology, general chemistry, organic chemistry, and physics. Format includes text for review, questions and answers for mastery of content, discussion of answers, and vocabulary and concepts checklists. In the 1988 edition, drawings have been added, physics and biology expanded, and a few short sections included for the purpose of gaining familiarity with the data and vocabulary of some current topics in science and medicine as they pertain to the MCAT.

Volume 1 remains more comprehensive than most first-year biology review courses, and it helps MCAT candidates to select review material from first-year chemistry and physics course topics that may be covered in the MCAT.

> **•*Volume 2--Skills Development for the Medical College Admission Test:***
> The change to a more generalized title reflects several new sections added to the 1988 edition of this volume. The new chapter "Introduction to Science Problems" includes a glossary of mathematics and science definitions. Writing and the reading chapter have been augmented, including new reading passages and questions; the quantitative analysis section is strengthened with the addition of advanced material written to test stamina and speed; and a review of high-speed math techniques is now included.

Volume 2 provides instruction in writing, analytical reading skills, and practice with reading passages similar to those in the MCAT. It provides content material needed for an understanding of the mathematics and quantitative procedures that are essential to a complete preparation for the MCAT, as well as practice in reasoning skills for the MCAT *Science Problems* Subtest.

*A Complete Preparation for the MCAT* also provides abundant review material for DAT, GRE, and CLEP exams in science and mathematics.

In addition to the original science text by Dr. Flowers, authors Angelica Braestrup and Aftab Hassan, who also served as senior technical editor on both volumes, have contributed their talent over the years to the final form of this 1988 edition. In closing, we also extend our thanks to Karen Aronson and Eric Jackson, whose new drawings now enhance this study guide.

*Chapter 1:*

# Introduction

# to

# Science

# Knowledge

## 1.1 THE ROLE OF THE MCAT IN THE ADMISSION PROCESS

The Medical College Admission Test is a standardized test designed to measure knowledge and cognitive skills important for medical education. An objective measure, MCAT scores can be reviewed and compared rapidly to more lengthy recommendations and the personal interview.

There is a positive correlation between MCAT scores (especially the science subtest) and success in the basic sciences (or preclinical phase of medical school), although numerous studies have shown no correlation between MCAT scores and success in the clinical phase of medical school or competence as a practicing physician. Nevertheless, most medical colleges have used and will continue to use this device as an entrance requirement because of the important information about candidates that it provides to admissions committees.

As mentioned above, the MCAT is only one part of the complex requirements and considerations inherent in the process of admission to medical school. Grade point average (and science GPA), letters of evaluation, major, quality of undergraduate education, work record, health related work experience, extracurricular activities, and research, in addition to the personal interview, personality and other non-cognitive factors, all play an important role. Attention should not be paid to the MCAT review to the exclusion of these and other important measures.

Books, guides, and pamphlets on the process of admission to medical school are available, including several from this publisher. Consult Betz Publishing's booklist, your campus bookstore, premedical advisor or premedical association, and obtain a premedical admissions planning manual to use as a supplement to your appointments with your premedical advisor.

## 1.2 STRUCTURE OF THE MCAT

The following information is to be found in *The MCAT Student Manual* (AAMC, 1984), which may be purchased from our booklist or obtained directly from:

> Association of American Medical Colleges
> One Dupont Circle NW
> Washington, D.C. 20036

The AAMC also makes an MCAT interpretive studies series available to educators. Information about registration, on the other hand, should be obtainable from your premedical advisor or from:

> MCAT Registration
> The American College Testing Program
> P.O. Box 414
> Iowa City, Iowa 52243

The MCAT is a day-long test divided into a morning session and an afternoon session (see Fig. 1.1). The morning session includes: Science Knowledge Subtest, Science Problems Subtest, and a written essay (although the essay may also be given after lunch, as reported by MCAT examinees from some states). The afternoon session includes the Skills Analysis: Reading Subtest and the Skills Analysis: Quantitative Subtest.

The Science Knowledge Subtest involves separate tests of approximately 40 questions each in biology, chemistry (general and organic), and physics. These questions are directed both to the content of your knowledge in the stated subject areas and to your understanding of the principles at the core of this knowledge. The Science Problems Subtest consists of approximately 60 questions. The questions apply the knowledge and principles learned in biology, chemistry, and physics to specific examples that are presented in short paragraphs, as a chemical structure, as an experiment, or as a chart or graph. The questions on any one example may be drawn from any combination of the physical sciences. To reemphasize, the questions are direct applications to specific examples of what you have learned in physics, biology, and chemistry. You need no new knowledge to do this section, but only the science knowledge you have already learned, integrated with your reasoning skills.

Since April 1985 the MCAT has included an essay module. The essay was first included experimentally as a pilot project, but as of this writing indications are that it will remain in the test. (The 1984 edition of *The MCAT Student Manual*, current as of January 1988, includes no information on the essay portion of the exam).

The reading subtest and quantitative subtest each has 68 questions. The companion volume to the book you are using is entitled (*A Complete Preparation for the MCAT*) *Volume 2: Skills Development for the Medical College Admission Test*. Volume 2 provides thorough guidance to prepare students for these afternoon subtests. In the exam the reading test contains selections drawn from medical and health related topics, the natural sciences, and social science passages from psychology, history, anthropology, economics, and so forth. The questions test analytical comprehension of material presented in each selection and your ability to draw logical conclusions. These require no prior knowledge. The quantitative test presents information in the form of graphs, tables, charts, maps, and equations. Once again, you are required to interpret and draw valid conclusions. *The MCAT Student Manual* explores each of these subtests in detail and provides examples.

## 1.3 HOW TO PREPARE FOR THE MCAT IN HIGH SCHOOL AND COLLEGE

The MCAT *accentuates the importance of developing good reading and data interpretive skills*. These are skills that take a long time to acquire and cannot be crammed into a month or so of preparation. For this reason, what you do in college, in high school, and even before, will help prepare you for the MCAT (and the medical profession) as much as any review manual or review course. If you feel your reading/study/interpretive skills are weak and your school or college offers a course specifically directed at this, then take it. If you can select your own courses, select those courses that demand interpretive reading (such as literature, philosophy, or history courses). And select those science courses that require you to understand and apply principles and to interpret data, rather than those that demand only memorization.

Speed reading will not help you unless you are already getting the right answers. When you read newspapers, journals, magazines, or watch TV news shows, for example, force yourself to draw conclusions about what is being presented, interpret the graphs and charts, predict trends in data, and assay the limitations and errors present in the data or opinions. By constantly forcing yourself to do these types of things, the skills necessary to do well on the skills analysis subtests will be developed and sharpened.

By taking the required courses for admission into medical school, you will have covered most of the information on the Science Knowledge Subtest. The following courses are suggested in addition to the basic requirements (if you have the time to take them, they will not only make the test easier, but they will also ease the shock of med school):

| | |
|---|---|
| Preferred: | physiology, biochemistry, microbiology |
| Useful: | genetics, anatomy (of any type), embryology |
| Luxury: | human anatomy, histology |

But understand that these courses *are not needed* before you take the test if your basic biology, chemistry and physics preparations are adequate.

In addition to the above long-term preparations, short-term "crash" courses are available. MCAT review courses are useful, they do raise scores; they tend to be expensive, but provide motivation to follow through for those who need it. MCAT manuals other than the ones mentioned above vary in their effectiveness. Some have good questions, whereas others are nearly irrelevant. None, to date, provides a systematic review of topics as they are presented in *A Complete Preparation for the MCAT*, the workbook you are using. One book, *How to Prepare for the Medical College Admission Test* (Harcourt Brace Jovanovich, 1987) contains three high-quality MCAT test simulations that may be used as a supplement in that area. *The MCAT Student Manual* is a valuable adjunct mainly because it is written by the organization that administers the MCAT, but also because it provides sample tests that are probably as close to the real one as you will find. Review the material you find in this book and its companion *Volume 2* and follow up with practice exam experience from the "Student Manual" and "How to Prepare" to see how well you have learned the material covered.

## 1.4     RATIONALE AND STRUCTURE OF *VOLUME 1* AND *VOLUME 2*

The main purpose of *Volume 1: Knowledge and Comprehension of Science,* is to provide a concise and thorough review in preparation for the complete science knowledge and science problems subtests of the Medical College Admission Test. The Science Knowledge Subtest (biology, chemistry, and physics) and the Science Problems Subtest will be adequately prepared for by studying chapters 2, 3, 4 and 5 of *Volume 1.*

The main purpose of *Volume 2: Skills Development for the Medical College Admission Test,* is to provide instruction and practice in writing, analytical reading skills, and practice with reading passages similar to those in the MCAT. In addition, the content material in Volume 2 provides for an understanding of the mathematics and quantitative procedures that are essential to a complete preparation for the MCAT. A brief "workout" has also been included for additional practice in science problems.

The structure of both volumes is organized around topics or skills as presented in *The MCAT Student Manual*. The general structure of both volumes of *A Complete Preparation for the MCAT* is exemplified in the following discussion of *Volume 1.*

To prepare chapters 2 through 5 of *Volume 1*, the outline presented in *The MCAT Student Manual* was used as a guide. This material is presented in more or less the same order as it exists in the *Student Manual*. The actual content of any section in chapters 2 through 5 reflects the author's interpretation of what is relevant to the stated topic. This material should in no way be construed as the only material to be presented in the exam, nor should it be inferred that the exam at some other time will include all the material discussed herein.

It is assumed that students will have taken the appropriate premedical courses before attempting to review from this book. The author assumes that most students will have seen most (not necessarily all) of the material presented, so that studying this book will be a true *review*. Nevertheless, for information beyond the scope of the book, appropriate bibliographical information is included at the end of each chapter. It is possible that a student, who has not had a major science course, could use the material presented here as a primary review text, but this will require considerable time and effort. If used in a course to review for the MCAT, the book provides material essential to gaining a better and clearer picture of the scope of the test. The book may also be used along with the appropriate coursework as a text for a pre-course or prep course in any of the areas presented (such as Chapter 2: Review of Biology during a biology course), and for a variety of other similar purposes.

An important aspect of using *Volume 1* for MCAT review is the clear, simple and comprehensive sketches and schematic drawings of various physiologic systems and their fundamental operation. For extra practice, use them to construct your own science problems. ("What happens to the renal system if you suddenly ingest 200 ml of salt water through the digestive system?" "Compare the biological and chemical effects of drinking milk, mineral water, or black coffee on the digestive and/or nervous system.") A feature of using Volume 2 is the addition of the new "Science Problems Workout" section. As the name implies, a workout suggests daily practice as a means to improve problem-solving ability. Problem-solving methods, the special skills that can be acquired to solve problems, and ways to use them in conjunction with basic biology, chemistry, and physics knowledge, are given.

The numbering of sections in *Volume 1* is based on the following system: the last number in a series separated by decimal points represents a division of the number (or section) prior to it. The first number is also the chapter number. The second number is the major section within each chapter. The third number represents divisions or subsections within each of those sections, as in 3.2.5. (This series represents the fifth subsection of the second major section of the third chapter.) The value of this system is that it allows for an infinite number of divisions of any level (such as chapter or section) without running out of symbols or having to change symbols such as letters, numbers, or roman numerals.

Each of the major sections of any given chapter (as an example, Atomic Structure, 3.1) is subdivided in a stereotyped way. In 3.1.1. a review of the topic is presented. This, again, is the author's interpretation of the relevant material and it is presented in a way to give it maximum meaning yet simplicity of presentation for review. Many statements are given as facts without much explanatory material because students generally have covered this in their primary course. But difficult concepts and key concepts are usually presented in slightly greater detail to make comprehension easier. In 3.1.2. questions are given for review of the material discussed. These questions are arranged in a specific sequence. The first questions may be answered by rote and merely ask the student to recall what was read. Their purpose is to emphasize important facts that need to be remembered and to help assess comprehension. They will, in general, cover the whole section. The second group of questions is problematic in nature. Their purpose is to allow the student to apply principles or concepts discussed in the section, and they emphasize what the student should be able to do with the information presented. These questions should be treated as "mini" science-problems. Depending on the specific topic, the number of rote or problematic questions will vary. Some sections have no problematic questions.

Notice that rote questions are similar to the MCAT Science Knowledge Subtest questions and problematic questions are similar to those on the Science Problems Subtest. (Remember that *similar* means *like* not *identical*.) The questions are not as difficult as the questions on the actual test. The questions in this manual are intended to review the material presented and not to mimic a true test situation.

The third subsection, 3.1.3, lists all the answers to the questions given. The fourth subsection, 3.1.4, is a discussion of the answers to the questions. The rote questions are not discussed because they are explained in the section. The problematic questions, however, are discussed in detail. The fifth subsection, 3.1.5, is a vocabulary checklist. This is a listing of all the terminology you should try to master. The sixth subsection, 3.1.6, which may be combined with the fifth in some chapters, is a checklist of concepts and principles. It attempts to list the concepts you should understand and the types of problems you should be able to do. In summary, the structure of this book is designed to deliver a maximum of relevant information in a concise manner and to provide a means of learning it well.

## 1.5     SUGGESTIONS ON HOW TO USE *VOLUME 1* EFFECTIVELY

As explained previously, the book you are now using was written to a uniform format designed to maximize speed of review and learning. Use of the book may be approached in many different ways based upon this format. One way is simply to review it cover to cover if it is felt that a comprehensive review is required. But if a student feels confident in a given subject, or specific topic within that subject, it is reasonable to skim or even pass over it. This is done best by going over the checklists or questions before reading the narrative and deciding if complete study of the section is required.

This book can also be used along with the corresponding college course (for example, the physics chapter with a physics course). It should be observed that much less information is required for the MCAT than is required for the course. But the value of using the book is in knowing what to focus on for the test. Of course, do not focus on the MCAT to the point that grades are jeopardized and course perspective is lost.

If the explanation on a given topic is not adequate for your needs, refer to a general text for a more detailed explanation. Bibliographies are given at the end of each chapter as "References for Review."

Take notes as you study. You may want to refer to *Volume 2: Skills Development for the Medical College Admission Test* for a system and practice in notetaking. The page layout of this workbook is designed with notetaking in mind, as the right-hand column headings on each page of this chapter show. Also prepare your own index cards for key definitions and concepts to help you randomize your review.

## 1.6     PREPARATION FOR THE MCAT

It is important to reemphasize that the best background for taking the MCAT is good preparation in high school and college. But even if this is lacking, a well-planned review can improve your performance on the exam.

One way to prepare your MCAT review is to organize it into three phases. The first phase precedes the test by months and should be concerned with the work of hard study. The second phase may be the three- or four-week period before the test and should be concerned with a final systematic review and some relaxation. Taking the test is the third phase. A rough timetable covering these three areas should be established to suit your individual needs.

While the most common complaint of a premedical student is "where do I get the spare time to prepare for the MCAT," a good study schedule is one that lets you set priorities based on requirements. Strongly recommended for learning time management skills is an excellent book, *Plan for Success: Time Management for the Pre-Med Student*, written by Charles E. Kozoll. This book is published by the National Association of Advisors for the Health Professions, P.O. Box 5017, Station A, Champaign IL 61820, and may be purchased directly from them or from Betz Publishing Company.

### 1.6.1     Months/Weeks Before the Test Date

For the first phase, the following are important considerations:

1. Determine strengths and weaknesses by subject or sub-subject areas. If you are unsure of what they are, take a practice test to identify your strengths and weaknesses; some resources for practice tests are identified below (item 4).

2. Spend more time on weak subjects, but enough time should also be spent on strong subjects to keep them strong.

3. Taking your strengths and weaknesses into account, establish a loose timetable for a systematic and thorough review of the following:

— biology
— general chemistry
— organic chemistry
— physics
— preparation for essay
— reading problems
— quantitative problems

4. Build into your schedule time to take practice tests, for example:

— *The MCAT Student Manual* (AAMC)
— *PreMedical Achievement Test—PMAT* (Betz Publishing Company)
— *How to Prepare for the MCAT* (Harcourt Brace Jovanovich)

5. Approximate a timetable by estimating the number of sections of the manual that can be done each week and the total number of sections that need to be studied. For example, if you decide to do three sections per week for a total of 54 sections, you will require 18 weeks; time required for other activities must be added to this.

6. As the review progresses, make notes of questions and points in the section that must be reviewed again and plan the time to review them. For example, 4 weeks to review again what has already been studied.

7. During the semester the MCAT will be taken, register for a *reasonable* course load to allow time for review.

8. Course texts should be consulted for points that need additional discussion.

9. An example of a suggested timetable follows:

| | |
|---|---|
| — time to review 54 sections at a rate of 3 per week | 18 weeks |
| — time to practice skills from *Volume 2* (reading problems, quantitative material, and preparation for the essay) | 12 weeks |
| — time to study and take practice tests | 2 weeks |
| — time to review materials again | 4 weeks |
| Total preparation time: | 36 weeks |

## 1.6.2    Weeks/Days Before the Test Date

The second phase covers the weeks and days just prior to the test. Relaxation and last-minute reviews are indicated. Relaxation does not mean partying, however. It means sufficient rest and activity to keep anxiety and tension at a healthy level, since there is no way they can be eliminated. If a solid preparation has been made, there is no need for last-minute panic. Knowledge will not fade away so rapidly. To alleviate some anxiety, it may be useful to attempt unhurried, relaxed reviews of certain areas that are of special concern.

These reviews should not be at the expense of rest. The night before the test, a good night's sleep is essential. Drugs of any type should be avoided unless medically indicated. Also, the last week is a good time to take additional practice tests and review test-taking techniques and strategy. The checklists and notes made in the margins of this workbook are a valuable means of rapid review during this time, and relaxation tapes may reduce further stress.

During the last week, remember to keep on the MCAT schedule, that is, 8 a.m. to 6 p.m., and eat the various high-energy foods you like the most.

If possible, on a Saturday before the date of the MCAT, drive to the testing location at the same time as you will need to on the day the MCAT is given. Pay attention to route, traffic, parking, etc.

Prepare for the things you will take with you to the test: your watch, raisins or candy, 3 or 4 pencils, tissues, a sweater, and possibly a practice reading section. Many students find it helpful to do a practice reading set at the end of the lunch break so that when they start the Skills Analysis: Reading Subtest they are already warmed-up and focused.

### 1.6.3    Taking the Test

The third phase is the test itself. In the morning, eat a sustaining high-energy breakfast and get to the testing room in plenty of time to settle in.

Suggestions for during the test:

1. Take about 3 minutes to skim the total number of questions, and, briefly, their types. Look over the answer sheet to be certain of its format. From this, a little relief in tension may occur and an estimate of how fast to progress through the questions may be made.

2. Estimate what questions you should be working about one-quarter, one-half, and three-quarters through the time period, and when the "first pass" should be completed. Remember that time should be left available to go over missed answers. For example, suppose a section has 45 questions and the time limit is 30 minutes. The first pass through the test may require 20 minutes; therefore, by 10 minutes into the test 22-23 questions should be completed; the final 10 minutes (of the total 30 minutes) may be spent going over the more difficult questions that were skipped. The time allocation is highly individual and should be established through practice. Always use good guessing techniques on totally unfamiliar questions. **Do not leave any questions unanswered.**

3. During the first pass, all questions should be answered that are definitely known (greater than 80% certain) or definitely not known (greater than 80% unsure). There will be many answers that will be known immediately—answer and then forget them. Equally, learn to recognize questions that there is no chance of answering and spend no more than 5-10 seconds on each. These should be marked on the same letter each time so that the maximum probability of getting them right is obtained (either B or C is a good choice).

4. **No answer should be filled in on the answer sheet, on the first pass, that has any chance of being changed later.** The answer sheet should be used as a means of rapid assessment of those questions that need to be gone over. This also ensures that all questions are answered—which they should be. See items 3 and 5.

5. After spending approximately 30 seconds on any one question, it should be passed over and that space on the answer sheet left blank. If this much time is spent on a question, there should be some chance of getting it right. Consider all answer choices. If there are options that are definitely wrong, they should be crossed out. This means when the question is gone over again, time is not wasted on those options. Key objectives of this approach is enhancement of the probability of getting the question right and an increase in time efficiency in going over it a second time.

6. If arithmetic operations or problem solving questions pose particular difficulties, and these types of questions do not form a large part of the subtest, it is reasonable to go over the other questions first. Don't get bogged down on one problem because it seems like you should be able to solve it. Save this for last and go on to other questions. Set up arithmetic operations (adding, dividing, etc.) on scrap paper to be sure no stupid mistake is made in arithmetic after setting up the problem correctly.

7. Make sure the question is being answered as it is stated and that a different question has not been consciously or unconsciously imposed upon it. This requires constant, diligent checking by the test-taker.

8. There is no prize for finishing early. Take enough time to go through the test and stick to your planned strategies throughout.

9. One of the primary distinguishing characteristics of the poor test-taker is the tendency to misread the question. Read actively. Use your pencil to mark questions. Underline key words. Circle negative words or key qualifiers. Periodically make sure your mark on the answer sheet corresponds to the number of the question you are answering. Consider all answer choices.

10. Just before the test or during breaks, make sure physiological needs are satisfied. Time lost during the test for bladder, bowel, hunger or thirst is unfortunate.

11. During lunch break, do not talk to other test-takers about the test.

### 1.6.4    Study and Test-taking Strategies

The points recommended for the day of the test should also be practiced during your review of the workbook sections. Set time limits and practice them as you prepare for the test day. Since the test is long, you want to do everything possible to optimize your time and energy resources, so included here are a few more study and test-taking suggestions you may want to consider as you plan your overall MCAT preparation.

While preparing for the MCAT, and insofar as your schedule permits, keep to the "MCAT day." If you regularly go to bed at 3 a.m. and rise at noon, changing your schedule at the last minute to start the MCAT at 8:30 a.m. and finish at 5:30 p.m. will not be easy.

When working science problems, do only 10 or so random questions at a time. (When analyzing your errors, you need to be able to remember the reasoning pattern you used as you worked the incorrect problem. A first step in correcting errors is to identify accurately where your reasoning is wrong.)

Remember, on the actual test, the reading portion follows lunch, so you will have to decide what you should eat in the middle of the day to give you energy and not put you to sleep. The quantitative portion is even harder in this regard than reading, since it usually starts around 4:15 in the afternoon, for many people a "dead" time of day. Try to practice for the reading and quantitative subtests at the appropriate times of day whenever possible, so you can work out the best strategies for countering fatigue, drowsiness, boredom, etc. (You might even want to try practicing reading/quantitative skills late at night to see how you do at a time when you are tired.)

When you analyze your errors, use the Answers to Questions (sections ending in .3, the answer key) *first*. Only use the Discussion of Answers to Questions (sections ending in .4) as a last resort and if you really cannot figure out why the book's answer is better than your own.

Keep a written record of your errors, even if only by making a check mark next to the appropriate outline entry in *The MCAT Student Manual*. This "error journal" will help you to use your available study time most efficiently, since you will know where you need to review the most.

As a further guide to efficiency, find out which topics appear most frequently in the MCAT. For example, there are many genetics problems both in the biology knowledge section and in the biology questions of the science problem section. Therefore, you will need to review Mendelian genetics and the application of the Hardy-Weinberg principle with some care. Conversely, you do not need to take a course just so you can answer a single obscure question from a topic that appears only once.

Study at least one topic in each of the three sciences every day—even if you spend the bulk of your study time on one topic. Do not set a schedule that reserves a week for biology, a week for physics, a week for chemistry. Do not even schedule single days devoted to one subject. **Instead spend at least some time on each subject each day.** The reason: you need to put this basic information into your long-term memory, and the best long-term memory technique available is constant review. Remember to leave enough time to analyze your answers.

While you are studying, try to predict and design MCAT-type questions. Don't forget to think about what is false, or the exception, as well as memorizing what is true. This is especially important when the text provides a concept and one or two examples. It is also good practice to estimate reasonable answers. If you usually work with a calculator, you may find that making rapid, reasonable estimates requires some practice. (*Volume 2* now has a section called "High-Speed Math Techniques" that will help.) At any rate, stop using calculators well before the MCAT.

If possible, find someone to study with. Explaining difficult material to someone who knows it better is a good idea. When your study partner is having difficulty, you be the listener. It is the job of the critical listener to make sure that what the speaker says is accurate, complete, precise and to the point.

While studying, try to distinguish short-term memory tasks from long-term memory tasks. For example, learning the entire circulatory system is a long-term memory task. Really understanding what is going on at each step will help your memory. Drawing it as you explain it to another person will also help your memory.

Alternately, examples of short-term memory tasks include seldom-used physics equations, or a chart showing the similarities and differences (comparison/contrast) between smooth, skeletal, and cardiac muscle. During the last few days of your study time commit to your short-term memory what you have identified as short-term memory tasks.

Remember, certain principles are basic to the development of test-taking skills; console yourself with them:

1. Knowledge of the subject is fundamental; a good preparation will pay dividends.
2. There is a finite amount of time to answer a finite number of questions.
3. No one (repeat, *no one*) will answer all the questions right and no one will answer all the questions wrong.

## 1.7    CORRELATION OF *VOLUME 1* AND *VOLUME 2* CONTENT WITH THE ACTUAL MCAT

*The MCAT Student Manual* published by the Association of American Medical College does not yet (January 1988) reflect recent changes incorporated into the test in the science knowledge, science problems, and writing subtests. These changes are explained below in Fig. 1.1. Actual exam time exceeds 6 and a half hours (see below).

Questions on the sample MCAT in the manual were analyzed for the biology, physics, chemistry, and science problems subtests only. If a question on the sample test was found verbatim or nearly verbatim in this book, that question was labeled *direct*. If a question on the sample test could be answered directly from a concept or something explained in this book, then it was labeled *indirect*. A question in the sample MCAT that was not covered in this book was labeled *not in book*. However, many of these questions could be answered from information present in the question itself. Fig. 1.1 illustrates the correlation between the sample questions and the material covered in this book. The data in Fig. 1.1 mean that if this book is studied and all the information in it is correctly applied, an average of 80-90 percent of all questions on the actual MCAT could be answered.

## AAMC PRACTICE MCAT: SAMPLE TEST (6.5 hours)

| Subtest | Total No. Questions | No. Direct Questions | No. Indirect Questions | No. Questions Not in Book | % Covered in this edition of A COMPLETE PREP |
|---|---|---|---|---|---|
| Biology | 38 | 26 | 11 | 1 | 97.0 |
| Chemistry | 38 | 24 | 6 | 8 | 79.0 |
| Physics | 33 | 28 | 5 | 0 | 100.0 |
| Science Problems | 60 | 10 | 30 | — | 67.0 |

Percent covered ("% Covered") equals Number of Direct Questions plus Number of Indirect Questions, divided by Total Number of Questions, times 100; or, the sum of the questions (Direct plus Indirect) that can be answered correctly by studying this book, divided by the total questions, times 100.

## AAMC ACTUAL MCAT (6.8 hours)

| Subtest | No. of Questions | Time Allocated | Comments |
|---|---|---|---|
| Science Knowledge | | 115 min. | Total questions: 109 |
|   Biology | 38 | | |
|   Chemistry | 38 | | |
|   Physics | 33 | | |
| *Rest Period* | — | *10 min.* | — |
| Science Problems | 60 | 78 min. | Total sets: 20 (Biology 6, Chemistry 10, Physics 4) |
| Writing | 1 essay | 45 min. | May be given before or after lunch; check with proctor on day of exam. |
| *Lunch Break* | — | *60 min.* | — |
| Reading Skills | 68 | 85 min. | — |
| *Rest Period* | — | *10 min.* | — |
| Quantitative Skills | 68 | 85 min. | — |

Fig. 1.1—Correlation of This Book with "Sample Test" from
*The MCAT Student Manual*

*Chapter 2:*

# Review

# of

# Biology

## 2.1    ENZYMES

### 2.1.1    Review of Enzymes

Enzymes are the agents by which organisms make (anabolism) needed molecules, break down (catabolism) unneeded molecules, produce energy, and, in general, maintain homeostasis (e.g., by regulating entry and exit of molecules and ions). A key aspect of their function is that they can be regulated to function as needed.

The total enzyme (holoenzyme) may be composed of a protein (apoenzyme) part with or without an associated molecule called a *prosthetic group* (nonprotein organic molecule) also called a *cofactor or coenzyme* or a *metal ion*. The enzyme molecule *catalyzes* (by lowering the activation energy) chemical reactions at the conditions found in living organisms—conditions under which these reactions would not ordinarily occur. Note that the protein part passes through the reaction unchanged (like a true catalyst), but the prosthetic groups, etc., which function as donors or acceptors of chemical groups, may or may not pass through the reaction unchanged. Some enzymes exist as zymogens and need to be activated by the cleaving of certain peptide bonds. A portion of the molecule may or may not be lost, but a conformational change usually occurs to expose the active site of the enzyme. An example is the conversion of trypsinogen to trypsin by enterokinase.

A key feature of enzyme function is their *specificity*. This means that enzymes are able to recognize certain molecules and not others due to minor chemical differences between them. A microenvironment is created by the tertiary structure of the protein that creates distinctive requirements of spatial and electrical organization (distribution of positive/negative charges or polar groups) that a molecule must possess in order to be bound by the molecule. This microenvironment need not be rigid as in the lock (enzyme) and key (molecule or substrate) idea, but may be inducible in the enzyme by the substrate as in the "induced fit hypothesis." Specificity may be *absolute* (only one molecule acceptable to the enzyme) or *relative* (a series of molecules acceptable, but some more than others). Note that since enzyme reactions are reversible, an enzyme can still have absolute specificity by reacting with one molecule in one direction and with another molecule in the opposite direction. The bonding is of a non-covalent type (hydrogen, ionic, van der Waals, hydrophobic).

Another key aspect of enzyme function is the *active site* idea. The substrate (molecule) is bound as discussed under specificity above. The appropriate chemical reaction is then catalyzed by structures in this active site. Note that for a reaction to occur the molecule bound must be able to undergo the reaction catalyzable by the enzyme. It is doubtful that the active site functions by causing mechanical bond strain in appropriate bonds, such that they are broken and new ones are made. Rather, the active site has the appropriate side groups of the amino acids, appropriate prosthetic groups, etc., and a microenvironment all conducive to lowering the activation energy of the reaction. The combination required varies with the type of reaction being catalyzed. For example, a reaction that involves a hydrolysis reaction of an ester may have serine (with its $-OH$ group) to displace the alcoholic part of the ester, aspartic acid (with its $-CO_2H$) and/or histidine (acts as acid or base) for acid-base catalysis, and a hydrophilic microenvironment (versus a hydrophobic one) because ions are produced during the reaction.

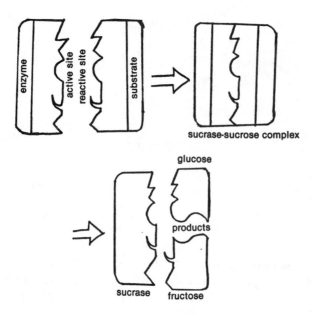

*Fig. 2.1—Enzyme and Substrate Model*
*(two parts of a jigsaw puzzle)*

In 1958, the induced fit theory was introduced. This theory states that the active site of an enzyme must adjust to fit the reactive site of the substrate. As the enzyme and the substrate join, the enzyme may change slightly in shape to fit the substrate better.

In both the lock and key hypothesis and the induced fit theory, a specific interaction occurs between the enzyme's active site and the substrate's reactive site. During the interaction, the enzyme and the substrate are joined by weak chemical bonds that are made and broken easily. Look at the equation for the breakdown of sucrose by sucrase, shown below:

$$\text{sucrase} + \text{sucrose} \rightarrow \text{sucrase-sucrose complex} \rightarrow$$
$$\text{sucrase} + \text{glucose} + \text{fructose}$$
$$\text{enzyme} + \text{substrate} \rightarrow \text{enzyme} - \text{substrate complex} \rightarrow$$
$$\text{enzyme} + \text{product.}$$

Enzymes are controlled in a number of ways. *Feedback inhibition* (FI) is a basic and effective method of enzyme control. In FI, the product of the enzyme reaction feeds back and blocks the enzyme from converting more substrate to product. In this manner, excessive product is not produced. Similarly, when the product is present in low amounts, there is no enzyme inhibition and the enzyme can convert substrate to product. Graphically:

Enzyme Reaction:     Substrate (S) $\xrightarrow{\text{Enzyme (E)}}$ Product (P)

Excess Product:
(1) Excess product present: S $\xrightarrow{E}$ P
(2) Enzyme binds product: E $\cdots\cdots$ P
(3) Reaction is blocked: S $\overset{E}{\cdots\blacktriangleright}$ P

Insufficient Product:
(1) Low amounts of product: S $\xrightarrow{E}$ P
(2) Enzyme does not bind product
(3) Reaction proceeds: S $\xrightarrow{E}$ P

## Names of Enzymes

Enzymes are usually named for the reaction they cause or for their substrate. A substrate is the substance upon which the enzyme acts. Most enzyme names end in the letters -ase. The enzyme sucrase is named for the substrate sucrose. Some enzymes are named for the reaction they cause and their substrate, such as the enzyme DNA polymerase, which helps make the molecules of DNA.

Enzymes that were named before the late nineteenth century do not have the -ase ending. Some of these names are still used today, such as pepsin and trypsin. These two enzymes break down proteins in the digestive system.

*Enzyme Cofactors or Coenzymes*

Many enzymes are made up of protein and a nonprotein part. A nonprotein molecule found in some enzymes is called a coenzyme. Coenzymes are organic molecules that work with enzymes. A coenzyme bonds weakly to the protein part of an enzyme, and can join and leave it easily. Coenzymes are needed for certain chemical reactions to take place.

Some coenzymes are made of vitamins or their parts. Organisms cannot make most vitamins and must take them in as part of their food. If vitamins are lacking, certain coenzymes cannot be made and the organism's metabolism does not function normally.

## 2.1.2    Questions to Review Enzymes

(1)    Enzymes probably play a direct role in all of the following except:

(a) maintenance of resting membrane potential by extrusion of $Na^+$ from cells
(b) synthesis of mRNA from DNA
(c) storage of hereditary information
(d) production of ATP

(2)    Since enzymes are proteins, they are affected by the same factors that affect proteins. An enzyme is "designed" to function under a certain set of conditions. Which of the following conditions would be most conducive to the normal function of a human cellular enzyme?

(a) Temperature = $25\,^\circ C$
(b) Temperature = $37\,^\circ C$
(c) pH = 1.0
(d) pH = 10.0

(3)    $NAD^+$ is a non-covalently bound coenzyme for the enzyme $\alpha$-glycerol-phosphate dehydrogenase. $NAD^+$ picks up an $H^{-1}$ (hydride) and becomes NADH; the enzyme is not affected by the reaction. The activation energy was lowered by the system.

(a) This is not true catalysis because the $NAD^+$ was changed in the reaction.
(b) This is true catalysis because the $NAD^+$ was not covalently bound to the enzyme.
(c) This is true catalysis because the activation energy of the reaction was lowered by the enzyme which was unchanged in the reaction.
(d) None of the above.

(4)    Succinate dehydrogenase catalyzes the following reaction:

$$succinate \rightleftharpoons fumarate.$$

This is the only reaction it catalyzes.

(a) The specificity of the enzyme is relative because it binds more than one substrate.
(b) The specificity of the enzyme is absolute because it catalyzes only one reaction of one pair of substrates.
(c) The specificity of the enzyme is absolute because it has only one substrate, succinate.
(d) None of the above.

(5) D-amino acid oxidase catalyzes the following reaction:

$$\begin{array}{c} (1)\ (2) \\ R\text{-CH-CO}_2H + \frac{1}{2}\ O_2 \longrightarrow R\text{-C-CO}_2H + R'NH_2. \\ | \qquad\qquad\qquad\qquad \| \\ HNR' \qquad\qquad\qquad\quad O \end{array}$$

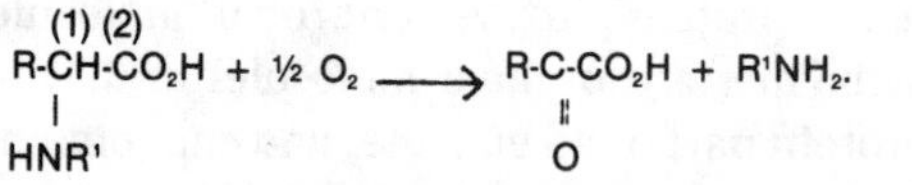

Following are some relative rates of reaction of various substrates with this enzyme.

| Substrate | Relative Rate | R | R' |
|---|---|---|---|
| D-Tyrosine | 13.6 | 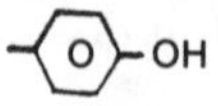 ⬡—OH | H |
| D-Alanine | 4.6 | -CH₃ | H |
| D-Isoleucine | 1.6 | -C-CH₂-CH₃ (CH₃) | H |
| D-Leucine | 1.0 | -CH₂-CH(CH₃)(CH₃) | H |
| L-Tyrosine | 0 | 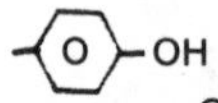 ⬡—OH | H |
| L-Leucine | 0 | -CH₂-CH(CH₃)(CH₃) | H |
| D-Leucylalanyltyrosine | 0 | 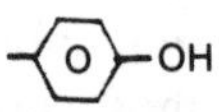 ⬡—OH | 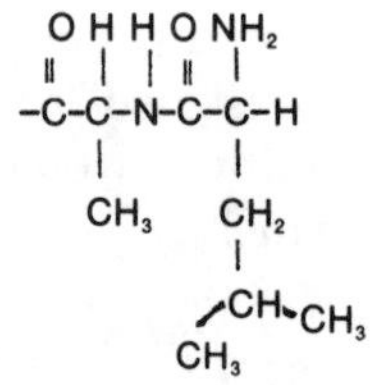 (peptide) |

The above information implies that

(a) the specificity of D-amino acid oxidase is absolute because D-tyrosine has a much higher rate of reaction than other substrates
(b) the configuration of carbon #1 is not important for the reaction to occur
(c) from the data given, the group at R has more effect on the outcome of the reaction than the group at $R^1$
(d) the specificity of the enzyme is relative because several molecules may react with the enzyme

(6) Enzymes usually combine readily with substrates in order for a reaction to occur. When the reaction is over, the product (derived from the substrate) usually readily dissociates from the enzyme. This is in spite of only minor changes in the substrate. A reason for this might be (the best of those given):

(a) Although the site of attachment for the substrate has not changed, the overall conformation of the enzyme may be made unfavorable to the product by the reaction.
(b) Minor differences in spatial or electrical organization of a molecule are all that are required to make a molecule unacceptable to the enzyme.
(c) The enzyme is forced into an unnatural conformation and this causes it to forceably expel the product.
(d) The substrate is covalently bound to the enzyme because of the enzyme's specificity, whereas the product is not.

(7) Malonate blocks (inhibits) the catalysis of the following reaction by succinate dehydrogenase:

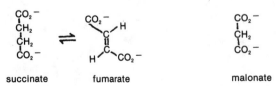

succinate     fumarate     malonate

Diethyl malonate will not block the reaction. Nor will the diethyl esters of succinate or fumarate undergo the reaction. The above information implies that

(I)   inhibition of the enzyme may be brought about by molecules that resemble the substrate but cannot undergo the reaction

(II)  the active site of the enzyme may contain positive ions or at least require the presence of $- CO_2^-$ on the substrate

(III) monoethyl malonate will not inhibit the reaction

(a) (I) only
(b) (II) and (III) only
(c) (I) and (II) only
(d) all are implied by the data

## 2.1.3    Answers to Questions in Section 2.1.2

(1) c    (2) b    (3) c    (4) b    (5) d    (6) b    (7) c

## 2.1.4    Discussion of Answers to Questions in Section 2.1.2

*Question #1* (Answer: c) The storage of hereditary information is a function of DNA, enzymes play no direct role in this. All of the other processes require direct involvement of enzymes.

*Question #2* (Answer: b) The function of a cellular enzyme should be maximal at those conditions found in the internal milieu of a cell or a particular compartment of a cell. This would generally be conditions similar to the whole organism. The temperature of 37°C is the normal human body temperature and the normal pH of blood is 7.40. The other conditions are extreme, but there are enzymes that can function at or near most of these—some in the human, some not.

*Question #3* (Answer: c) True catalysis occurs when the activation energy is lowered and this lowering is accomplished by the enzyme's active site environment. Coenzymes serve the accessory function of transferring chemical groups.

*Question #4* (Answer: b) Nearly all enzymatic reactions are truly reversible. The product occupies the same site occupied by the substrate, so the enzyme can recognize it, and the substrate-product can be considered as a pair.

*Question #5* (Answer: d) The relative specificity of the enzyme should be clear from the several different substrates undergoing the reaction. A case might be made for the "absolute" specificity for D-amino acids which is supported by the data. The configuration of carbon #1 is essential to the reactivity of the substrate because this is the carbon about which the *D* or *L* configuration is determined (see $\alpha$-amino acids in Section 4.13.1). The *R* group represents the side chains of the various amino acids, if the configuration is D at the $\alpha$-carbon (#1 in diagram), the reaction can still occur although variable. The $R^1$ could represent a second amino acid (or more), as in D-leucylalanyltyrosine, which does not react at all. Hence, with the limited information given, the presence of a group (other than H) appears critical in the reaction.

*Question #6* (Answer: b) Although the other options may sound reasonable, the simplest reason is as in (b) which serves to emphasize that only small differences in substrate structure can affect enzyme recognition and reaction.

*Question #7* (Answer: c) The structures not given are

$O = \overset{|}{\underset{|}{C}}\text{-O-CH}_2\text{-CH}_3$
$\overset{|}{\text{CH}_2}$
$O = \overset{|}{C}\text{-O-CH}_2\text{CH}_3$
Diethyl malonate

$O = \overset{|}{\underset{|}{C}}\text{-OCH}_2\text{CH}_3$
$\overset{|}{\text{CH}_2}$
$\overset{|}{\text{CH}_2}$
$O = \overset{|}{C}\text{-OCH}_2\text{CH}_3$
Diethyl succinate

$O \approx \overset{|}{\underset{|}{C}}\text{-O}^-$
$\overset{|}{\text{CH}_2}$
$O = \overset{|}{C}\text{-O-CH}_2\text{CH}_3$
Monoethyl malonate

$\text{CH}_3\text{CH}_2\text{O-C} \overset{\nearrow O}{\underset{\diagdown}{}} \overset{\diagup H}{C}$
$H \overset{\diagup}{\underset{\diagdown}{C}} \text{-OCH}_2\text{CH}_3$
$\overset{\|}{O}$
Diethyl fumarate

Statement (I) is reasonable given that malonate and succinate are similar and since specificity is based upon similarity in structure. Also this reactions requires the group,

$$\overset{\diagdown}{\underset{\diagup}{\text{CH}_2}} \quad \longrightarrow \quad \overset{\diagdown}{\underset{\diagup}{\text{CH}}} \; + \; H^+, H:^{\ominus}$$

for the reaction to occur and malonate does not have this. So, malonate will bind at the active site and block succinate; but it will just sit there and not react. It appears that only molecules with two (or one?) $-CO_2^-$ (which is negative) are attracted to the active site. There is no evidence one way or the other about a molecule with one $-CO_2^-$ and one $-CO_2CH_2CH_3$.

## 2.1.5    Vocabulary Checklist for Enzymes

_____ anabolism
_____ catabolism
_____ holoenzyme
_____ apoenzyme

_____ prosthetic group
_____ cofactor
_____ coenzyme
_____ catalysis

## 2.1.6    Concepts, Principles, etc. Checklist for Enzymes

_____ general role of enzymes
_____ specificity of enzymes
_____ Active Site Concept
_____ feedback inhibition

_____ induced fit theory
_____ maltase
_____ amylase
_____ trypsin

## 2.2    BIOENERGETICS

### 2.2.1    Review of Bioenergetics

Energy production involves the step-wise degradation of organic molecules *from more reduced to more oxidized states* (reduced means abundance of hydrogen atoms and lack of, or few, oxygen atoms). The process may be *aerobic* (in the presence of oxygen) or *anaerobic* (without the presence of oxygen). *Fermentation* is a type of anaerobic respiration where the final acceptor of electrons is an organic molecule. In aerobic respiration, $O_2$ is the final acceptor of electrons producing $H_2O$ (fate of hydrogens in organic molecules being oxidized) and $CO_2$ is also produced (the fate of carbon). (See Section 2.11.1 for the fate of nitrogen.)

Key organic molecules in energy production are:

(1) *ATP* (adenosine triphosphate). The bonds between the phosphates are high energy $(P \sim P)$, and when hydrolyzed (split by adding water), this energy (about 7-8 kcals/mole) is released. ATP is the main short term energy storage molecule.

(2) *NAD$^+$ and NADP$^+$* (nicotinamide adenine dinucleotide and nicotinamide adenine dinucleotide phosphate). These carry two electrons and one hydrogen to form, respectively, NADH and NADPH. NADH transfers its electrons to the electron transport system. NADPH is used for synthetic purposes and is the major product of the Pentose Shunt in which glucose-6-phosphate dehydrogenase is a key enzyme. Niacin is a part of NAD$^+$ and NADP$^+$.

(3) *FAD* (Flavin adenine dinucleotide). FAD carries two electrons and two hydrogens as FADH$_2$ to the electron transport chain. Its most important role is in the breakdown of fatty acids. Riboflavin is a component of FAD.

(4) *Cytochromes* (b, c, a). They transfer electrons (which are attached to iron) and they are part of the electron transport chain. The iron is in a porphyrin ring (together called heme) which is bound by a protein.

The *four key processes* of energy production are glycolysis, the citric acid cycle (Kreb's cycle, Tricarboxylic Acid Cycle or TCA cycle), the electron transport system (ETS), and oxidative phosphorylation. *Glycolysis* (Fig. 2.2) takes glucose (C$_6$) and converts it to two pyruvates (C$_3$). This produces 2ATPs and 2NADHs. If no oxygen is around, the NADH converts pyruvate to lactic acid (as in exercise) which may be converted to alcohol (as in a type of fermentation). The latter process (to pyruvate) is *anaerobic glycolysis*. In the presence of oxygen, the pyruvate (C$_3$) is converted to acetyl CoA (C$_2$) and CO$_2$ with 2NADHs produced per original glucose. CoA (Coenzyme A) is an acyl carrier and the vitamin pantothenic acid is a key component. Acetyl CoA may also arise from fatty acid and amino acid breakdown. The acetyl CoA (C$_2$) enters the *citric acid cycle* (Fig. 2.3) by combining with oxaloacetic acid (C$_4$) to form citrate (C$_6$). This is degraded step-wise to oxaloacetic acid again producing 3NADHs, 1FADH$_2$, and 1ATP (from GTP) for each cycle (must double to get production per original glucose) as well as CO$_2$ and H$_2$O. The NADH and FADH$_2$ enter the *ETS* in this sequence:

$$\overset{(1)}{\text{NAD}} \rightarrow \overset{\hspace{3.5cm}(2)}{\text{FAD} \rightarrow \text{ubiquinone (CoQ)} \rightarrow \text{Cyt b} \rightarrow \text{Cyt c} \rightarrow} \overset{(3)}{\text{Cyt a} \rightarrow \text{O}_2}$$

Each intermediate is first reduced (receives electrons from) by the preceding and oxidized (gives electrons to) by the following, with oxygen as the final acceptor being converted to water. ATPs are produced at 1, 2, and 3 by the process called *oxidative phosphorylation*. Each NADH produces 3ATPs and each FADH$_2$ produces 2ATPs. Malonate is a potent inhibitor of the citric acid cycle. Cyanide is a potent inhibitor of the ETS at Cyt a. An exception is the NAHD produced outside the mitochondria from glycolysis. The electrons of NADH are transported by a shuttle to ubiquinone and only 2ATPs per NADH (of glycolysis) are produced.

*Anaerobic glycolysis* yields a net of 2ATPs per glucose. *Aerobic glycolysis* (because it proceeds to the citric acid cycle and ETS) yields a total of 38ATPs per glucose as follows:

| STEP | Molecules Produced | ATP Yield |
|---|---|---|
| Glycolysis | 2ATP | 2ATP |
|  | 2NADH | 6ATP |
| Pyruvate to acetyl CoA | 2NADH | 6ATP |
| Citric Acid Cycle (2 turns) | 2ATP | 2ATP |
|  | 6NADH | 18ATP |
|  | 2FADH$_2$ | 4ATP |
|  |  | 38ATP |

Of the 686 kcals (for glucose $\rightarrow$ $CO_2$ + $H_2O$), aerobic processes store 308 kcals (for 45% efficiency) as ATP; anaerobic efficiency is much less.

Fats store the most energy (9.1 kcals/gm), whereas proteins (about 4.1) and carbohydrate (approximately 4) are about the same.

Glycolysis occurs in the cell cytoplasm. The citric acid cycle occurs in the matrix of the mitochondrion. Electron transport and oxidative phosphorylation occur on the inner membrane of the mitochondrion.

*Metabolic Pathways and their Interconnection:*

In animals the primary site for gluconeogenesis or formation of glucose is the liver. The involvement of oxaloacetate in the initial steps of gluconeogenesis provides a connection between this process and the Krebs cycle. All of the intermediates of the Krebs cycle may thus serve as precursors of glucose.

Gluconeogenesis requires a supply of pyruvate. In animals the primary source is the lactate and pyruvate produced by the glycolysis occurring in active skeletal muscle. Lactate and pyruvate can easily penetrate cell membranes and enter the blood for transport to the liver.

The transfer of electrons down the respiratory chain from NADH to molecular oxygen is the primary source of the energy utilized for the formation of ATP by the coupling of ADP phosphorylation.

The net product in the linking of electron transport and oxidative phosphorylation can be expressed by,

$$NADH + H^+ + 3ADP + 3 P_i + \frac{1}{2}O_2 \rightarrow$$
$$NAD^+ + 3ADP + 4H_2O$$

The sketches for each pathway should be carefully reviewed and integrated in a convenient manner, using the four individual sketches for each key process.

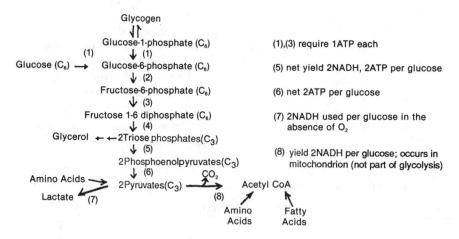

*Fig. 2.2—Glycolysis*

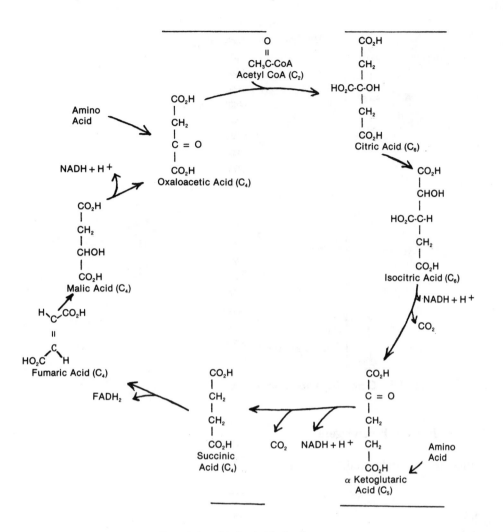

**Fig. 2.3—Citric Acid Cycle**

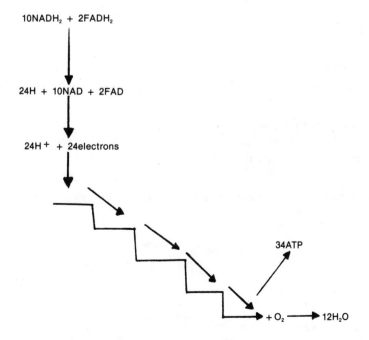

**Fig. 2.4—Electron Transport Chain**

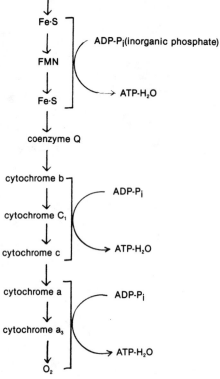

*Fig. 2.5—Oxidative Phosphorylation*

### 2.2.2    Questions to Review Bioenergetics

(1)    Which substance has the highest energy content per gram?

    (a) proteins
    (b) fats
    (c) carbohydrates
    (d) phospholipids

(2)    The cytochromes are involved in:

    (a) citric acid cycle
    (b) oxidative phosphorylation
    (c) glycolysis
    (d) electron transport system

(3)    In the biological production of energy from chemical molecules, the step-wise degradation is

    (a) by addition of hydrogens to molecules
    (b) by removal of oxygen from molecules
    (c) from more oxidized to more reduced states
    (d) from more reduced to more oxidized states

(4)    Select the substance which is not an electron carrier in cellular energy production:

    (a) NAD +
    (b) ATP
    (c) FAD
    (d) ubiquinone

(5)    Select the *incorrect* association:

    (a) ATP - adenine
    (b) NAD - nicotinamide or niacin
    (c) FAD - folic acid
    (d) cytochromes - porphyrin ring

(6)  Select the *incorrect* statement concerning glycolysis:

(a) End product may be lactate.
(b) If anaerobic, no ATPs are produced.
(c) If aerobic, the ATP yield can be 38ATPs because its products enter the citric acid cycle and electron transport system.
(d) It occurs in the cytoplasm.

(7)  Select the *incorrect* statement regarding the citric acid cycle:

(a) The first step is the combination of acetyl CoA and oxaloacetate to form citrate.
(b) It is not a true cycle because $CO_2$ and $H_2O$ are net products of it.
(c) Each turn of the cycle yields 3NADHs, 1FADH$_2$, and 1ATP (from GTP).
(d) It occurs in the mitochondrion.

(8)  Select the *incorrect* statement:

(a) The final receptor of electrons in the electron transport system is oxygen.
(b) Oxidative phosphorylation (production of ATPs) occurs only at certain steps in the electron transport system.
(c) The electron transport system can produce ATPs without oxidative phosphorylation occurring.
(d) Both electron transport and oxidative phosphorylation occur on the inner membrane of the mitochondrion.

(9)  Cyanide blocks cellular production of energy at which stage?

(a) glycolysis
(b) citric acid cycle
(c) electron transport system
(d) oxidative phosphorylation

(10)  Below are structures of a typical fatty acid and a hexose:

Fatty Acid

Hexose

If both were degraded bioenergetically to $CO_2$ and $H_2O$, equal weights of fatty acid would yield

(a) more energy because it is more reduced than the hexose
(b) less energy because it is more oxidized than the hexose
(c) less energy because it is more reduced than the hexose
(d) more energy because it is more oxidized than the hexose

## 2.2.3  Answers to Questions in Section 2.2.2

(1) b    (2) d    (3) d    (4) b    (5) c    (6) b    (7) b    (8) c    (9) c    (10) a

## 2.2.4  Discussion of Answers to Questions in Section 2.2.2

*Questions #1 to #9* Answers found or discussed in reading.

*Question #10* (Answer: a) A reduced compound has all (or mostly) hydrogens and not oxygens. The fatty acid has many more hydrogens and fewer oxygens so it is more reduced. The more reduced a compound, the higher the energy that can be released when it is oxidized to $CO_2$ and $H_2O$. The factor of the number of atoms in each molecule is eliminated by considering the substances on a weight basis.

### 2.2.5    Vocabulary Checklist for Bioenergetics

_____ aerobic

_____ anaerobic

_____ fermentation

_____ ATP

_____ high energy bonds

_____ acetyl CoA

_____ $NAD^+$, $NADP^+$

_____ FAD

_____ cytochromes

_____ pyruvate

_____ glucose

### 2.2.6    Concepts, Principles, etc. Checklist for Bioenergetics

_____ energy content of reduced vs. oxidized organic molecules

_____ molecules that serve as electron acceptors

_____ glycolysis

_____ citric acid cycle

_____ electron transport system

_____ oxidative phosphorylation

_____ localization of the processes of energy production in the cell

_____ interrelationships of the pathways above

_____ energy production (ATPs) by the various pathways from glucose

_____ relative energy content of proteins, fats, carbohydrates

## 2.3    NUCLEIC ACIDS

### 2.3.1    Review of Nucleic Acids

Nitrogen bases (NB) combine with five carbon sugars (S) to form *nucleosides* which combine with *inorganic phosphate* (P) to form *nucleotides* which polymerize to form *nucleic acids* (Fig. 2.6).

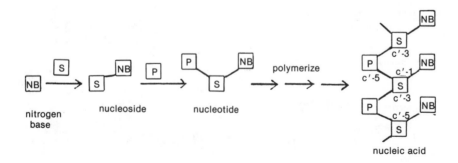

*Fig. 2.6—Relation of Nucleotides, Nucleosides, and Nucleic Acids*

An example of a nucleotide is deoxyadenylic acid:

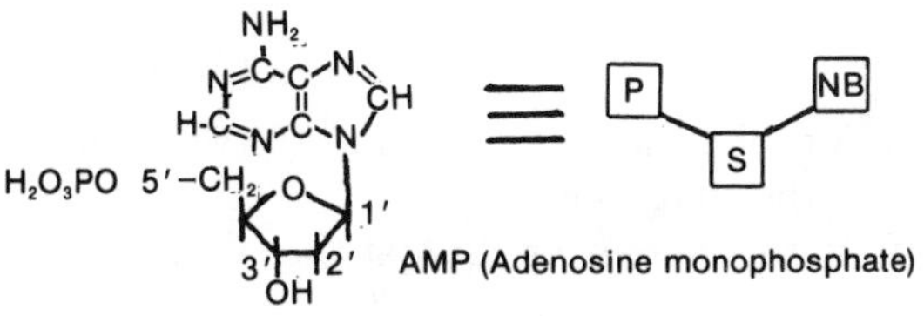

AMP (Adenosine monophosphate)

The *nitrogen bases* are the substituted *purines* (two rings) and *pyrimidines* (one ring), see Fig. 2.7. *Guanine (G)* and *adenine (A)* are purines. *Thymine (T), cytosine (C),* and *uracil (U)* are pyrimidines.

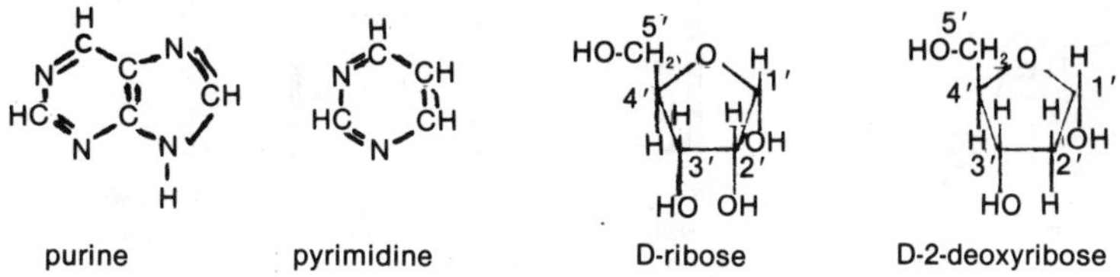

purine          pyrimidine          D-ribose          D-2-deoxyribose

*Fig. 2.7—Components of Nucleotides*

The sugars are *ribose* and *2-deoxyribose* (Fig. 2.7) The nitrogen bases bond at C'-1 to form nucleosides. Then one, two, or three phosphates attach at C'-5 of the sugar and nucleotides result (Figs. 2.6 and 2.7).

The triphosphate nucleotides then polymerize to form nucleic acids by eliminating two phosphates in the process. The phosphate of one nucleotide is bound to the C'-3 hydroxyl of the sugar of the next. If the sugar is ribose, then the nucleic acid is *ribonucleic acid (RNA)*. If the sugar is deoxyribose, then the nucleic acid is *deoxyribonucleic acid (DNA)*.

DNA has a *helical structure* with sugar-phosphates as the backbone with the nitrogen bases sticking off at more-or-less right angles (Fig. 2.8). It is composed of two strands of nucleic acids running in antiparallel fashion (i.e., one strand goes 5' → 3' and the other 3' → 5'). The nitrogen bases pair by hydrogen bonding and this holds the strands together. The nitrogen bases that pair are dictated by the matching up of hydrogen bonding sites and by space limitations in the double helix (proposed by Watson-Crick), which require a purine (two rings) and pyrimidine (one ring) to bond to each other. Adenine and thymine pair forming two hydrogen bonds. Guanine and cytosine pair forming three hydrogen bonds. Uracil replaces thymine in RNA which may occasionally have pairing of strands. The more hydrogen bonds, the more stable the nucleic acid. Hydrophobic bonds between the stacked nitrogen bases also stabilize the double helix.

DNA is *duplicated* in a semi-conservative fashion. That is, each strand serves as the template upon which a new complementary strand is made (Fig. 2.9). Note that the actual process is very complicated and may occur at multiple sites along the DNA strand simultaneously.

## 2.3.1.1   RNA STRUCTURE

RNA is involved in the manufacture of proteins. The RNA molecules are much shorter but there are structural similarities between DNA and RNA. The important differences between DNA and RNA structures are:

(a) RNA usually has only *one* strand of nucleotides. The strand does not bond to a complementary strand as in a DNA molecule and hence does not form a helix.

(b) The four bases in RNA are *uracil, guanine, cytosine,* and *adenine*. The base *thymine* is not found in RNA. Instead, uracil forms a complementary pair with adenine.

(c) RNA nucleotides contain ribose sugars instead of deoxyribose sugars. The ribose sugars contain an extra oxygen atom.

There are three different types of RNA:

1. *mRNA:* Messenger RNA transfers the DNA code from the nucleus to the ribosomes.
2. *rRNA:* Ribosomal RNA makes up a part of the ribosomes.
3. *tRNA:* Transfer RNA carries amino acids to the messenger RNA at the ribosomes.

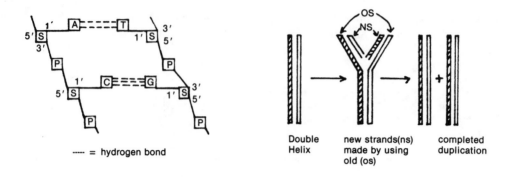

*Fig. 2.8—Base Pairing*          *Fig. 2.9—Semiconservative Duplication*

### 2.3.2 Questions to Review Nucleic Acids

(1)    Which of the pairs below do not normally hydrogen bond in nucleic acids?

(a) adenine-thymine
(b) adenine-guanine
(c) guanine-cytosine
(d) adenine-uracil

(2)    Both DNA and RNA contain all the nitrogen bases except:

(a) guanine
(b) adenine
(c) cytosine
(d) thymine

(3)    The sugar found in DNA is:

(a) deoxyribose
(b) ribose
(c) dextrose
(d) deoxyglucose

(4)    Nucleic acids are composed of repeating units of:

(a) nucleotides
(b) nucleosides
(c) nitrogen bases
(d) adenines

(5)    Which is not a pyrimidine?

(a) guanine
(b) thymine
(c) cytosine
(d) uracil

(6)     DNA always differs from RNA by

    (a) forming hydrogen bonds between strands
    (b) having thymine and not uracil
    (c) being found only in the nucleus
    (d) having a sugar-phosphate backbone

(7)     The following is one strand of a double helix of DNA (showing only nitrogen bases). What is the structure of its complementary strand? (A = adenine, G = guanine, T = thymine, C = cytosine, U = uracil)

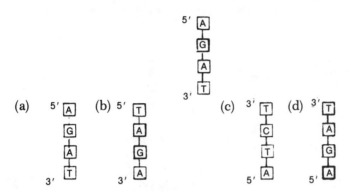

(8)     Given the following data, which organism *probably* has the most heat stable DNA?

| Organism | $(A + T)/(G + C)$ ratio |
| --- | --- |
| Mycobacterium phlei | 0.49 |
| Escherichia coli | 1.02 |
| Calf Thymus | 1.29 |
| Bacteriophage T2 | 1.90 |

    (a) Mycobacterium phlei
    (b) Escherichia coli
    (c) Calf thymus
    (d) Bacteriophage T2

(9)     Methods to differentiate between DNA and RNA might involve all of the following except

    (a) reaction of ribose with orcinol under suitable conditions
    (b) ultraviolet absorption by nitrogen bases at 260nm
    (c) chromatography to separate the different nitrogen bases
    (d) $^{14}C$ labeled uracil


## 2.3.3     Answers to Questions in Section 2.3.2

(1) b    (2) d    (3) a    (4) a    (5) a    (6) b    (7) c    (8) a    (9) b


## 2.3.4     Discussion of Answers to Questions in Section 2.3.2

*Questions #1 to #6* Discussion in Section 2.3.1.

*Question #7* (Answer: c) The complementary DNA strand is the opposite of the given strand and must be 3' → 5'. The base pairing is as discussed in the reference.

*Question #8* (Answer: a) The higher the percentage of G + C pairs, the higher the heat stability because more hydrogen bonds (three per G + C pair vs. two per A + T pair) are present making it more difficult to disrupt the double helix. This means the smaller the ratio $\dfrac{A + T}{G + C}$, the larger the G + C so the answer is (a).

*Question #9* (Answer: b) One must look for chemical differences between DNA and RNA and exploit them. (a) uses the fact that RNA contains ribose and DNA contains deoxyribose. (c) and (d) use the fact that RNA contains uracil and DNA doesn't. The selection (b) measures nitorgen bases, in general, and does not distinguish between them and, therefore, could not distinguish between RNA and DNA. This method does distinguish between proteins and nucleic acids.

## 2.3.5    Vocabulary Checklist for Nucleic Acids

_____ nitrogen bases           _____ thymine
_____ cytosine                 _____ DNA
_____ adenine                  _____ guanine
_____ pyridimine               _____ purine
_____ deoxyribose              _____ nucleotide
_____ nucleic acid            _____ ribose
_____ nucleoside              _____ RNA
_____ uracil

## 2.3.6    Concepts, Principles, etc. Checklist for Nucleic Acids

_____ structure of DNA          _____ composition of DNA vs. RNA
_____ replication of DNA        _____ pairing of the nucleotides

## 2.4    BIOSYNTHESIS

### 2.4.1    Review of Biosynthesis

DNA has the information that is the key of life. This information codes for the sequence of amino acids in proteins and is the sequence of nucleotides (see Section 2.3.1) in DNA. The *genetic code (triplet code)* is 64 sets of sequences of three nucleotides each. Sixty-one of these code for amino acids and three are punctuation marks (terminate protein chains). Some amino acids have only one triplet (methionine, tryptophan) while one has six (leucine).

The *genetic code is universal* (all living organisms have the same code). A *gene or cistron* is the sequence of triplets that codes for a single polypeptide chain. DNA is *duplicated* semi-conservatively (using each strand as a template for the new DNA strand) by DNA polymerase from 3' to the 5' end (see Section 2.3.1). Information on DNA is passed to mRNA (messenger RNA) by the process called *transcription*. Only one of the DNA chains is used, the enzyme is called RNA polymerase, and the direction of syntheses is 3' to 5'. The mRNA is then used as a guide to make proteins by a process called *translation*.

Once the mRNA is synthesized from DNA, it moves out of the nucleus (eukaryotes) through pores and into the cytoplasm. There it attaches to the *small subunit* of the ribosome (composed of rRNA and protein). The large subunit is then attached and a complete ribosome is formed. Meanwhile, an amino acid in the cytoplasm is being activated by phosphorylation with ATP by an *activating enzyme* (there is one enzyme for each amino acid). Another type of RNA called tRNA (transfer RNA), specific for the amino acid (AA) and activating enzyme is first bound by the enzyme, and then the amino acid is transferred to it by enzymatic action (Fig. 2.10). The tRNA ~ AA dissociates from the enzyme and moves to a specific position on the large subunit. Another position on the large subunit is occupied by the last tRNA to attach and which binds the carboxyl end of the growing peptide chain. The tRNA molecule has at least three recognition regions, one for the activating enzyme, and, hence, the AA, one for the ribosome, and a sequence of three nucleotides called the anticodon which pairs (hydrogen bonds) with the codon of the mRNA. So, the *anticodon* of tRNA pairs with the *codon* of mRNA and the next AA is in position for *peptide bond formation* which causes a transfer of the growing peptide to this new tRNA. After the peptide bond is formed, a *translocation* occurs moving the newly attached tRNA peptide into the position previously occupied by the old tRNA-peptide. This latter tRNA is now displaced. A new codon is exposed on the mRNA for another tRNA-AA to attach and the process is repeated. The protein is made from the free amino end to the free carboxyl end. More than one ribosome may "read" a mRNA at a time—this creates polyribosomes (polysomes). Synthesis stops when one of the punctuation mark codons is reached. *Note* that a gene (three nucleotides in this case) is on DNA, a codon is on mRNA and an anticodon is on tRNA (Fig. 2.11).

$$AA + AE \rightarrow AE - AA \sim Pi \xrightarrow{+ \underline{RNA}} AE \begin{smallmatrix} \nearrow AA \sim \\ \searrow tRNA \end{smallmatrix} Pi \xrightarrow{- AE} t\text{-}RNA \sim AA$$

~ = energy bond

*Fig. 2.10—Activation of Amino Acid (AA) by Activating Enzyme (AE)*

*Protein Synthesis and the DNA Code:*

Cells manufacture the proteins they need. The making of proteins is called protein synthesis. The sequence of DNA bases determines the code for protein synthesis. The bases of one chain attach to those of the other according to the "base-pairing rule". The base-pairing rule states that:

    (1) Adenine always pairs with thymine (A:T or T:A)
    (2) Cytosine always pairs with guanine (G:C or C:G)

Scientists found that at least 20 different amino acids are used to make proteins. The following reasoning was used to justify that each codon is made up of 3 bases. If a codon was only 1 base long, messenger RNA could code for only 4 amino acids (both DNA and RNA have 4 bases). If a codon was 2 bases long, only $2^4 = 16$ amino acids could be coded. However, if a codon is 3 bases, $4^3 = 64$ arrangements are possible. Review Volume II: *Skills Development for the Medical College Admission Test* under the section on permutations, combinations, and probability to understand the fundamental principles of arranging 4 letters, 3 at a time. Scientific experiments also support the concept of a 3-base codon.

*List of Amino Acids and DNA Codons*

| | |
|---|---|
| 1. Termination Codons: | ATT, ATC, ACT |
| 2. Valine: | CAA, CAG, CAT, CAC |
| 3. Tyrosine: | ATA, ATG |
| 4. Tryptophan: | ACC |
| 5. Threonine: | TGA, TGG, TGT, TGC |
| 6. Serine: | AGA, AGG, AGT, AGC, TCA, TCG |
| 7. Proline: | GGA, GGG, GGT, GGC |
| 8. Phenylalanine: | AAA, AAG |
| 9. Methionine: | TAC |
| 10. Lysine: | TTT, TTC |
| 11. Leucine: | AAT, AAC, GAA, GAG, GAT, GAC |
| 12. Isoleucine: | TAA, TAG, TAT |
| 13. Histidine: | GTA, GTG |
| 14. Glycine: | CCA, CCG, CCT, CCC |

| 15. Glutamine: | GTT, GTC |
| 16. Glutamic Acid: | CTT, CTC |
| 17. Cysteine: | ACA, ACG |
| 18. Aspartic Acid: | CTA, CTG |
| 19. Asparagine: | TTA, TTG |
| 20. Arginine: | TCT, TCC, GCA, GCG, GCT, GCC |
| 21. Alanine: | CGA, CGG, CGT, CGC |

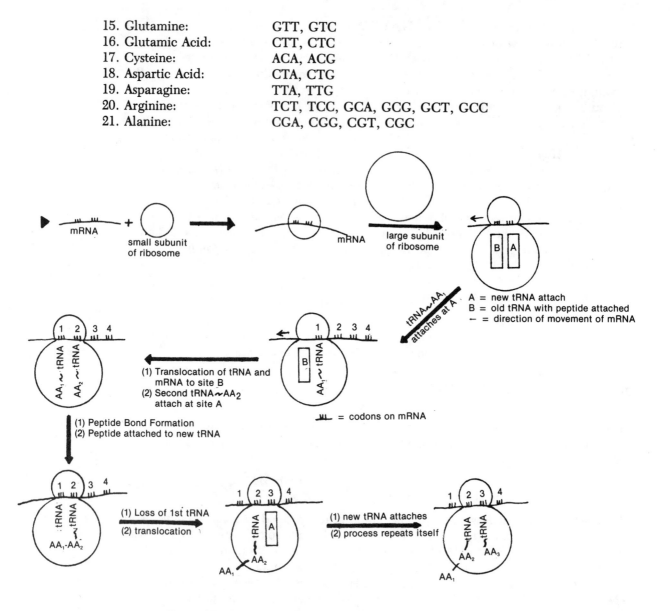

*Fig. 2.11—Protein Synthesis on Ribosome*

## 2.4.2 Questions to Review Biosynthesis

(1) The genetic code is composed of sequences of:

(a) three nucleotides
(b) three nucleosides
(c) three amino acids
(d) two amino acids

(2) The genetic code (triplet code) consists of 64 sets of three nucleotides each. Which statement is *incorrect* concerning the triplet code?

(a) The code is universal (i.e., all living organisms have the same code).
(b) All 64 triplets code for amino acids.
(c) More than one triplet can code for the same amino acid.
(d) A triplet may code for only one amino acid or termination codon.

(3)  Select the *correct* association:

(a) duplication-synthesis of DNA using DNA as a template;
(b) transcription-synthesis of RNA using DNA as a template;
(c) translation-synthesis of proteins using information on RNA;
(d) all are correct.

(4)  Translation of the genetic code does *not directly* require:

(a) activated tRNA ~ AA
(b) ribosomes
(c) mRNA
(d) DNA

(5)  Select the *incorrect* association:

(a) DNA-codon
(b) mRNA-anticodon
(c) tRNA-gene
(d) all are incorrect

(6)  Translation is the synthesis of proteins using mRNA as a guide. All are correct concerning translation *except*

(a) mRNA initially binds to the small ribosomal subunit
(b) the codon of tRNA pairs with the anticodon of mRNA
(c) protein synthesis is from the free amino to the free carboxyl end of the protein chain
(d) more than one ribosome may read a given mRNA at a time

(7)  All of the following processes occur on the ribosome *except*

(a) binding of mRNA to be "read" by tRNAs
(b) activation of tRNA and its amino acid
(c) peptide bond formation
(d) all of the above occur on the ribosome

### 2.4.3    Answers to Questions in Section 2.4.2

(1) a    (2) b    (3) d    (4) d    (5) d    (6) b    (7) b

### 2.4.4    Discussion of Answers to Questions in Section 2.4.2

All are adequately discussed in the Section.

### 2.4.5    Vocabulary Checklist for Biosynthesis

_____ gene              _____ mRNA             _____ codon
_____ cistron           _____ tRNA             _____ anticodon
_____ ribosome subunits _____ rRNA             _____ translation
_____ activating enzymes


### 2.4.6    Concepts, Principles, etc. Checklist for Biosynthesis

_____ genetic code
_____ duplication of DNA
_____ production of RNA from DNA – transcription
_____ process of translation (overall)
_____ ribosomal role in translation
_____ types of RNA and roles

## 2.5    EUKARYOTIC CELL

### 2.5.1    Review of the Eukaryotic Cell

Eukaryotes differ from prokaryotes (see Section 2.6.1) primarily by virtue of membrane bound structures in the former. The eukaryote is, thus, conveniently divided into a cell membrane, cytoplasmic region, and nuclear region. The special characteristics of fungi are considered separately.

### 2.5.1.1    THE CELL MEMBRANE AND TRANSPORT

Cell membranes are composed of phospholipids and proteins. Two major propositions for the structure of the cell membrane are the unit membrane model and the fluid mosaic model. The unit membrane model proposes a bilayered structure with two internal lipid layers surrounded by protein layers. "Pores" (ill-defined) are supposed to be present for movements of large and/or non-lipid molecules (Fig. 2.12). The fluid mosaic model proposes a continuous lipid bilayer with the phosphate ends of the phospholipids in contact with water. The hydrophobic (lipid) tails are contained within the lipid bilayer and are not in direct contact with water. Globular proteins are thought to "float" in this sea of lipids. Some of these proteins may stretch from the outside to the inside of the membrane (Fig. 2.13).

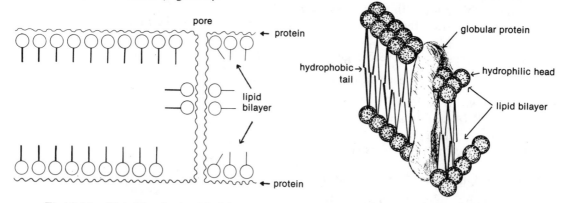

Fig. 2.12—Unit Membrane Model          Fig. 2.13—Fluid Mosaic Model in Three Dimensions

Substances move through the membrane by diffusion, osmosis, facilitated diffusion, active transport, phagocytosis, or pinocytosis. *Diffusion* is the random movement of free molecules or ions or particles in solution or suspension under the influence of thermal motion toward a uniform distribution throughout the available volume. This can occur through cell membranes if the substance diffuses through the cell "pores." In diffusion, the net movement of solute is from the region of higher concentration to that of lower concentration. Small organic molecules (ethanol, glycerol) and some ions ($Cl^-$) and $H_2O$ are moved by diffusion.

*Osmosis* is diffusion through a semi-permeable membrane. In osmosis, a solute cannot cross the membrane in order to equalize its concentration on both sides. This then creates a concentration difference for water across the membrane and the water diffuses in response to this to the side with the lower concentration of water (which is the side with the highest concentration of solute). *Tonicity* refers to relative concentrations of solute in two solutions. *Isotonic* means the two are equal. A *hypertonic* solution has more solute per unit volume than the reference. Osmosis (flow of solvent) occurs from hypotonic to hypertonic solution. If an RBC is placed in a solution less concentrated than itself (RBC is hypertonic), it swells until it hemolyzes (bursts). If it is placed in a solution more concentrated than itself (RBC is hypotonic), it crenates (shrinks). *Osmotic pressure* is the hydrostatic pressure needed to oppose the movement of the solvent.

*Facilitated diffusion* is a process by which substances insoluble in a membrane are carried across the membrane with the concentration gradient by means of a carrier substance. Saturation kinetics are observed; that is, as the substrate concentration rises relative to the number of carrier molecules, the rate of transport levels off. Some sugars and amino acids are transported in this fashion.

*Active transport* is the process of moving molecules uphill against an electrochemical gradient. A carrier molecule is involved as well as the expenditure of energy (ATP). This system exhibits saturation kinetics and inhibition by inhibitors of energy production (e.g., cyanide or 2,4-DNP). An important active transport system is the Na-K pump which is responsible for maintaining the electrical gradient of various membranes and neurons. Other locations of active transport include the gut (for sugars and amino acids) and the kidney tubules (for secretion and reabsorption of ions and small molecules).

*Phagocytosis* is a process by which particulate matter adhering to the cell membrane cause the membrane to invaginate around the particle forming a vesicle which is released to the interior of the cell. The vesicle then may combine with a lysosome whose enzymes digest its contents. This is an energy requiring process.

*Pinocytosis* is similar to phagocytosis but occurs in response to proteins or strong solutions of electrolytes. It involves the uptake of liquids and for this reason is also called "cell drinking." This is an energy requiring process.

## 2.5.1.2    THE CYTOPLASM AND CYTOPLASMIC ORGANELLES

The cytoplasm is composed of a matrix containing membrane bound organelles and various other structures such as microtubules. (See Fig. 2.14)

The *endoplasmic reticulum* (ER) is a double membrane system running throughout the cell. It probably breaks up and reforms and is continuous with the cell membrane and nuclear envelope. In this way it is probably a precursor for other membrane systems and peroxisomes. Rough (granular) ER contains ribosomes on its surface and is concerned with protein synthesis. Smooth ER (SER) is devoid of ribosomes and may serve several functions, a primary one being steroid synthesis. In the liver, SER plays an important role in the metabolism of endogenous small organic molecules, exogenous drugs, and toxins. In muscle, SER is called the sarcoplasmic reticulum and plays a role in impulse conduction and muscle contraction via calcium regulation. It may also serve a storage function--starch in plants, glycogen in animals.

The *Golgi complex* is a collection of smooth membranes probably continuous with the SER. Its primary function is in packaging and secretion of proteins and polysaccharides. It also plays a role in synthesis of complex polysaccharides.

*Mitochondria* are double membraned organelles which produce ATP. The inner membrane is folded into cristae which contain the enzyme systems of electron transport and oxidative phosphorylation. The matrix contains a circular DNA molecule, procaryotic type ribosomes, elementary bodies (ionic crystals), and enzymes of the Kreb's Cycle. Mitochondria replicate independently of the cell.

*Chloroplasts* carry out photosynthesis and photophosphorylation. They have a double membrane. The inner membrane is highly folded into grana which contain chlorophyll. DNA and prokaryotic-like ribosomes are also present. Found in green plants.

*Lysosomes* are single membraned organelles containing acid hydrolases (digestive enzymes). Functions of lysosomes include digestion of the cell at death (autolysis), digestion of substances within the cell, and digestion of substances taken in by phagocytosis (heterolysis). Storage diseases result when one or more of the hydrolytic enzymes are absent or defective. Lysosomes are produced from the rough ER.

*Peroxisomes* are single membraned, are part of a group of organelles called microbodies and contain enzymes for the metabolism of oxygen and/or hydrogen peroxide.

*Cilia* have the structure of centrioles (see Section 2.5.1.3), and are at the cell surface bound to the cell by a basal body (kinetosome). Cilia may function in locomotion but more commonly are used to move fluids and particulates past the cell surface.

*Flagella* are longer than cilia, are used for locomotion, and are composed of a cylinder of nine paired tubules with two unpaired centrally.

*Microfilaments* are aggregated proteins with no lumen and may be important for maintenance of cell structure and cytoplasmic streaming.

*Microtubules* are aggregated proteins with a lumen, may be important for intracellular transport and strucure, and are inhibited by colchicine.

*Ribosomes* are important in protein synthesis, composed of rRNA and protein, and are divisible into a large subunit and a small subunit (see Section 2.4.1).

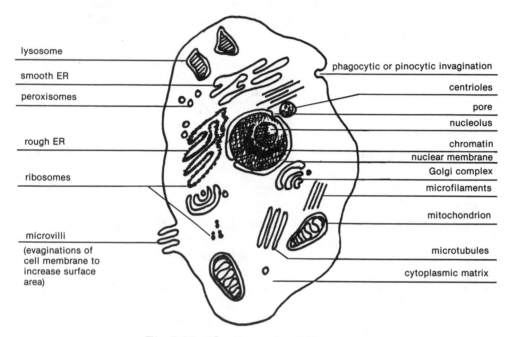

*Fig. 2.14—The Composite Cell*

## 2.5.1.3   THE NUCLEUS AND CELL DIVISION (MITOSIS)

The nucleus is surrounded by a double layered *membrane* interrupted regularly by pores. Inside the nucleus is DNA in a form called *chromatin* (DNA, histones, non-histone protein) which becomes visible as *chromosomes* during cell division. A specific region of the chromatin is called the nucleolus where rRNA is made.

*Mitosis* occurs to maintain an optimal nucleocytoplasmic to volume ratio, allow growth, differentiation, and specialization of cells in a multicellular organism. There is one division of the cell into two identical diploid (2n, n = number of different chromosomes in a set) daughter cells from one parent cell (assuming these were diploid also).

This cell division involves the processes of *cytokinesis* (division of the cytoplasm, not discussed) and *karyokinesis* (division of the nucleus). When a cell becomes *specialized*, it generally loses its ability to divide or reproduce itself (nerve cells, muscle cells, red blood cells, e.g.). Therefore, most cell division occurs in *"stem cells"* which are highly undifferentiated, multipotential cells with a high rate of cell division (e.g., bone marrow stem cells, crypt cells of the gut).

The *cell cycle* is divided into four phases. $G_1$ (Gap) is the first period of cell growth. It immediately follows cell division and precedes DNA duplication (Phase S). $G_2$ follows DNA replication and precedes cell division; further growth occurs. *M (mitosis)* is the period of cell division. The cycle is thus:

$$M \nearrow G_1 \searrow S \\ \nwarrow G_2 \swarrow$$

*Interphase* comprises G₁, S, and G₂. Prophase, metaphase, anaphase, and telophase are part of the M period. *Prophase* — the DNA coils tightly and becomes visible as chromosomes, and the nuclear envelope disappears. The *centrioles* (structure is a cylinder of nine sets of three tubules each, found near the nucleus in a region called the centrosome; the centrosome contains a pair of centrioles at right angles to each other) have moved to opposite poles of the nucleus and spindle fibers (microtubule structure) are forming from them. *Metaphase* — the chromosomes arrange radially along the equatorial plane of the cell and the spindle fibers are attached to the centromeres of each chromosome (now being composed of two chromatids, each of which becomes a new chromosome after the centromere divides). *Anaphase* — individual chromosomes divide at their centromeres and each new resulting chromosome migrates to the opposite pole being guided by the spindle fibers. Note that each chromatid of the chromosome at metaphase gives rise to a complete new chromosome after the centromeres divide. *Telophase* — the chromosomes uncoil, the nuclear membrane reforms, cytokinesis occurs, and the centrioles replicate themselves. The cell now enters *interphase*. See Section 2.18.1.2 to contrast mitosis and meiosis. The above concepts are diagrammed in Fig. 2.15.

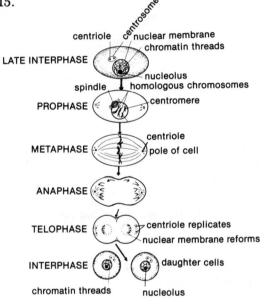

**Fig. 2.15—Mitosis**

### 2.5.1.4 GENERAL CHARACTERISTICS OF FUNGI AND THEIR LIFE CYCLE

Fungi are composed of *eukaryotic cells*, are plant-like, but contain *no chlorophyll*. They are *unicellular* (e.g., yeast) or *multicellular* (e.g., molds, mushrooms) with little differentiation into tissue types. They are *parasitic* (survive upon living organisms) or *saphrophytic* (survive upon dead organic matter), and they can *digest food* extracellularly by the secretion of digestive enzymes before absorbing them or can *absorb* already digested foods. Multicellular fungi tend to be filamentous with individual filaments called *hyphae*. Masses of hyphae are called mycelia. Fungi are important as causes of disease, in spoilage of food and materials, as decomposers of dead organic matter, as sources of food (mushrooms), in food production (bread yeast, cheese molds), and in alcohol production.

*Reproduction* is by *sexual* and/or *asexual* means with the latter predominating. The specific cycles vary among the different groups of fungi. Various *sexual stages* include ascus formation (has haploid spores), basidium (2n) formation, or just fusion of special cells to form zygotes (2n). *Asexual structures* or stages include the spores (n), the sporangium (n), and the conidia (n). These are either spores or give rise to spores. The sporangium and conidia arise from specialized hyphae. A general scheme for the life cycle of a typical fungus is in Fig. 2.16.

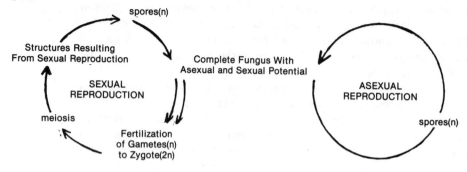

(Note that the spores can result from sexual or asexual reproduction.)

*Fig. 2.16—Life Cycle of a Typical Fungus*

## 2.5.2    Questions to Review the Eukaryotic Cell

(1)    The correct sequence of steps in mitosis is:

(a) Prophase, Metaphase, Interphase, Anaphase, Telophase
(b) Interphase, Anaphase, Metaphase, Prophase, Telophase
(c) Interphase, Prophase, Metaphase, Anaphase, Telophase
(d) Anaphase, Prophase, Interphase, Metaphase, Telophase

(2)    Which is not a feature of the unit membrane model of the cell membrane?

(a) continuous lipid bilayer present
(b) globular proteins floating in lipids
(c) hydrophobic ends of lipids not in contact with water
(d) continuous protein bilayers outside lipid layer

(3)    "Cell Drinking":

(a) phagocytosis
(b) pinocytosis
(c) both
(d) neither

(4)    The substance below not ordinarily found in cell membranes is (are):

(a) globular proteins
(b) phospholipids
(c) DNA
(d) all are found in cell membranes

(5)    Active Transport:

(a) diffusion
(b) with the concentration gradient
(c) phagocytosis
(d) Na-K-ATPase

(6)    Which of the following is *not* a function of smooth endoplasmic reticulum?

(a) metabolism of drugs and toxins in the liver
(b) synthesis of proteins
(c) conduction of impulses in muscle
(d) synthesis of steroids

(7)  Chloroplasts:

   (a) found only in prokaryotes
   (b) vestigial structures in animal cells
   (c) produce negative ions
   (d) photosynthesis

(8)  Mitochondria (best answer):

   (a) transport of molecules
   (b) protein synthesis
   (c) cell replication
   (d) energy production

(9)  Synthesis of Proteins:

   (a) lysosomes
   (b) Golgi bodies
   (c) mitochondria
   (d) rough endoplasmic reticulum

(10)  Centrioles:

   (a) found in the nucleus
   (b) found on chromosomes
   (c) make microvilli
   (d) form spindle fibers during cell division

(11)  Which is not true about the cell cycle?

   (a) there are typically four phases $G_1$, $G_2$, S, and M
   (b) interphase corresponds with the M phase
   (c) S is the phase of DNA synthesis
   (d) M is the phase of cell division

(12)  Which is not true about mitosis?

   (a) It can maintain an optimal nucleocytoplasmic to volume ratio.
   (b) It can allow growth of organisms.
   (c) It has phases of karyokinesis and cytokinesis.
   (d) It results in haploid daughter cells when the parent cells are diploid.

(13)  The chromosomes become coiled and visible and the nuclear membrane disintegrates. This is what phase of mitosis?

   (a) interphase
   (b) prophase
   (c) metaphase
   (d) telophase

(14)  Facilitated diffusion:

   (a) carrier substances carry molecules across the membrane
   (b) can go against a concentration gradient
   (c) requires energy
   (d) saturation kinetics is not observed

(15)  Fungi:

   (a) are prokaryotic
   (b) may be unicellular
   (c) contain chlorophyll
   (d) hyphae are unicellular stages

(16)   In the Fungus

(a) the haploid phase tends to dominate
(b) the diploid phase tends to dominate
(c) there is only asexual reproduction
(d) spores are sexual structures only

(17)   All are associated with reproductive functions in fungi except:

(a) conidia
(b) sporangium
(c) basidium
(d) mesenchymal

(18)   A key difference in the mechanism of mitosis and meiosis is

(a) mitosis has crossing over of homologous chromosomes during prophase
(b) meiosis has a second duplication of DNA during interphase I
(c) meiosis has alignment of homologous chromosomes in metaphase I and separation of homologous chromosomes in anaphase I
(d) mitosis has a reductional division

(19)   The main difference in the outcome of mitosis versus meiosis is

(a) meiosis produces identical daughter cells and mitosis produces different daughter cells
(b) mitosis occurs only in vertebrates
(c) meiosis produces somatic cells
(d) meiosis results in haploid cells and mitosis results in diploid cells when the parent cells are diploid

(20)   If container A has a higher concentration of a solute than container B, and they are separated by a semipermeable (to solute) membrane, then:

(a) nothing happens because membrane is only semipermeable
(b) solute particles move from B to A
(c) solvent moves from B to A
(d) solvent moves from A to B

(21)   What probably limits the size a cell may attain?

(a) surface area
(b) volume of a cell
(c) balance of surface area and volume
(d) specialization of the cell

(22)   Which structure below is found in eukaryotes but not prokaryotes?

(a) ribosomes
(b) mesosomes
(c) cell walls
(d) mitochondria

(23)   Which structure or molecule is *not* found or made in the nucleus of eukaryotes?

(a) nucleolus
(b) microsomes
(c) tRNA
(d) chromatin

(24)   If red blood cells are put into a hypertonic solution, they will:

(a) remain the same size
(b) hemolyze
(c) swell up
(d) shrink

(25)    Which structure does not play a part in motion of cells?

    (a) microvilli
    (b) cilia
    (c) flagella
    (d) pseudopods

(26)    Which of the following substances probably would not cross a membrane by simple diffusion?

    (a) ethanol
    (b) chloride ion
    (c) glucose
    (d) water

## 2.5.3    Answers to Questions in Section 2.5.2

( 1) c  ( 2) b  ( 3) b  ( 4) c  ( 5) d  ( 6) b  ( 7) d  ( 8) d  ( 9) d  (10) d  (11) b
(12) d  (13) b  (14) a  (15) b  (16) a  (17) d  (18) c  (19) d  (20) c  (21) c  (22) d
(23) b  (24) d  (25) a  (26) c

## 2.5.4    Discussion of Answers to Questions in Section 2.5.2

*Questions #1 to #17* Discussed adequately in Section.

*Questions #18, #19* Answers obtained by comparing Section 2.5.1.3 (Nucleus and Cell Division) and Section 2.18.1.3 (Meiosis). These differences should be understood well.

*Question #20* (Answer: c) The solvent moves across the semipermeable membrane from the side *it* is more concentrated, and the solute is less concentrated (which is side B), to the side where it is less concentrated (and the solute is more concentrated) which is side A. This is osmosis.

*Question #21* (Answer: c) This is not discussed in the Section. The reasoning is as follows: the nutritional and energy requirements and waste production are proportional to the volume of the cell. The volume of a cell is proportional to a linear dimension (l = length) cubed, i.e., $l^3$. The flux (i.e., the exchange rates) of materials in (nutrients) and out (wastes) is proportional to the surface area of a cell. The surface area is proportional to a linear dimension squared, i.e., $l^2$. As the cell increases in size (as volume increases), the requirements, given by $l^3$, increase much more rapidly than supply and waste removal, given by $l^2$. Hence, a balance between surface area and volume is required such that supply (and waste removal) can keep in balance with cell requirements.

*Question #22* (Answer: d) Membrane bound organelles are not found in prokaryotes, e.g., the mitochondrion. The cell walls (also in plants) and mesosomes (invaginations of cell membrane) are found in prokaryotes. Ribosomes are found in both, although the structures are different.

*Question #23* (Answer: b) Microsomes are artifacts produced from the endoplasmic reticulum during cell homogenization and centrifugation. Nucleolus and chromatin are parts of DNA. All RNA, including tRNA, are made from the DNA template in the nucleus.

*Question #24* (Answer: d) This is discussed in the Section. The solvent (water) flows from the hypotonic (red cells) to the hypertonic solution by osmosis.

*Question #25* (Answer: a) Microvilli and pseudopods were not discussed in the Section. The latter are cytoplasmic extensions that aid in motion as found in amoeba. Microvilli are evaginations (out pouches) of the cell membrane which increase its surface area. Its function is to permit more area for flux of materials in and out of cells, as in the gut.

*Question #26* (Answer: c) This is alluded to in the Section. Some ions, lipid soluble substances, and very small molecules (such as ethanol, glycerol, urea) can diffuse through membranes. Polar molecules, ions (especially cations), and larger molecules must enter by other processes.

### 2.5.5 Vocabulary Checklist for Eukaryotic Cell

| | |
|---|---|
| _____ unit membrane model | _____ microfilaments |
| _____ fluid mosaic model | _____ microtubules |
| _____ osmotic pressure | _____ ribosomes |
| _____ diffusion | _____ chromatin |
| _____ osmosis | _____ chromosomes |
| _____ tonicity | _____ nucleolus |
| _____ facilitated diffusion | _____ cytokinesis |
| _____ active transport | _____ karyokinesis |
| _____ phagocytosis | _____ cell cycle |
| _____ pinocytosis | _____ interphase |
| _____ endoplasmic reticulum | _____ prophase |
| _____ Golgi complex | _____ centrioles |
| _____ mitochondria | _____ metaphase |
| _____ lysosomes | _____ anaphase |
| _____ peroxisomes | _____ telophase |
| _____ cilia | _____ hyphae |
| _____ flagella | |

### 2.5.6 Concepts, Principles, etc. Checklist for Eukaryotic Cell

_____ differences between prokaryotes and eukaryotes
_____ models of cell membrane structure
_____ functions of cell organelles
_____ mechanism of mitosis
_____ characteristics of Fungi and Life Cycle

## 2.6 PROKARYOTIC CELL (Bacteria and Viruses)

### 2.6.1 Review of Bacteria and Viruses

*Prokaryotes (bacteria and blue-green algae) differ from eukaryotes* (Section 2.5) by the latter having (1) genetic material in a nucleus and DNA conjugated with proteins, (2) organelles bound within membranes, (3) subcellular structural units to carry out specific functions (ATP production, photosynthesis, e.g.), and (4) presence of cell walls made of cellulose of chitin versus murein (amino sugars and amino acids) as in prokaryotes. The DNA of prokaryotes is found in a non-membrane region called the nucleoid. Enzymes for metabolism and energy production are either free in the cytoplasm or bound to the cell membrane, and the ribosomes are smaller than in eukaryotes. Viruses are not prokaryotes or eukaryotes but constitute a group unto themselves.

### 2.6.1.1 BACTERIA

The general characteristics of bacterial *structure* are discussed above under prokaryotes. More specifically, from outside in, a bacteria may have a *capsule* which is usually made of a polysaccharide mucoid-like material and protects the bacteria from phagocytosis. Inside the capsule is the cell wall, and this prevents the hypertonic bacteria from bursting. Inside the cell wall is the cell membrane which may contain invaginations called *mesosomes* where localization of enzymes concerned with similar functions may be found. The cytoplasm and nucleoid are as described above. The DNA is circular and is haploid. Some bacteria contain flagella or cilia for locomotion—these are structurally different from their eucaryotic counterparts.

Bacteria have three common *shapes: Cocci* (spherical or ovoid), *bacilli* (cylindrical or rod-like), and *spirillia* (helically coiled). The cocci are often found in clusters: diplococci (two bacteria together), *streptococci* (linear chains of cocci), or *staphylococci* (grape-like clusters of cocci). All of these are made up of individual bacteria with distinct cell walls.

*Metabolically,* bacteria are aerobic or anaerobic. Anaerobic bacteria may use fermentation (where an organic molecule such as pyruvate or lactate is the final electron acceptor) or inorganic substances as final electron receptors (such as $S \rightarrow H_2S$). An *obligate anaerobe* is one that is killed if exposed to oxygen. This is usually because they cannot handle the peroxides (very toxic) produced in oxidative metabolism. A *facultative anaerobe* can survive in the presence or absence of oxygen. Bacteria may use a great variety of molecules as nutrients. Some are photosynthetic, other heterotrophic (using organic molecules made by other organisms) and others are chemosynthetic (making organic molecules and energy from inorganic precursors). The last group are important in fixation of nitorgen for use by all organisms. The variety of metabolic nutrients required and products produced are extremely important in studying basic questions of genetics, as well as biochemistry, and also in differentiating between the different types of bacteria.

Most bacteria *reproduce asexually* by the process of *binary fission* which produces two identical haploid daughter cells by the simple process of mitosis. Genetic recombination, (e.g., transfer and rearrangement of genetic informtion) may occur by three distinct means: transformation, transduction, and conjugation. *Transformation* involves a bacterium picking up free DNA from a medium; the free DNA being from a different bacterium. *Transduction* is the transfer of parts of DNA between bacteria by bacteriophages. In *conjugation* there is pairing of "male" and "female" forms. DNA is passed sequentially between them via structures called pili. All or a fraction of the DNA may be passed in this way. The above three genetic mechanisms allow extraordinary adaptability and variability of bacteria. Since bacteria can reproduce in a span as short as twenty minutes, a new trait such as drug resistance can spread rapidly in a given population.

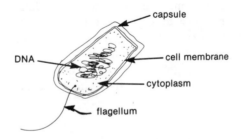

*Fig. 2.17—A Typical Bacterial Cell*
*(about 1 micrometer in diameter)*

### 2.6.1.2   VIRUSES

Viruses are usually called "non-living" and *differ from bacteria and other "living" organisms* because they, (1) don't contain both DNA and RNA, (2) have no metabolic machinery for energy production or protein synthesis, (3) do not arise directly from other viruses but depend on the host's metabolic machinery to synthesize them, and (4) have no membranes to regulate exit and entry. *Structurally,* most viruses consist of a protein coat surrounding a core (center) of either DNA or RNA.

There are many variations of the basic *life cycle* of a virus given below. A cell may have a special receptor or region that is recognized by the virus. The virus attaches and may enter via a process similar to phagocytosis. In the cell, the central core of DNA or RNA and occasionally special enzymes or proteins take over the host's metabolic machinery to produce new coat proteins and new viral DNA or RNA. This may occur in the nucleus or the cytoplasm or both. The viral coat and viral core (DNA or RNA) then combine to form complete viral particles. At a certain point, the host cell lyses (bursts) and releases the new viral particles as well as uncombined viral coats and viral cores. Sometimes the viral particles exit by a process similar to reverse phagocytosis and incorporate part of the host's cell membrane onto their protein coat in doing so. The above is typical of a virus that attacks an animal or plant cell.

Viruses that attack bacteria are called *bacteriophages*. Bacteriophages, in general, consist of a *head* made of a protein coat and a core as before, and they also contain a *tail* made of protein which is specialized for attaching to bacteria. A bacteriophage attaches to the surface of a bacteria, the core of RNA or DNA is injected into the bacteria, and the protein coat remains on the surface. Then the cycle may proceed as described for viruses above and is called *lytic* or *virulent*. However, the bacteriophage nucleic acid may become combined with the bacterial nucleic acid and remain as such for long periods before new bacteriophages are produced and cell rupture occurs. In this case, the bacteriophage is called *lysogenic* or *temperate*. The nucleic acid from the bacteriophage is called a *prophage*. Newly released bacteriophages may contain some bacterial nucleic acid which may be passed onto other bacteria when they are attacked by these bacteriophages. This is the mechanism of *transduction*.

*Rickettsiae* are intracellular parasites intermediate between bacteria and viruses. They can only reproduce in host cells similar to viruses, e.g., typhus.

*AIDS*

AIDS stands for "Acquired Immune Deficiency Syndrome" and is transmitted by the human immunodeficiency virus (HIV). As reported by the surgeon general, this virus that causes AIDS is a "lentivirus." Lentiviruses are special because they cause slow virus infections. They frequently have a lengthy incubation period before symptoms develop. The HIV has two main parts. There is an outer shell made of protein—actually three shells, one inside another. Inside the shells are the virus's genes, which carry its genetic code. When the virus invades a human cell, it makes copies of its genes and splices them permanently into the genes of the cell. The genes force the cell to make many new human immunodeficiency viruses. The immune system normally responds to a virus infection by sensing the protein coat of an invading virus. Then the immune system makes special molecules called "antibodies." In the case of AIDS, however, the immune system is too slow. The virus splices its genes into blood cells before there are enough antibodies to stop it. Antibodies cannot attack a virus once it is inside a cell. Scientists are currently trying to develop a vaccine to help in stopping the spread of AIDS.

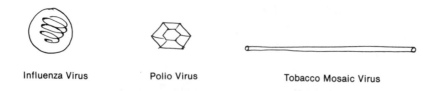

Influenza Virus          Polio Virus          Tobacco Mosaic Virus

*Fig. 2.18—Several Common Viruses*
*(about 100 nanometer in diameter)*

## 2.6.2 Questions to Review Viruses and Bacteria

(1) Bacteriophages:

(a) cause disease in humans
(b) are viruses
(c) are bacteria
(d) can reproduce by binary fission

(2) Select the substance not ordinarily found in viruses:

(a) carbohydrates
(b) proteins
(c) RNA
(d) DNA

(3) Viruses:

(a) are considered to be living organisms
(b) consist of protein, lipids, and carbohydrates only
(c) do not arise from other viruses directly
(d) have an incomplete metabolic machinery for energy production

(4) Eukaryotes are characterized by all except:

(a) genetic material in a nucleus
(b) organelles bound within membranes
(c) presence of cell walls made of murein
(d) subcellular structural units to carry out specific functions

(5) "Contains DNA or RNA, no means of energy production, cannot reproduce self directly" would be a description of a(an):

(a) animal cell
(b) plant cell
(c) bacteria
(d) virus

(6) In the replication of a virus in a host cell,

(a) the virus directs the metabolic machinery of the host
(b) the host directs synthesis of new viral particles
(c) viral particles are made as a single unit (i.e., coat and core)
(d) coat and core structures are released from the host and then combined

(7) Structurally, bacteriophages differ from the usual virus by

(a) having a protein coat
(b) having a core of DNA or RNA
(c) being able to replicate independently of a host cell
(d) having a tail region made of protein for attaching to cells

(8) The part of the cycle of a bacteriophage that may be different from that of a typical virus is

(a) taking over of host cell's metabolic machinery
(b) incorporation of its nucleic acid into the host cell's nucleic acid
(c) lysis of host cell
(d) synthesis by host cell of coat and core separately and then combining to form complete particle

(9) Which structure may protect a bacteria from phagocytosis by white blood cells?

(a) mesosome
(b) capsule
(c) nucleoid
(d) cell wall

(10)   Select the incorrect association:

(a) *cocci*-spherical
(b) *bacilli*-rod-like
(c) *diplococci*-two cocci
(d) *staphylococci*-linear combinations of cocci

(11)   The process whereby a bacterium picks up DNA from a medium and incorporates it into it's own DNA is called:

(a) binary fission
(b) conjugation
(c) transformation
(d) transduction

(12)   Bacteria transfer (exchange) genetic information between themselves by all except:

(a) transformation
(b) transduction
(c) budding
(d) conjugation

(13)   Methods used to distinguish between bacteria may include all of the following except:

(a) shape
(b) nutrient requirements
(c) products of metabolism
(d) all are possible

(14)   A form of hepatitis (inflammation of the liver) is caused by a virus. The serum of patients with hepatitis may contain antigens from the virus, $HB_SAg$ (hepatitis B surface antigen) and $HB_CAg$ (hepatitis B core antigen). (An antigen is a substance foreign to the body capable of eliciting an immune response.) Select the correct statement:

(a) This information is inconsistent with what is known about modes of viral replication.
(b) The $HB_CAg$ is probably a lipid.
(c) The $HB_SAg$ is probably a protein.
(d) Enzymes found in liver cells probably do not increase in the serum during the acute disease.

(15)   Which of the following would interfere most with the replication of a virus? Assume all agents can only affect the host cell and its contents.

(a) an agent that blocks synthesis of lipids
(b) an agent that blocks synthesis of carbohydrates
(c) an agent that blocks synthesis of proteins
(d) all of the above

(16)   In the treatment of viral infections, a drug is discovered that directly blocks the synthesis of the viral protein coat. This drug

(a) probably adversely affects protein synthesis by the host cell and hence may cause side affects in the host
(b) probably does not affect host protein synthesis

(17)   Given a bacterial population without resistance to a certain drug, all of the following may cause introduction of bacterial resistance except (excluding mutations):

(a) transformation
(b) binary fission
(c) transduction
(d) conjugation

## 2.6.3 Answers to Questions in Section 2.6.2

( 1) b  ( 2) a  ( 3) c  ( 4) c  ( 5) d  ( 6) a  ( 7) d  ( 8) b  ( 9) b  (10) d  (11) c
(12) c  (13) d  (14) c  (15) c  (16) a  (17) b

## 2.6.4 Discussion of Answers to Questions in Section 2.6.2

*Questions #1 to #13* Adequately discussed in Section.

*Question #14* (Answer: c) From the knowledge about viral replication, the coat (protein) and core (nucleic acid) are synthesized separately and then combined. When cell lysis occurs, complete viral particles as well as coat (e.g., HB$_S$Ag) and core (HB$_C$Ag) may be released. Since, the cells do lyse, their contents would also appear (e.g., the liver enzymes). And, since the antigens are found in the serum, it is not unreasonable to expect the liver enzymes to be there also. In fact, a rise in certain liver enzymes are key to the diagnosis of hepatitis. Also, since incomplete viral particles are liberated into the serum, it might be expected that other viral products might also appear as antigens. Some do, for example the "e"-antigen and viral DNA-polymerase.

*Question #15* (Answer: c) Viruses need the synthesis of proteins by the host cell machinery to make their protein coats as well as enzymes necessary to make nucleic acids.

*Question #16* (Answer: a) It is the host's metabolic machinery that makes viral protein. Therefore, if the synthesis of viral coat protein is blocked, it is likely, not absolutely necessary, that this is due to a blockage of host protein synthesis.

*Question #17* (Answer: b) Without new mutations, binary fission can only produce identical non-resistant daughter cells. The other mechanisms allow the introduction of new nucleic acid which may contain drug resistant genes.

## 2.6.5 Vocabulary Checklist for Viruses and Bacteria

_____ bacteriophage
_____ virulent
_____ temperate
_____ transduction
_____ mesosomes
_____ bacilli
_____ diplococci
_____ staphylococci
_____ facultative anaerobe

_____ transformation
_____ conjugation
_____ rickettsiae
_____ HIV
_____ lytic
_____ lysogenic
_____ prophage
_____ capsule
_____ cocci

_____ spirillia
_____ streptococci
_____ obligate anaerobe
_____ binary fission
_____ transduction
_____ AIDS
_____ flagellum

## 2.6.6 Concepts, Principles, etc. Checklist for Viruses and Bacteria

_____ differences between prokaryotes and eukaryotes
_____ difference of viruses from other organisms
_____ structure of a virus
_____ life cycle of a virus
_____ difference between viruses and bacteriophages in structure and life cycle
_____ structure of a bacterium
_____ shapes of bacteria
_____ metabolism of bacteria
_____ reproduction of bacteria

## 2.7    EMBRYOLOGY

### 2.7.1    Review of Embryology

*Fusion of the gametes* produced by meiosis (see Section 2.18.1 for details) involves first the penetration of the ovum by the sperm. The acrosome (part of sperm that contains hydrolytic enzymes) dissolves the *corona radiata* (collection of follicle cells and zona pellucida around ovulated ovum), and only the head of the sperm (contains the DNA) penetrates the ovum. Upon penetration, a reaction in the ovum occurs preventing additional sperm from entering. The ovum now completes meiosis II (see Section 2.18.1.3). Then the male and female pronuclei fuse and cleavage of the fertilized egg (zygote) begins.

*Growth, differentiation, and morphogenesis* occur together after the first few cleavages. The amount of *yolk* in the egg is an important determinator of the cleavage pattern but will not be discussed. Note, though, that the egg has polarity (i.e., is asymmetrical) by virtue of the yolk distribution. The first few cleavages (4-5) result in a grape-like cluster of cells called the *morula*. These divisions occurred without cell growth, and, hence, the morula is not much larger than the zygote. The morula develops into a *blastula* which is a hollow sphere one-cell thick with a cavity called the blastocoel. From this point *morphogenesis* (movements of cells to delineate shape and function) begins with the invagination of the blastula. What results is a two-layered structure with a new cavity called the *archenteron* that opens to the outside via the *blastopore* (site of invagination); this structure is the *gastrula*. Cells from the lip of the blastopore migrate between the two layers of cells to form a third layer. The gastrula then becomes a three-layered structure composed of *ectoderm* (outside), *mesoderm* (middle), and *endoderm* (inside). The blastopore cells induce the overlying ectoderm to form a neural groove and the embryo is now called a *neurula*. The neural groove forms the *neural tube*. At the margins of the neural tube detachment are a group of cells called the *neural crest* cells which form the adrenal medulla, melanocytes, and myelin sheaths among other tissues. The neural tube develops into the central nervous system (spinal cord and brain). Ventral to the neural tube, mesodermal tissue forms somites which gives rise to the vertebral column (formed on, but not from, the notochord) and associated muscles. The *ectoderm develops into* the nervous system, the epidermis of the skin and its derivatives, the lens of the eye, and the linings of the mouth and anus. The *endoderm will develop into* the gut (esophagus, stomach, intestines), associated organs (liver, gallbladder, pancreas), the lung, and the thyroid gland. *The mesoderm develops into* the skeleton, muscles, kidney, circulatory system (heart and vessels), blood, and dermis of skin. A schematic summary of the sequence above is in Fig. 2.19.

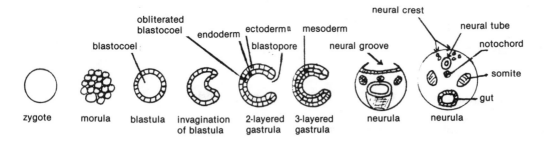

*Fig. 2.19—Early Development of the Embryo*

The question of how a single egg develops into a complex organism is not completely answered. The concepts of differentiation, determination and induction are integral to understanding the changes which occur. *Differentiation* is the process whereby a cell can change into more specialized cells to become a tissue. A *tissue* is a set of similar cells which carries out a specific function, such as muscle. The magnitude of this process is appreciated when one realizes that all the varied cells of the human body (muscle, bone, skin, nerve, etc.) arise from the same zygote. What is it about the zygote that allows this differentiation to occur? It is generally accepted that *all cells in an organism contain the same genetic information* (sequences of genes on DNA). What probably makes one cell different from another is which of these genes is activated. The *set of activated genes is responsible for each cell's characteristics*—the structural components, metabolic machinery, and general composition of the cell. So, in some way, as the zygote divides (cleavages), different sets of its *daughter cells must have different sets of genes activated.*

Differentiation is not brought about by the daughter cells having different genes (i.e., different sets of genetic material), in general. If the cytoplasm of the zygote was totally homogeneous, then each daughter cell, resulting from the cleavage, would be identical with regard to the nucleus and the cytoplasm and would remain undifferentiated. But, if there were an asymmetrical distribution of cytoplasmic constituents, and the cleavage results in daughter cells with different distributions of these constituents, then the daughter cells would be different. That is, a small amount of cytoplasmic differentiation would have occurred. If these cytoplasmic differences led to the activation of different sets of genes in their respective nuclei, differences between the cells would be perpetuated in their daughter cells, and some degree of true differentiation (production of daughters different from parent cells) will have occurred. So, asymmetrical distribution of cytoplasmic constituents is one way differentiation may be brought about. Then, in general, if a factor can affect the cells' cytoplasmic composition (which can affect the set of activated genes) or if it can affect the nucleus directly to activate (or inactivate) genes, and this effect is unevenly distributed among the cells, differentiation of the cells along different lines can be brought about.

Other factors which cause cells to differentiate are: (1) *Neighboring cells* (by contact inhibition of growth by secreting a diffusible chemical that stimulates or inhibits the cytoplasm or nucleus). An example is *tissue induction* in which a given tissue can induce cells in contact with it to develop along a certain line. For example, the dorsal lip of the blastopore induces the overlying ectoderm to become neural tissue as mentioned above. (2) *Physical environment* (by differences in light, temperature, pressure, humidity, pH, etc.). As the embryo develops, some cells are internal, some are on the surface, some have lots of yolk, some a little yolk, etc., so more opportunities occur for agents to act on cells in a differential manner. In general, the more specialized a cell becomes (i.e., the more differentiated), the less likely it is to differentiate to perform other functions or even divide. Certain cells remain at low levels of differentiation such that they may differentiate as they are needed. Examples are the mesenchymal cell found throughout the body and the bone marrow stem cell which can give rise to all the blood elements. Occasionally, a cell may dedifferentiate (i.e., revert to a less differentiated form), and, thus, its potential to divide increases. This is what happens in many cancers.

The concept of *determination* is related to that of differentiation in that, as a cell differentiates, fewer options become available. That is, at certain points a cell or tissue may be "determined" to become one of a certain set of cells and not others. For example, the surface cells of the gastrula are "determined" to become ectodermal structures and not endodermal or mesodermal structures. So, although in the blastula all the cells were surface cells and, apparently, had the option of becoming ectodermal cells, only those that did not invaginate became so. The mechanism of determination is probably also related to the environmental differences of cells and their interaction with preset sequences of gene activation and inactivation. Occasionally, the cells resulting from cleavage of a zygote are not "determined" until after 3 divisions (8 cells). Up to this point each cell can develop into a complete organism. After this point, only incomplete organisms would develop from each cell. Cleavages up to this point are called indeterminate because each cell has all the options available. The next cleavage is called determinate because the daughter cells no longer have all options available. In some instances the first cleavage may be determinate.

## 2.7.2    Questions to Review Embryology

(1)    The blastula is generally preceded by the:

(a) gastrula
(b) morula
(c) neurula
(d) both (a) and (b)

(2)    The three germ layers—the ectoderm, the mesoderm and the endoderm—are found at which stage?

(a) morula
(b) gastrula
(c) blastula
(d) neurula

(3)    Select the one that is not derived from the ectoderm germinal layer:

(a) nerve
(b) muscle
(c) lens of eye
(d) epidermis of skin

(4)    Select the organ/tissue *not* derived from the mesodermal germinal layer:

(a) muscle
(b) kidney
(c) intestines
(d) bones

(5)    Select the organ/tissue not derived from the endodermal germinal layer:

(a) nerve
(b) liver
(c) intestines
(d) lung

(6)    The individual cells resulting from the cleavage of a fertilized egg may occasionally give rise to complete organisms up to the *third* cleavage. Select the correct statement.

(a) Cleavages prior to the *third* were determinate cleavages.
(b) The number of cells resulting from the third cleavage is 16.
(c) Determinate cleavages cannot occur, in general, prior to the third cleavage.
(d) The cells resulting after the next cleavage are probably different in the set of activated genes and/or cytoplasmic composition.

(7)    Once the sperm head penetrates the _____, a reaction ensues that _____.

(a) corona radiata; causes the pronuclei to fuse
(b) corona radiata; prevents the penetration of additional sperm
(c) ovum; causes the pronuclei to fuse
(d) ovum; prevents the penetration of additional sperm

(8)    All of the following processes occur during the process of fertilization of the egg by the sperm except

(a) acrosome dissolves the corona radiata
(b) only the head of the sperm enters the ovum
(c) the sperm nucleus completes its second meiotic division
(d) the ovum nucleus completes its second meiotic division

(9)    The correct sequence of the early stages of development is:

(a) morula, gastrula, blastula, neurula
(b) morula, blastula, gastrula, neurula
(c) blastula, morula, gastrula, neurula
(d) neurula, blastula, gastrula, morula

(10)  Which of the following stages is essentially the same size as the zygote?

(a) gastrula
(b) blastula
(c) morula
(d) all are larger

(11)  The first stage of development in which a cavity appears is the:

(a) neurula
(b) morula
(c) gastrula
(d) blastula

(12)  Morphogenesis begins at which stage?

(a) morula
(b) blastula
(c) gastrula
(d) neurula

(13)  Factors important in the differentiation of cells include:

(a) cytoplasmic composition and distribution of constituents
(b) characteristics of neighboring cells
(c) physical environmental agents
(d) all of the above

(14)  As a cell becomes more specialized for a particular function, the opportunity for it to become specialized for other functions:

(a) decreases
(b) increases
(c) remains the same

(15)  A cell found in the middle layer of the three-layered gastrula has probably lost the option to become:

(a) epidermis
(b) kidney
(c) muscle
(d) blood

(16)  Select the following situation(s) that have the best likelihood of leading to differentiated daughter cells after a cleavage occurs:

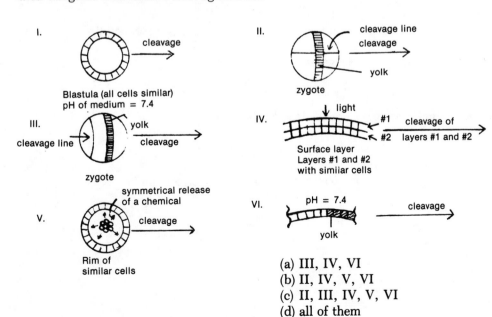

(a) III, IV, VI
(b) II, IV, V, VI
(c) II, III, IV, V, VI
(d) all of them

2-37

(17)    Which of the following cells or cell types is the most differentiated?

   (a) mesenchymal cell
   (b) nerve cell
   (c) cancer cell
   (d) bone marrow stem cell

## 2.7.3    Answers to Questions in Section 2.7.2

( 1) b   ( 2) b   ( 3) b   ( 4) c   ( 5) a   ( 6) d   ( 7) d   ( 8) c   ( 9) b   (10) c   (11) d
(12) b   (13) d   (14) a   (15) a   (16) a   (17) b

## 2.7.4    Discussion of Answers to Questions in Section 2.7.2

*Questions #1 - #5, #7-#15, #17* All discussed adequately in reference.

*Question #6* (Answer: d) This is discussed in the Section. The implication of the question being that the divisions after the third are determinate and result in cells that are somewhat differentiated. The cells resulting from the nth cleavage is $2^n$ assuming at each cleavage all cells divide (not always true). Then $2^3 = 2 \cdot 2 \cdot 2 = 8$ and not 16 as in option (b).

*Question #16* (Answer: a) The point stressed in the Section was that differentiation is possible if a factor can affect a group of similar cells in an unsymmetrical or unequal manner. In (I), the pH affects all the similar cells equally. In (II), the cleavage results in two cells with similar yolk distributions. In (III), the cleavage results in different yolk distributions so the daughter cells are different cytoplasmically and this can lead to differentiation. In (IV), the light may either affect the surface layer only or affect the surface layer (#1) more strongly than the underlying layer (#2). This can potentially affect gene activation and can lead to differentiation between the cell layers. In (V), the rim of similar cells are probably affected similarly by the symmetrically diffusing chemicals, and the daughter cells will probably be similar. In (VI), although the pH is constant, this can have different effects on cells with and without yolks, and, hence, result in potentially differentiated daughter cells.

## 2.7.5    Vocabulary Checklist for Embryology

_____ acrosome            _____ corona radiata        _____ blastocoel
_____ morula              _____ blastula              _____ gastrula
_____ archenteron         _____ blastopore            _____ endoderm
_____ ectoderm            _____ mesoderm              _____ neural crest
_____ neurula             _____ neural tube
_____ tissue induction    _____ cleavages

## 2.7.6    Concepts, Principles, etc. Checklist for Embryology

_____ fertilization of the ovum and related changes in the egg
_____ sequences of stages of development
_____ development of the ectoderm, mesoderm, endoderm into organs and/or organ systems
_____ morphogenesis
_____ concept of determination
_____ concept of differentiation
_____ concept of induction

## 2.8 RESPIRATORY SYSTEM

### 2.8.1 Review of Respiratory System

In humans, air enters through the *mouth or nose* where it is cleaned, warmed and moistened. It then passes down the *trachea* to two main *bronchi* and then to *bronchioles* then to *alveoli*. Gas exchange occurs in the alveoli. Incomplete *cartilage rings* hold the trachea, bronchi, and bronchioles open. *Mucus* traps particles which are then moved out of the respiratory tract by *ciliary action* of the lining cells. *Coughing* is a reflex action mediated by the medulla. The reflex is initiated by a stimulation (e.g., by particles) of the tracheo-bronchial tree, followed by expulsion of these particles and mucus as sputum (or phlegm). *Sneezing* is a reflex mediated by the medulla also, but the intial stimulation is in the nose followed by forceful expulsion of the irritating substance and naso-oral secretions.

The act of *inspiration* is accomplished by the contraction of the diaphragm (via impulses from the *phrenic nerve*) which moves downward and/or by certain rib muscles lifting the rib cage up. These mechanisms create a negative pressure inside the chest cavity which causes the lungs to expand and pull in air. *Expiration* is a passive process due to the elastic recoil of the chest wall and lung tissue itself. Respiration is largely *involuntary*, but some voluntary control is possible over the rate and depth of respiration. The *control center* of respiration is in the medulla of the brainstem. It causes an increase in the rate of respiration when there is a fall in pH (e.g., more acidic), an increase in $CO_2$ tension (which causes a drop in pH), or a decrease in oxygen tension in the blood. Also impulses from the cerebrum can affect ventilatory rate, as in anxiety, when the rate increases.

A key substance for the function of lungs is *surfactant* (dipalmitoyl lecithin—a phospholipid). This substance coats the alveoli and creates a variable surface tension in them. As the alveoli get smaller, the surface tension decreases due to surfactant. This prevents the alveoli from collapsing during expiration, because high surface tension would cause alveoli to collapse. In the absence of surfactant, collapsed alveoli require fairly high inspiratory forces to re-expand them. This is what happens in *RDS* (Respiratory Distress Syndrome) of the newborn in whom there is an absence of surfactant. The infant is not strong enough to re-expand the collapsed alveoli.

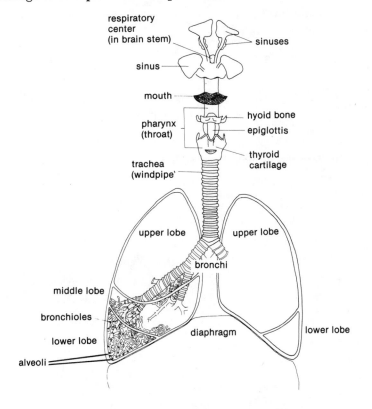

*Fig. 2.20—Respiratory System*

*In summary,* the respiratory system functions mechanically to move air in and out of the lungs (highest $O_2$ and lowest $CO_2$ tension) and to allow diffusion of gases in and out of the body. *Oxygen* moves into the blood (lower $O_2$ tension and highest $CO_2$ tension) where it is taken up and utilized. In the tissues, *carbon dioxide* ($CO_2$) is produced by oxidation of nutrients. The $CO_2$ then diffuses into the blood where it dissolves in the serum, is converted to carbonic acid ($CO_2 + H_2O \rightarrow H_2CO_3$) and then to bicarbonate ($HCO_3^-$), or combines with hemoglobin. Next it circulates to the lungs where the above reactions are reversed and the $CO_2$ is expired. Note that in all cases the gases go from higher tensions (pressures) to lower. By regulating the amount of carbonic acid and bicarbonate in the serum, the lungs are important in the regulation of acid-base balance in the body.

*Effects of Smoking*

Tobacco smoke consists of gases such as carbon dioxide and tiny unburned carbon particles. These substances harm the *cilia* and *mucous membranes* that line the breathing passages. Many smokers cough frequently. The cough is the body's effort to clear the breathing passages. Healthy cilia and mucous membranes accomplish the cleaning process automatically. Smoke also damages the lungs. Long-term smoking can cause the walls of the alveoli to rupture, or break. As a result, the surface area for *gas exchange* decreases considerably. This condition, called *emphysema* interferes with oxygen intake.

### 2.8.2    Questions to Review the Respiratory System

(1)    The path of air into the lungs of humans is:

    (a) alveoli, trachea, bronchi, bronchioles
    (b) trachea, bronchi, bronchioles, alveoli
    (c) bronchi, bronchioles, trachea, alveoli
    (d) trachea, bronchioles, brochi, alveoli

(2)    Expiration of air from the lungs

    (a) is a passive process
    (b) causes negative pressure in the chest cavity
    (c) requires contraction of the diaphragm
    (d) both (b) and (c)

(3)    During inspiration of air into the lungs

    (a) the chest cavity has a positive pressure
    (b) the diaphragm moves upward
    (c) the diaphragm contracts
    (d) the rib cage moves down

(4)    What structure(s) is(are) used to prevent the bronchi from collapsing?

    (a) cartilage rings
    (b) bony rings
    (c) fibrous tissue
    (d) none of the above

(5)    Surfactant:

    (a) dipalmitoyl lecithin
    (b) decreases surface tension
    (c) deficiency may result in RDS
    (d) all of the above

(6) Which reflex moves secretions out of the tracheobronchial tree?

  (a) cough
  (b) sneeze
  (c) baroceptor
  (d) pH

(7) The control center of respiration is in the:

  (a) cerebrum
  (b) cerebellum
  (c) medulla
  (d) thalamus

(8) All of the following may cause an increase in respiratory rate except:

  (a) increased hydrogen ion concentration
  (b) increased carbon dioxide tension
  (c) increased oxygen tension
  (d) anxiety

(9) Carbon dioxide may be present in all of the following forms except:

  (a) dissolved in the blood
  (b) bound to hemoglobin
  (c) as dimers
  (d) as bicarbonate

## 2.8.3 Answers to Questions in Section 2.8.2

( 1) b   ( 2) a   ( 3) c   ( 4) a   ( 5) d   ( 6) a   ( 7) c   ( 8) c   ( 9) c

## 2.8.4 Discussion of Answers to Questions in Section 2.8.2

All questions are adequately discussed in the Section.

## 2.8.5 Vocabulary Checklist for the Respiratory System

| | | |
|---|---|---|
| _____ trachea | _____ mucus | _____ surfactant |
| _____ alveoli | _____ cartilage rings | _____ control center of respiration |
| _____ sneeze | _____ phrenic nerve | _____ emphysema |
| _____ ciliary action | _____ bronchioles | _____ bronchial tubes |
| _____ bronchi | _____ cough | |

## 2.8.6 Concepts, Principles, etc. Checklist for the Respiratory System

_____ structure/function of the respiratory system
_____ mechanism of inspiration and expiration
_____ factors that affect rate of respiration
_____ role of surfactant in lung function
_____ functions of lung in $O_2$ and $CO_2$ homeostasis
_____ effects of smoking

## 2.9  CIRCULATORY SYSTEM

### 2.9.1  Review of the Circulatory System

The elements of the circulatory system in humans are the heart, the blood vessels, blood and the lymphatics (Section 2.10.1).

### 2.9.1.1  THE HEART

The *heart* consists of two *atria* (left-LA and right-RA) and two *ventricles* (LV and RV). Between the RA and RV is the *tricuspid valve* (TV, 3 leaflets). Between the RV and the pulmonary artery (PA) is the *pulmonic valve* (PV). Between the LA and LV is the *mitral valve* (MV, 2 leaflets). Between the LV and the aorta is the *aortic valve* (AV). The PV and AV valves are called *semilunar valves*—these prevent reflux of blood back into their respective ventricles during diastole. See Fig. 2.21. The TV and MV are attached via *chordae tendinae* to *papillary muscles* on their respective ventricles to prevent reflux into the corresponding atria during systole. Improper functioning of the valves is one of the causes of heart murmurs. A schematic of the heart and circulation is:

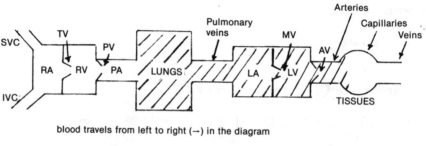

blood travels from left to right (→) in the diagram

SVC = superior vena cava            //// = oxygenated blood

IVC = inferior vena cava

*Fig. 2.21—Schematic of the Circulatory System*

The heart is made of cardiac muscle. This differs from skeletal muscle (Section 2.15.1) by: (1) being made of distinct cells, (2) having specializations of cell membranes called *intercalated discs* to decrease resistance to impulse conduction, (3) being able to initiate beats without the need of a nerve impulse, and (4) being largely involuntary. The microscopic structures are similar (see Section 2.15.1).

*Heart beats* are divided into systole (contraction) and diastole (relaxation) on the basis of the state of the ventricles. *Beats* originate in the *sinus node* which is considered the pacemaker of the heart. Impulses from here activate the atria to contract (diastole), then pass to the *atrioventricular (AV) node*. From this point, impulses pass down the *bundle of His* to the left and right branch bundles to the *Purkinje fibers* which activate the left and right ventricles causing them to contract (systole). Beats can originate in other parts of heart if the sinus node fails. Also, some of the bundles or fibers may become injured so that they cannot conduct impulses—then the impulses find alternate paths. *Sympathetic* nerves serve to increase the heart rate and force of contraction. *Parasympathetic* nerves (e.g., the *Vagus nerve*) decrease the heart rate. During *systole* the ventricles are ejecting blood into the large vessels (PA, aorta), and during *diastole* the ventricles are being filled with blood from the atria. Note that the RV pumps blood to the lungs and the LV pumps blood to the rest of the body.

## 2.9.1.2   THE BLOOD VESSELS

*Blood vessels* consist of arteries, arterioles, capillaries, and veins. Vessels are made of (to different degrees), from the inside out, an *intima* (endothelial cell lining), a *media* (consisting of muscle and elastic tissue), and an *adventitia* (connective tissue covering). *Arteries* contain a lot of muscle and/or elastic tissue and deliver blood from the heart (not always oxygenated blood). The contraction of the ventricles in systole imparts energy and pressure to the blood as they enter the arteries. This causes expansion (elastic nature) of the arteries during systole which stores the energy part. During diastole the elastic recoil converts the stored energy to pressure and maintains the pressure. The blood pressure is higher during systole than diastole in the arteries. But because of the recoil of the arteries and the effect of the arterioles (see below) the diastolic blood pressure remains well above zero in the arteries. An average blood pressure is 120/80 (systolic/diastolic) measured in mm Hg. *Arterioles* connect arteries and capillaries and are the location of the greatest *resistance* to blood flow. Blood pressure varies directly as the flow of blood (amount of blood pumped by the heart) and directly as the resistance to flow.

$$\text{blood pressure} \propto (\text{heart output}) \times (\text{resistance}).$$

Resistance to flow varies inversely as the fourth power of the radius (r) of the vessel: resistance $\alpha$ $1/r^4$

Arterioles can change their radii greatly. So, arterioles are very important determinators of blood pressure. Sympathetic nerves can constrict the arterioles, that is, make the radius smaller. *Capillaries* contain only endothelial cells which allow transport of substances across them. Nearly all the transfer of substances between the blood and the tissues occur across the capillaries. The *hydrostatic pressure*, generated by the heartbeat, tends to push fluid and molecules (not cells) out of the capillary. The *oncotic pressure*, due primarily to the presence of proteins like albumin in the blood, tends to pull fluid and molecules into the capillary. Hence, the *net transfer of fluid* depends on the balance of these two. On the arterial side of the capillary, the hydrostatic pressure dominates and fluid, etc., leaves the capillary and enters the tissue space (not cells directly). At the venule end of the capillary, the oncotic pressure dominates and this draws fluid, etc. (different substances than exited), back into the capillary (Fig. 2.22). Not all the fluid and proteins are pulled back in; these are returned to the blood vessels via the lymphatics (Section 2.10.1).

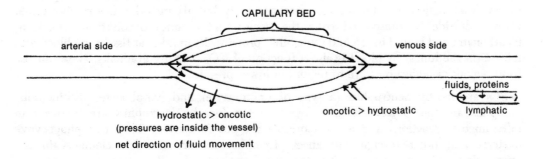

*Fig. 2.22—Capillary Fluid Exchange*

The *veins* have less muscle and elastin than arteries, some have valves to prevent backward flow of blood away from the heart, and they carry blood to the heart. Veins can contain a lot of blood under low pressure, i.e., they have a high capacitance (can act as a reservoir). Veins are assisted by the action of skeletal muscle contractions to move blood forward (the heart valves prevent backward movement). *Anatomically,* the blood vessels consist of three main divisions. (1) The *systemic circulation* supplies blood to the head, extremities, and trunk. The main artery is the aorta and the main veins are the inferior and superior vena cavas. (2) The *pulmonary circulation* supplies blood to the lungs. (3) The *coronary circulation* supplies blood to the heart. The coronary arteries arise at the base of the aorta at the aortic valve. The arteries give rise to the coronary veins that enter the coronary sinus (on the atria), which empties into the RA.

## 2.9.1.3    THE BLOOD

Blood consists of *formed elements:* (1) red blood cells (RBC or erythrocytes), (2) white blood cells (WBC), and (3) platelets; and many *non-formed elements:* proteins, lipids, hormones, dissolved gases, ions, carbohydrates.

*RBCs* contain hemoglobin (made of four proteins called globin, and heme, which is a porphyrin ring, and iron—II) and are biconcave discs (    &#9683;   ◉   ).

The *hematocrit* is the percentage of whole blood that is RBCs. The *plasma* is whole blood minus the formed elements. *Serum* is plasma after clotting has occurred. *Hemoglobin* (Hb) carries oxygen ($O_2$) attached to iron (Fe). $O_2$ is picked up slowly by Hb at low $O_2$ tension, but this rapidly accelerates as $O_2$ tension increases, and it eventually levels off at high $O_2$ tension (Fig. 2.23). (The tension of a gas is the pressure of the gas.)

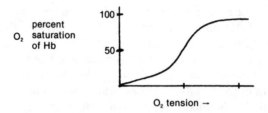

*Fig. 2.23—Hemoglobin-Oxygen Saturation Curve*

This is due to the *allosteric nature* of the Hb molecule. The first subunit binds $O_2$ slowly, but once bound, the bound $O_2$ causes a conformational change in the second subunit which causes it to pick up the next $O_2$ faster. This is repeated in the third and fourth subunits until the Hb is saturated. Hb releases $O_2$ more readily at low pH than at high pH—the *Bohr effect*. Hb picks up $O_2$ in the lung and releases it in the tissues. Release and uptake is primarily a function of $O_2$ tension (pressure) gradients, but pH and other factors play a role. Carbon dioxide is transported from the tissues to the lungs dissolved in blood, as bicarbonate, and bound to Hb and some other proteins. Its uptake (at tissues) by blood and release (in the lungs) by blood is also a function of $CO_2$ pressure gradients. Gases diffuse from regions of higher pressure to regions of lower pressure.

*WBCs* are mostly neutrophils (a type of granulocyte) and lymphocytes. Eosinophils, basophils and monocytes are also found in the blood. Neutrophils are involved in inflammatory reactions and are responsible for pus formation. They can phagocytize bacteria and other foreign substances. Lymphocytes are the key elements in the immunologic response system. *Platelets* are fragments of cells called megakaryocytes (located in the bone marrow). They play a part in the clotting of blood. All of the formed elements arise from precursor cells in the bone marrow.

*Proteins* in the blood are albumin (maintains oncotic pressure and acts as a nonspecific carrier protein) and globulins. Globulins include the immunoglobulins which are antibodies, carrier proteins, and the coagulation factors (fibrinogen, prothrombin, etc.). Calcium is also required for clotting; agents like EDTA and oxalate complex calcium and may prevent clotting. *Vitamin K* is responsible for formation of some of the clotting factors, and, thus, the clotting of blood.

### 2.9.1.4 FUNDAMENTAL PRINCIPLES OF BLOOD CIRCULATION

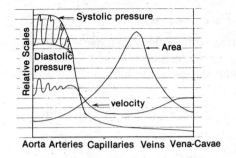

*Fig. 2.24—Fundamental Principles of Blood Circulation*

As shown in Fig. 2.24, generally the velocity of blood flow in any segment of the cardiovascular system is inversely proportional to the total cross-sectional area of the vessels of the segment. Efficient circulation requires an adequate volume of circulating blood. Blood encounters resistance as it flows through blood vessels. Resistance to blood flow is affected by physical and biological variables such as viscosity, temperature, diameter, etc. Four equations are provided below for studying the relationships among various circulation variables. (The MCAT Science Problems and Quantitative Analysis subtests will test your skills in "proportional reasoning" for a typical situation.)

1. Resistance (R) $= \dfrac{\text{Pressure Gradient } (\Delta P)}{\text{Flowrate } (Q)}$

    This equation is analogous to Ohm's law in electric circuits,

    $$R = \frac{V}{I} = \frac{\text{Voltage}}{\text{Current}}$$

2. Ejection fraction (EF) $= \dfrac{\text{Stroke Volume (SV)}}{\text{End-Diastolic Volume (EDV)}}$

    The ventricles eject only a portion of their contained blood with each beat. The ejection fraction is that fraction of the end-diastolic volume that is ejected during systole. Normally EF > 0.5.

3. Critical velocity $(v_C) = \dfrac{R\eta}{\varrho r}$

    R = Reynolds number
    $\eta$ = blood viscosity
    $\varrho$ = blood density
    r = tube or vessel radius

    This equation is used to study heart murmurs (vibrations set up within the heart and great vessels by turbulent blood flow).

4. Cardiac output (CO) $= \dfrac{60I}{Ct}$

    I = indicator or dye in mg

    C $= \dfrac{I}{V}$ the mean concentration in mg/$l$

    V = Volume of liquid in which dye is injected in liters
    t = Passage time in seconds

### 2.9.1.5 SUMMARY

The function of the circulatory system is to maintain tissue oxygenation, supply nutrients and remove wastes. This function is compromised when the heart, blood vessels, or blood fail to perform as intended. Also, the lungs are critical in $O_2$ and $CO_2$ homeostasis. Malfunction in these systems can lead to a decreased flow of suitable blood (e.g., enough $O_2$) to tissues and this can lead to their death. Also, a fall in blood pressure or loss of blood volume can have similar effects.

### 2.9.2 Questions to Review the Circulatory System

(1) Which statement(s) is(are) correct?

(a) Veins and arteries carry both oxygenated and deoxygenated blood.
(b) Veins carry only deoxygenated blood.
(c) Arteries carry only oxygenated blood.
(d) Both (b) and (c).

(2) Which of the following is not part of the conduction system of the heart?

(a) atrioventricular node
(b) chordae tendinae
(c) Bundle of His
(d) Purkinje fibers

(3) Cells in the blood are normally derived from precursor cells in the:

(a) liver
(b) spleen
(c) bone marrow
(d) connective tissue

(4) All are types of white *blood* cells *except*:

(a) megakaryocyte
(b) neutrophil
(c) eosinophil
(d) lymphocyte

(5) The mitral valve is located between the

(a) left atrium and left ventricle
(b) left and right ventricles
(c) left and right atria
(d) superior vena cava and the heart

(6) Which agent below chelates calcium and may prevent clotting of blood?

(a) Vit D
(b) EDTA
(c) Vit K
(d) $NH_3$

(7) All of the following are true about albumin except:

(a) found in the plasma
(b) plays a role in immunologic reactions
(c) made in the liver
(d) plays a role in maintaining the colloid oncotic pressure of the blood

(8) The beats of the heart are initiated by:

(a) the brain
(b) the sympathetic nerves
(c) the parasympathetic nerves
(d) the sinoatrial node

(9) Chordae tendinae:

(a) hold muscles to bones
(b) hold muscles to muscles
(c) hold bones to bones
(d) found in the heart

(10)   The Bohr Effect on hemoglobin function:

(a) The electrons in the hemoglobin are easily ionized.
(b) Hemoglobin can also carry $CO_2$.
(c) Affinity of hemoglobin for oxygen increases with altitude.
(d) Hemoglobin releases oxygen more readily at lower pHs.

(11)   Hematocrit:

(a) the number of red blood cells in the blood
(b) the percentage of blood that is red blood cells
(c) the amount of hemoglobin
(d) the total amount of blood in the body

(12)   Hemoglobin:

(a) does not carry carbon dioxide
(b) is normally free (not in cells) in the blood
(c) is composed of protein, porphyrin, and iron
(d) is normally found in the plasma portion

(13)   Which statement is correct concerning the heart?

(a) Right ventricle pumps blood to the body excluding the lung.
(b) Right ventricle pumps blood to the lung.
(c) Left ventricle pumps blood to the lung.
(d) Left ventricle pumps blood to the body including the lung.

(14)   Which is the correct sequence of blood passing through the heart? (R = right, L = left, A = atrium, V = ventricle, SVC = Superior Vena Cava, IVC = Inferior Vena Cava)

(a) RA to RV to SVC/IVC to LA to LV to lungs to aorta to RA
(b) SVC/IVC to LA to LV to lungs to RA to RV to aorta to SVC/IVC
(c) SVC/IVC to RA to RV to lungs to LA to LV to aorta to SVC/IVC
(d) RA to RV to LA to LV to lungs to aorta to IVC/SVC to RA

(15)   Systole refers to

(a) the contraction phase of the atria
(b) the relaxation phase of the atria
(c) the contraction phase of the ventricles
(d) the relaxation phase of the ventricles

(16)   Heart muscle differs from skeletal muscle in all the following except:

(a) having striations
(b) being made of distinct cells
(c) having intercalated discs
(d) having the capacity to originate beats without nervous impulses

(17)   Sympathetic impulses

(a) increase the heart rate
(b) decrease the heart rate
(c) do not affect the heart rate

(18)   In diastole

(a) the aortic valve is closed
(b) the tricuspid valve is closed
(c) the mitral valve is closed
(d) the ventricles are contracting

(19) Layers of blood vessels include all of the following except:

(a) tendinae
(b) media
(c) adventitia
(d) intima

(20) Arteries

(a) conduct blood toward the heart
(b) help maintain blood pressure due to their elastic recoil properties
(c) always carry oxygenated blood
(d) contain a large media, a small adventitia, and no intima

(21) The greatest resistance to blood flow is in the:

(a) capillaries
(b) veins
(c) arteries
(d) arterioles

(22) All of the following might increase blood pressure except:

(a) increase in sympathetic tone of vessels
(b) increase in the radius of a vessel
(c) increase in blood output by the heart
(d) increase in resistance of vessels

(23) Exchange of substances between tissues and the blood occurs in the:

(a) veins
(b) capillaries
(c) arterioles
(d) arteries

(24) The oncotic pressure of blood:

(a) has no effect on the movement of fluid
(b) causes fluid to move into the tissues from the blood vessels
(c) causes fluid to move into the blood vessels from the tissues

(25) On the venous side of the capillary

(a) hydrostatic pressure exceeds oncotic pressure and causes fluid to move into the tissues
(b) oncotic pressure exceeds hydrostatic pressure and causes fluid to move into the tissues
(c) hydrostatic pressure exceeds oncotic pressure and causes fluid to move into the blood vessel
(d) oncotic pressure exceeds hydrostatic pressure and causes fluid to move into the blood vessel

(26) Regarding the fluid that escapes from the blood on the arterial side of the capillaries:

(a) some of the fluid and proteins is carried off by lymphatics
(b) all of the fluid is returned to the blood at the venous end of the capillary
(c) the fluid normally contains red blood cells
(d) none of the above

(27) The coronary circulation supplies the:

(a) brain
(b) heart
(c) lungs
(d) trunk

(28) Select the following which is most likely a red blood cell:

(a)

(b)

(c)

(d)

(29) Hemoglobin

(a) binds $O_2$ uniformly at all $O_2$ tensions
(b) binds $O_2$ rapidly at low $O_2$ tensions
(c) binds $O_2$ slowly at low $O_2$ tensions
(d) does not become saturated at high $O_2$ tensions

(30) Which of the following is involved in the immune response?

(a) neutrophils
(b) lymphocytes
(c) platelets
(d) basophils

(31) Clotting:

(a) platelets
(b) neutrophils
(c) lymphocytes
(d) eosinophils

### 2.9.3 Answers to Questions in Section 2.9.2

( 1) a  ( 2) b  ( 3) c  ( 4) a  ( 5) a  ( 6) b  ( 7) b  ( 8) d  ( 9) d  (10) d  (11) b
(12) c  (13) b  (14) c  (15) c  (16) a  (17) a  (18) a  (19) a  (20) b  (21) d  (22) b
(23) b  (24) c  (25) d  (26) a  (27) b  (28) a  (29) c  (30) b  (31) a

### 2.9.4 Discussion of Answers to Questions in Section 2.9.2

All are adequately discussed in the Section except the following:

*Question #22* (Answer: b) Sympathetic tone means there is a decrease in the radius of the vessels. A decrease in the radius of the vessels means an increase in resistance (resistance $\propto$ $1/r^4$). This means that the pressure increases (pressure $\propto$ resistance). An increase in radius causes a drop in blood pressue:

> as radius increases, the resistance decreases
> (resistance $\propto 1/r^4$).
> as resistance decreases, the pressure decreases
> (pressure $\propto$ resistance)

Options (c) and (d) are straight from the Section.

### 2.9.5 Vocabulary Checklist for the Circulatory System

_____ atrium
_____ tricuspid valve
_____ mitral valve

_____ chordae tendinae
_____ intercalated discs
_____ diastole

_____ bundle of His
_____ systole
_____ intima
_____ adventitia
_____ vein
_____ ventricles
_____ pulmonic valve
_____ aortic valve
_____ papillary muscles
_____ sinus node
_____ atrioventricular node
_____ Purkinje fibers
_____ vagus nerve
_____ media
_____ artery
_____ arteriole
_____ capillary
_____ resistance
_____ oncotic pressure
_____ white blood cells
_____ hematocrit

_____ serum
_____ Bohr effect
_____ eosinophils
_____ lymphocytes
_____ albumin
_____ blood pressure
_____ hydrostatic pressure
_____ red blood cells
_____ hemoglobin
_____ plasma
_____ allosteric
_____ neutrophils
_____ basophils
_____ platelets
_____ globulins
_____ systolic pressure
_____ diastolic pressure
_____ ejection fraction
_____ critical velocity
_____ stroke volume
_____ cardiac output

## 2.9.6 Concepts, Principles, etc. Checklist for the Circulatory System

_____ structure-function relations of heart
_____ relation of heart muscle and skeletal muscle
_____ effects of nerves on heart rate
_____ changes in heart during systole and diastole
_____ structure of blood vessels in general
_____ structure-function of arteries, arterioles, veins, capillaries
_____ control of blood pressure
_____ fluid and particle transport across the capillary
_____ the different circulations in the body
_____ structure-function of red blood cells and hemoglobin
_____ blood circulation equations

## 2.10 LYMPHATIC SYSTEM

### 2.10.1 Review of the Lymphatic System

The lymphatic system consists of lymph nodes and lymphatic vessels. *Lymph nodes* are points of mergence of several different lymphatic vessels. They contain lymphocytes and macrophages. *Lymphocytes* are involved in the antibody response to antigens (foreign materials). Removing particulate (bacteria, dead cells, etc.) matter by phagocytosis and helping lymphocytes in the immune response are functions of the *macrophage* which performs a similar function all over the body (especially in the lung, liver and spleen). Lymph nodes often swell and become tender during infection or inflammation due to this function. The location of the swollen gland (e.g., at the angle of the jaw) is important in localizing the infection (e.g., the throat) or even a cancer (i.e., metastasis from the primary cancer) because nodes drain lymphatic vessels from given regions of the body.

*Lymphatic vessels* are generally one cell thick being made of endothelial cells (like the cells lining blood vessels). These vessels begin as blind pouches in all tissues of the body. They remove fluid, proteins, and particulate matter that arise in tissues directly or by extravasation from the blood vessels. Once in the lymphatics, the lymph (the above materials) is "filtered" at the lymph nodes and eventually re-enters the circulatory system by flowing into the large veins in the thorax (chest cavity) via the thoracic duct. Lymph flow is passive and requires muscle action (acting as a pump) to move lymph along the vessels. If lymph vessels are destroyed, if lymph nodes are blocked, or if there is no muscle action, the lymph does not flow and the fluid remains in the tissues and that tissue swells up (becomes edematous). Note also that gravity would tend to retard the flow of lymph back into the blood vessels. So, the return of fluid and proteins to the circulation from the tissues and protection against foreign materials are the key *functions* of the lymphatic system. A schematic is:

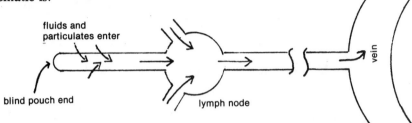

Fig. 2.25—*Lymphatics*

## 2.10.2    Questions to Review the Lymphatic System

(1)    The lymphatic system

   (a) returns fluid and proteins to blood vessels
   (b) has a direct connection to the heart
   (c) consists of vessels only
   (d) is not integral to the function of the body

(2)    Lymph nodes

   (a) are found in veins
   (b) contain lymphocytes only
   (c) may contain lymphocytes and macrophages
   (d) are not directly important in protecting the body against disease

(3)    Macrophages

   (a) are found in lymph nodes only
   (b) are phagocytic cells
   (c) are the lining cells of lymphatic vessels
   (d) all the above

(4)    An enlarged lymph node may mean:

   (a) infection
   (b) inflammation
   (c) cancer
   (d) all of the above

(5)    Lymph moves toward the veins due to:

   (a) tissue pressure
   (b) muscle action
   (c) pumping action of heart
   (d) gravity

**2.10.3    Answers to Questions in Section 2.10.2**

(1) a    (2) c    (3) b    (4) d    (5) b


**2.10.4    Discussion of Answers to Questions in Section 2.10.2**

All questions are adequately discussed in the Section.


**2.10.5    Vocabulary Checklist for the Lymphatic System**

_____ lymph node                         _____ lymphatic vessel
_____ lymph                              _____ macrophage
_____ lymphocyte


**2.10.6    Concepts, Principles, etc. Checklist for the Lymphatic System**

_____ structure of lymphatic system
_____ role of lymphatic system in disease prevention and recognition
_____ role of lymphatic system in fluid and protein homeostasis
_____ composition of lymph
_____ movement of lymph through the vessels


**2.11    RENAL SYSTEM AND BODY FLUID COMPOSITION**

**2.11.1    Review of Renal System and Body Fluid Composition**

**2.11.1.1    BODY FLUID COMPOSITION**

Human body fluids divide conveniently into an *intracellular (IC) compartment* and an *extracellular (EC) compartment*. The EC compartment is further divided into an *interstitial (I) compartment* (outside of cells and outside of the circulation) and a *plasma (P) compartment* (circulatory component). Each compartment has a particular substance that tends to maintain its volume. Potassium $(K^+)$ ion is the main molecule of the IC compartment. Sodium $(Na^+)$ ion is the main molecule of the EC compartment. And protein, in addition to $Na^+$, is important in the plasma compartment.

In the plasma there are *cations*, $Na^+$ and $K^+$ primarily, balanced by *anions*, chloride $(Cl^-)$ and bicarbonate $(HCO_3^-)$ primarily. Also, there are many small organic molecules such as glucose, amino acids, etc. Larger organic molecules such as proteins and fat complexes are also present.

The *acidity*, measured by the pH, is relatively constant at pH $\approx$ 7.40 for the plasma. The major sources of acidity are the $CO_2$ (produced in tissues) and acids from the oxidation of glucose, fats, and amino acids sch as pyruvate, lactate, or sulfur (from sulfur containing amino acids). Bicarbonate (basic) is produced by the kidney to balance these acids. The ratio of dissolved $CO_2$ and $HCO_3^-$ is the determinator of the pH. As $CO_2$ increases the pH decreases and as $HCO_3^-$ increases the pH increases:

$$pH \propto \frac{[HCO_3^-]}{P_{CO_2}}$$

where $P_{CO_2}$ is the partial pressure of $CO_2$. Remember that $CO_2$ undergoes this reaction with water,

$$CO_2 + H_2O \rightleftharpoons H_2CO_3$$
$$\text{carbonic acid}$$

and carbonic acid dissociates to give $H^+$, $H_2CO_3 \rightleftharpoons H^+ + HCO_3^-$ (remember $H^+$ is measured by the pH).

The plasma also contains waste products of the tissues, one of the most important being urea. *Urea*,

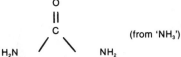

is the result of the breakdown of nitrogen containing organic molecules, especially amino acids. *Creatinine* is a product of muscle metabolism and is also continuously released into the plasma. Both are excreted by the kidneys.

### 2.11.1.2   THE KIDNEY (HUMAN)

The structure and function of the kidney will be described by following the path of blood through the kidney and the formation of urine by the kidney.

Blood from the renal artery passes to a tuft of capillaries called the *glomerulus* which sits in a space created by *Bowman's capsule*. *Filtration* of the blood occurs, but larger proteins and formed elements (i.e., cells) are not filtered through the glomerulus. This initial filtrate which contains water, ions, all non-polymeric organic molecules, and small proteins first passes into *Bowman's capsule (BC)* and then into the *proximal convoluted tubule (PCT)* which is continuous with BC. In the PCT, proteins, amino acids, sugars and other nutrients are *reabsorbed* by active transport by the tubular cells. Sodium, potassium and bicarbonate are reabsorbed as is most of the water. Hydrogen ion and ammonium ions are *secreted* into the tubular lumen by the PCT cells. Also, toxic substances and waste molecules are secreted into the lumen by the PCT cells. The fluid remaining in the lumen continues into the *descending limb of the loop of Henle (LOH)* where $Na^+$ is picked up from the medulla (inside of kidney) interstitium. The filtrate continues around the LOH to the *ascending limb of the LOH* where $Cl^-$ is being actively extruded into the medulla and $Na^+$ passively follows. A $Cl^-$ pump that requires energy as ATP is responsible for this extrusion against the concentration gradient. This *countercurrent multiplier system* between the limbs of the LOH maintains a high concentration of $Na^+$ in the medulla. The filtrate (urine) passes on to the *distal convoluted tubule (DCT)* where $Na^+$ in the lumen is exchanged for $K^+$ (and $H^+$) in the cells stimulated by *aldosterone* (from the adrenal gland). The filtrate (now urine) continues to the *collecting duct (CD)* which dips into the medulla with its large $Na^+$ concentration. The $Na^+$ in the medulla draws most of the water out of the CD into the medulla, where the water is picked up by a system of blood vessels called the *vasa rectae*. *ADH* (antidiuretic hormone; vasopressin) is synthesized in the hypothalamus and stored in and released from the posteior pituitary. It acts on the CD to increase water resorption and results in a more concentrated urine. The urine now passes to the *calyces* to the *pelvices* to the *ureter* to the *urinary bladder* to the *urethra* to the outside. *Excretion* is the passing of the urine to the outside.

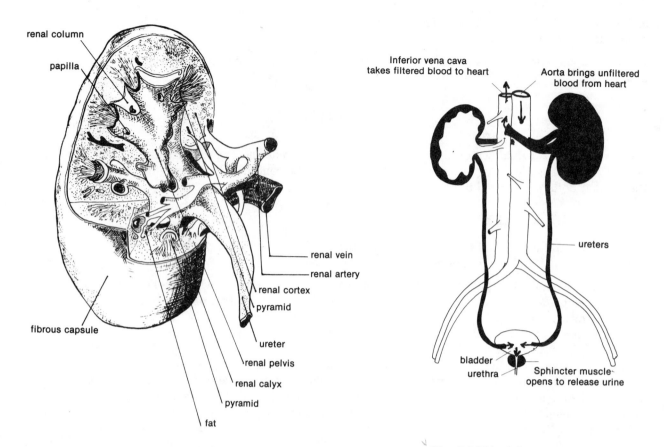

renal column
papilla

renal vein
renal artery
renal cortex
pyramid

fibrous capsule

ureter
renal pelvis
renal calyx
pyramid

fat

**Fig. 2.26(a)—The Kidney**

Inferior vena cava
takes filtered blood to heart

Aorta brings unfiltered
blood from heart

ureters

bladder
urethra

Sphincter muscle
opens to release urine

**Fig. 2.26(b)—The Renal System**

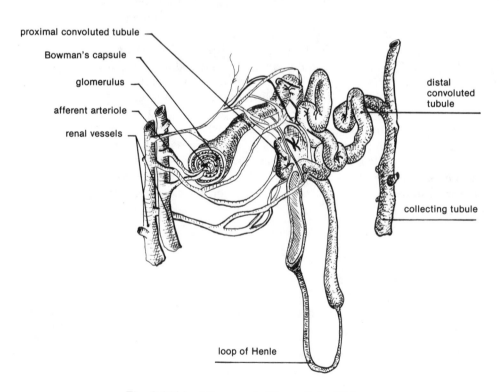

proximal convoluted tubule
Bowman's capsule
glomerulus
afferent arteriole
renal vessels

distal
convoluted
tubule

collecting tubule

loop of Henle

**Fig. 2.26(c)—Microscopic View of the Kidney**

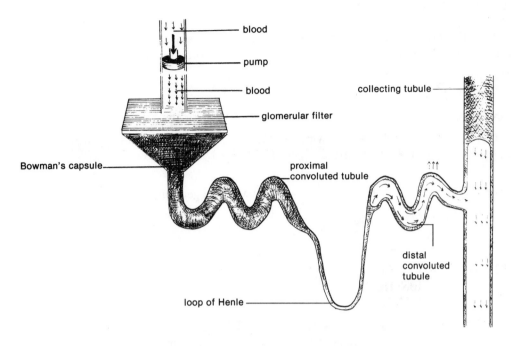

**Fig. 2.26(d)—Schematic of the Renal System**

## 2.11.1.3 SUMMARY OF HOMEOSTASIS OF BODY FLUIDS

The body regulates the composition of its body fluids within fairly narrow limits. This is because too much or too little of most substances is toxic to cells. The kidney is the central regulator. In general, substances taken into the body (by gastrointestinal tract, lungs, skin or directly into vessels) and substances made in the tissues are in balance with substances used by the tissues and *excreted* by the body (in the lungs, gastrointestinal tract, skin, and kidneys). That is, Input = Output. This results in fairly constant levels of most substances in the blood. Changes in the function or amount of the load imposed on any of the above can destroy homeostasis and cause changes in body fluid composition.

The *heart and blood vessels* (2.9.1) serve their part by keeping blood flowing to all the organs and tissues. This allows a constant exchange between the tissues and the blood. If cardiovascular function decreases, fluid nutrients can't get to tissues and wastes accumulate in tissues and the blood. Also, if the heart output falls too much the kidney cannot function. The *lymphatic vessels* (2.10.1) return fluid and protein to the cardiovascular system to help maintain its function. When lymphatic function decreases, fluid accumulates in the tissues, and the heart has less blood to pump which compromises its function. The *lungs* (2.8.1) remove $CO_2$ from the body and supply the $O_2$ needed. If lung function is affected, the acidity of blood is affected as well as the production of energy (need $O_2$). The *skin* (2.12.1) plays a role in the passage of water and ions ($Na^+$, $K^+$, $Cl^-$) in the form of sweat. If sweating is excessive, water and ion loss can compromise the circulation. The *gastrointestinal tract* (2.13.1) is responsible for the intake of nutrients and excretion of certain wastes and ions ($Na^+$, $K^+$, $Cl^-$, $HCO_3^-$) and water. So, malfunctions, as in diarrhea, can lead to body fluid abnormalities.

Finally, the *kidney* serves the role of fine tuning the body fluids. After the other systems have upset or tried to correct the homeostasis, the kidney, through the mechanisms described in Section 2.11.1.2, can return the body fluids to a new (not necessarily the same) homeostasis. When kidneys malfunction, substances collect in the blood (e.g., urea) and/or are excreted (e.g., sugar, excess $Na^+$) that would ordinarily not be retained or excreted.

## 2.11.1.4   BUFFERS IN THE RENAL SYSTEM

The main buffer in the ECF (extracellular fluid) is bicarbonate. Its interaction with hydrogen ions has been explained earlier in 2.11.1.1. In order to use the Henderson-Hasselbalch equation,

$$pH = pK + \log \frac{base}{acid}$$

we should use actual experimental values of an average person: pK = 6.1 for the ECF.

*Example:* Add 10m M/L of hydrochloric acid to 1L of water and to 1L of extracellular fluid. Assume that the ECF [$HCO_3'$] is 20m M/L and the [$H_2CO_3$] is 1.2mM. Study pH changes.

*Solution:* For water, 10mM HCl contains 10mM $= \dfrac{10}{1000} = 0.010$M hydrogen ion.

Therefore, by definition, $pH = -\log[H+]$
$$= -\log[.010]$$
$$= 2.00$$

For ECF, 10HCl + 20NaHCO$_3$ $\rightarrow$ 10NaCl +
$$10NaHCO_3 +$$
$$10H_2CO_3.$$

As seen, bicorbonate reduces the change in pH caused by addition of H +. Using Henderson-Hasselbalch equation, and noting that there is already 1.2 mM $H_2CO_3$ in the fluid,

$$pH = 6.1 + \log \frac{10}{10 + 1.2}$$

$$= 6.1 + \log \frac{10}{11.2} = 6.99$$

$HCO_3'$ is the most important physiologic buffer because its two components can be regulated by the kidneys and the lung.


## 2.11.2     Questions to Review the Renal System and Body Fluid Composition

(1)     Functions of the kidneys include all except

    (a) excretion of $NH_3$ from protein oxidation as urea
    (b) regulation of fluids and electrolytes
    (c) elimination of toxic substances
    (d) elimination of carbon dioxide directly

(2)     All are part of the human kidney except:

    (a) glomerulus
    (b) loop of Henle
    (c) Malpighian tubules
    (d) collecting ducts

(3)     Filtration of *blood* occurs at which structure in the kidney?

    (a) loop of Henle
    (b) collecting ducts
    (c) tubules
    (d) glomerulus

(4)     Select the correct statement concerning the antidiuretic hormone (ADH):

    (a) synthesized in the posterior pituitary gland
    (b) acts on the collecting duct of the kidney
    (c) also called aldosterone
    (d) all of the above are correct

(5)    Select the correct sequence of filtered blood through the kidney:

(a) Bowman's capsule, glomerulus, tubules, collecting duct
(b) glomerulus, Bowman's capsule, collecting ducts, tubules
(c) Bowman's capsule, collecting ducts, glomerulus, tubules
(d) glomerulus, Bowman's capsule, tubules, collecting duct

(6)    The volume of fluid in the plasma is maintained by

(a) protein
(b) $Na^+$
(c) $Na^+$ and protein
(d) $K^+$

(7)    The cations of $Na^+$ and $K^+$ are balanced in the plasma by

(a) $Cl^-$
(b) $HCO_3^-$
(c) $Cl^-$ and $HCO_3^-$
(d) proteins

(8)    The acidity of the plasma is caused by

(a) oxidation of glucose and fats
(b) metabolism of sulfur containing amino acids
(c) production of $CO_2$ by the tissues
(d) all of the above

(9)    Carbon dioxide when dissolved in water

(a) has base properties
(b) has acid properties
(c) is neutral

(10)    Urea

(a) is a product of protein metabolism
(b) contains only carbon, hydrogen, and oxygen
(c) is excreted by the lungs
(d) all of the above

(11)    The _____ is part of the circulatory system.

(a) Bowman's capsule
(b) loop of Henle
(c) medulla
(d) glomerulus

(12)    All of the following substances are filtered at the glomerulus except:

(a) platelets
(b) proteins
(c) glucose
(d) sodium

(13)    Reabsorption of most of the water, glucose, amino acids, sodium and other nutrients occurs at:

(a) loop of Henle
(b) collecting duct
(c) proximal convoluted tubule
(d) distal convoluted tubule

(14)    The high concentration of sodium in the medulla is maintained by the:

    (a) proximal convoluted tubule
    (b) distal convoluted tubule
    (c) loop of Henle
    (d) collecting duct

(15)    The movement of $Cl^-$ out of the ascending limb of the loop of Henle occurs by:

    (a) diffusion
    (b) active transport
    (c) osmosis
    (d) facilitated diffusion

(16)    In the distal convoluted tubule

    (a) $K^+$ moves into the lumen
    (b) $H^+$ moves into the tubular cells
    (c) $Na^+$ moves into the lumen
    (d) $Na^+$ is actively extruded into the medulla

(17)    Malfunction in which of the following systems might result in body fluid disturbances?

    (a) heart
    (b) skin
    (c) lung
    (d) all of them

## 2.11.3    Answers to Questions in Section 2.11.2

( 1) d  ( 2) c  ( 3) d  ( 4) b  ( 5) d  ( 6) c  ( 7) c  ( 8) d  ( 9) b  (10) a  (11) d
(12) a  (13) c  (14) c  (15) b  (16) a  (17) d

## 2.11.4    Discussion of Answers to Questions in Section 2.11.2

All questions are adequately discussed in the Section.

## 2.11.5    Vocabulary Checklist for Renal System and Body Fluid Composition

_____ intracellular compartment
_____ distal convoluted tubule
_____ extracellular compartment
_____ interstitial compartment
_____ plasma compartment
_____ proximal convoluted tubule
_____ descending limb of loop of Henle
_____ aldosterone
_____ collecting duct
_____ vasa rectae
_____ ADH
_____ urea
_____ calyx
_____ pelvis
_____ ascending limb of loop of Henle

_____ countercurrent muliplier system
_____ glomerulus
_____ medulla
_____ reabsorption
_____ excretion
_____ Henderson-Hasselbalch equation
_____ nephron
_____ creatinine
_____ cortex
_____ filtration
_____ secretion
_____ Bowman's capsule
_____ renal system
_____ kidney

## 2.11.6    Concepts, Principles, etc. Checklist for Renal System and Body Fluid Composition

_____ role of different substances in maintaining volumes of fluid compartments
_____ balance of cations and anions in fluids
_____ origin of acidity in plasma and role of $CO_2$ and $HCO_3^-$
_____ structure/function of kidney
_____ factors involved in body fluid composition homeostasis
_____ systems and their role in body fluid homeostasis
_____ buffers in the renal system

## 2.12    THE SKIN AND THERMOREGULATION

### 2.12.1    Review of the Skin and Thermoregulation

#### 2.12.1.1    THE SKIN

The layers of the skin are the epidermis, dermis, and subcutaneous tissue. The *epidermis* (Fig. 2.27) is a layer comprised of several types of related cells and melanocytes. The deepest layer of the epidermis, the basal layer, contains cells which are dividing. As these cells move toward the surface, they lose their nucleus and produce a protein called *keratin* (which is stable and water insoluble). At the surface, these cells have no nucleus, are dead, are essentially keratin and are called the *stratum corneum* which is the scaly dry surface layer of the skin. *Melanocytes* synthesize *melanin* (a black to dark-brown pigment) which is responsible for the color of the skin. It also responds to ultraviolet light to produce tanning of the skin.

The *dermis* is internal to the epidermis and contains most of the accessory structures of the skin. Blood vessels end in the dermis. Sensory endings for pain, temperature and touch are found here and in the subcutaneous tissue. Hair follicles and sebaceous glands (secrete an oily fat substance; if clogged cause acne), and sweat glands originate here. All of these exit at the epidermis. General connective tissue cells, fibroblasts, and macrophages among other cells may be found in the dermis.

The *subcutaneous tissue* contains primarily fat cells.

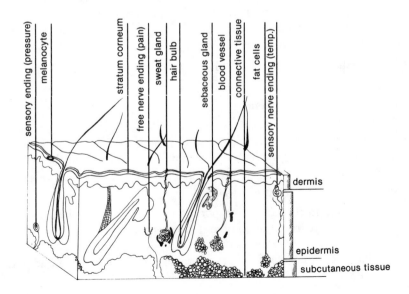

*Fig. 2.27—The Skin*

*Functions of the skin* include:

(1) protection from physical agents (wind, water, etc.)—afforded by the stratum corneum and melanocytes (radiation),

(2) protection from microbial agents especially bacteria—afforded by the stratum corneum and some secretions of the sebaceous glands,

(3) thermoregulation (see 2.12.1.2),

(4) waste removal (e.g., excess water, salts, urea, others)—via the sweat glands,

(5) site of the first activation of vitamin D—by ultraviolet light,

(6) sensation—by the many nerve endings.


## 2.12.1.2   THERMOREGULATION

Thermoregulation is the regulation of the internal body temperature between the narrow limits necessary for life. Too high or low a temperature can cause proteins (enzymes especially) to become less effective or totally inactive (denatured) and cause the protoplasm to gel (become more solid).

Normally, the body temperature is a balance between heat produced by metabolism and heat loss by the various means described below. Processes that increase body metabolism increase body heat, this is especially true of muscle activity (e.g., shivering). Regulation of body temperature is centered in the *hypothalamus* (in the brain).

*Pyrogens* released during bacterial infections, among other causes, can affect the hypothalamus in a way that it allows the body temperature to rise higher than normal, and fever results.

The <u>mechanisms of heat conservation</u> include those that are always present and those called upon in emergencies (note: * = most important):

(A)   Mechanisms always present:

* (1) subcutaneous fat as insulation;
   (2) presence of hair or fur (lower animals).

(B)   Mechanisms called upon as needed:

* (1) shivering—contractions of muscles produce heat;
* (2) constriction of vessels to skin—prevents heat loss from surface;
   (3) piloerection of hair on skin—traps air against skin that once warmed serves as an insulation;
   (4) increase in metabolic rate.

The <u>mechanisms of heat loss</u> include those that are always present and those called upon in emergencies:

(A)   Mechanisms always present:

(1) loss of heat by radiational cooling;
(2) low level of evaporation of moisture from skin—for a liquid to evaporate, heat must be supplied; this heat comes from the skin which is cooled.

(B)   Mechanisms called upon as needed:

* (1) sweating and consequent evaporation of water—the sweat itself removes heat from the body and more is lost when this evaporates;
* (2) dilation of vessels to the skin—increases the amount of radiational cooling.

## 2.12.2　Questions to Review the Skin and Thermoregulation

(1)　Layers of the skin include all except:

(a) epidermis
(b) dermis
(c) lamina propria
(d) subcutaneous tissue

(2)　Dead cells are found in the:

(a) subcutaneous tissue
(b) dermis
(c) epidermis
(d) no dead cells are in the skin

(3)　Melanocytes are found in the:

(a) dermis
(b) epidermis
(c) subcutaneous tissue
(d) none of the above

(4)　The dermis usually contains all of the following except:

(a) hair follicles
(b) sweat glands
(c) fat cells
(d) fibroblasts

(5)　All are functions of the skin except:

(a) exchange of gases
(b) thermoregulation
(c) activation site of Vitamin D
(d) protection from bacteria

(6)　The main effect of extremes of temperature is on the functions of:

(a) carbohydrates
(b) phospholipids
(c) proteins
(d) nucleic acids

(7)　Control of body temperature is localized in the:

(a) skin
(b) heart
(c) cerebrum
(d) hypothalamus

(8)　Select the mechanism that is *not* used to conserve heat:

(a) shivering
(b) dilation of blood vessels
(c) piloerection
(d) subcutaneous fat

(9)　Select the mechanism that is *not* used to lose heat:

(a) sweating
(b) increase in metabolic rate
(c) radiational cooling
(d) dilation of blood vessels

**2.12.3    Answers to Questions in Section 2.12.2**

(1) c    (2) c    (3) b    (4) c    (5) a    (6) c    (7) d    (8) b    (9) b


**2.12.4    Discussion of Answers to Questions in Section 2.12.2**

All questions adequately discussed in Section.


**2.12.5    Vocabulary Checklist for Skin and Thermoregulation**

_____ epidermis
_____ Vitamin D
_____ sebaceous glands
_____ stratum corneum
_____ pyrogens
_____ fibroblasts
_____ melanin
_____ piloerection
_____ fat cells

_____ hair follicles
_____ keratin
_____ hypothalamus
_____ sweat glands
_____ melanocytes
_____ shivering
_____ subcutaneous tissue
_____ dermis
_____ radiational cooling


**2.12.6    Concepts, Principles, etc. Checklist for Skin and Thermoregulation**

_____ structure of skin
_____ functions of the skin
_____ general concept of thermoregulation
_____ mechanisms of heat conservation
_____ mechanisms of heat loss


**2.13    DIGESTIVE SYSTEM**

**2.13.1    Review of the Digestive System**

**2.13.1.1    STRUCTURE/FUNCTION RELATIONSHIPS OF THE DIGESTIVE SYSTEM**

The structure and function of the digestive system will be discussed by following a bolus of food through it.

The _teeth_ and the _tongue_ are responsible for breaking food down into swallowable chunks (called boluses). Adults have 32 teeth, children have 20 (called deciduous teeth). Each quadrant (quarter) contains two _incisors_ (for cutting), one _canine_ (for tearing), two _premolars_ (for crushing), and 3 _molars_ (for grinding). _Salivary glands_ secrete alkaline _saliva_ to moisten food for swallowing, protect against bacteria, and begin digestion of starch. _Swallowing_ is initiated voluntarily but becomes involuntary as food enters the pharynx. The _swallowing center_ is located in the medulla, and the hypoglossal (XII) and glossopharyngeal (IX) nerves are responsible for the esophageal phase after the bolus passes from the pharynx. The bolus enters the _stomach_ from the esophagus where it may be stored for several hours. Grinding and liquefying the food are the main functions of the stomach accomplished by its strong muscles. _Hydrochloric acid_ and _intrinsic factor_ (for absorption of Vit $B_{12}$) are secreted by parietal cells, and _pepsin_ (digests proteins) is secreted by the chief cells of the stomach. _Mucus_ is secreted by goblet cells to protect the stomach from the acid. The acid kills many bacteria and its secretion is controlled by the vagus nerve and _gastrin_. Food (now _chyme_) is propelled to the duodenum by *peristalsis* (propulsive contractions in the gut) through a relaxed *pyloric sphincter*. Chyme entering the duodenum causes *secretin* (causes bicarbonate and fluid to be released from the pancreas) and *cholecystokinin-pancreozymin* (causes primarily enzymes and water to be released from the pancreas and bile to be released by the gall bladder) to be released. The *pancreas* secretes inactive enzymes called *zymogens*. *Trypsinogen* which is converted to *trypsin* by *enterokinase*, located in the duodenal mucosa, activates its precursor and other zymogens. Other enzymes: chymotrypsin, lipases and amylases. *Bile* is secreted by the liver and stored in and released from the gall bladder. *Bile salts* in bile emulsify lipids to make them more available for digestion. The duodenum has an alkaline pH. Chyme passes into the jejunum where the mucosa contains disaccharidases and peptidases for the final breakdown of nutrients before they are absorbed by active transport. The *small intestine* is composed of the *duodenum, jejunum* and *ileum* in that order. The duodenum is important for absorption of $Ca^{+2}$ and $Fe^{+3}$, the jejunum for most sugars, amino acids, fats, etc., and the ileum absorbs Vit $B_{12}$ (complexed to intrinsic factor) and bile salts. In the *colon (large intestine)* the remaining water from the small intestine is largely absorbed as are most ions—this compacts the chyme into feces. *Feces* are stored in the *sigmoid colon* and *rectum* until they are defecated. The *appendix* is attached to a part of the colon called the *cecum*.

The small intestines are thrown into folds called *villi*. Individual cells have convolutions of the cell membrane called *microvilli*. Both of these increase the surface area for absorption of nutrients. *Crypts* are regions at the base of villi where new cells are generated.

The *liver* is a vital organ reflected in its numerous functions. The major functions will be listed: (1) *syntheses and storage of glycogen* to be converted to glucose under the stimulation of epinephrine or glucagon; (2) *gluconeogenesis*—the synthesis of glucose from amino acids stimulated by glucagon and epinephrine via cAMP; by removal of storage glycogen and

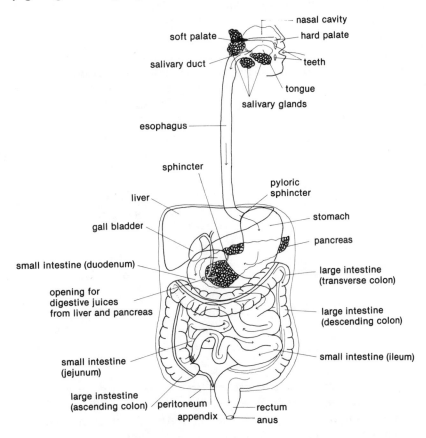

**Fig. 2.28—Structure of the Digestive System**

gluconeogenesis the liver plays an important role in *regulation of blood glucose;* (3) *proteins*—synthesizes coagulation factors, albumin, and various others; (4) synthesizes *bile and cholesterol;* (5) contains numerous *macrophages* (called *Kupffer cells*) for defense against foreign materials (e.g., bacterial); (6) contains a system for *detoxification and degradation* of toxins, drugs, and normal metabolites; (7) *fats*—packages fats for transport, oxidizes fatty acids to ketone bodies for use by other tissues; (8) *amino acids*—deaminates (removes nitrogen), produces urea; (9) can interconvert fats, carbohydrates, and amino acids, (10) *stores* substances such as iron and vitamin $B_{12}$; and (11) red blood cells—potential site for production of RBCs in the adult, site of destruction of old red blood cells.

## 2.13.1.2   THE DIGESTION OF KEY NUTRIENTS

The digestive functions will be reviewed by discussing each of the major nutrients in turn.

*Carbohydrates* (approximately 4 kcal/gm). A small amount of carbohydrate digestion occurs in the mouth (salivary *amylase*) and the stomach (acid digestion). *Pancreatic amylases* digest the starch to disaccharides (*maltose,* isomaltose) and *glucose.* These disaccharides and *sucrose* (cane sugar, sugar beets) and *lactose* (from milk) are broken down, respectively, by *maltases, sucrases,* and *lactases* located on the outer surface of *mucosal cells.* The resulting monosaccharides then enter by *active transport* (glucose and galactose) or *facilitated transport* (the above and fructose, mannose, xylose, arabinose). The active transport mechanisms involve a coupling with $Na^+$ via a Na-K-ATPase and a specific carrier for glucose both located in the mucosal cell. Carbohydrates are not essential (for life) to the diet. But, they normally provide (in the US) 50 + % of calories. Cellulose cannot be digested by humans.

*Lipids.* Triglycerides are hydrolyzed by *lipase* from the pancreas. *Bile salts* aid this by emulsifying and solubilizing the fat. Fatty acids, monoglycerides, diglycerides, and glycerol are the products of lipases. These products can diffuse across the mucosa. *Glycerol and short chain fatty acids* go directly to the liver via the venous portal system. *Long chain fatty acids, and the mono- and diglycerides* are resynthesized into triglycerides and packaged with proteins as *chylomicrons* which are absorbed into *lymphatics* and then go to the liver. In the liver, the lipids are reorganized into lipoproteins (lipid plus special proteins) and shipped to adipose cells primarily. Linolenic and linoleic acids are essential fatty acids (cannot be synthesized by humans). Fats are the long term energy storage compounds (approximately 9 kcal/gm). The molecules discussed above are in Figure 2.29.

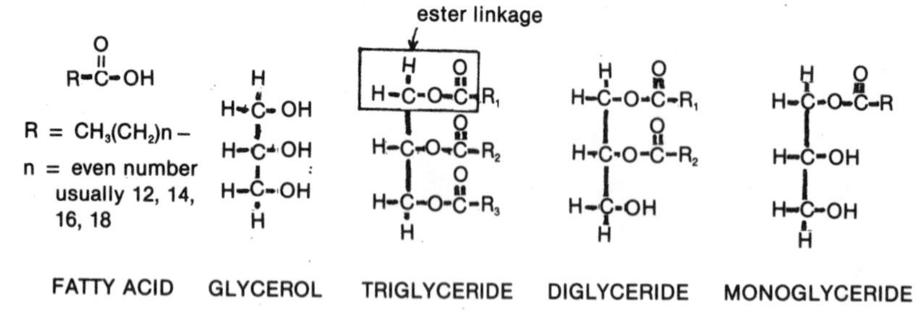

*Fig. 2.29—Lipids*

*Proteins.* Some protein digestion occurs in the stomach by *pepsin* (secreted as inactive pepsinogen which is activated by stomach acid or other pepsins). *Enterokinase* (intestinal enzyme) converts trypsinogen to trypsin which then converts trypsinogen and *chymotrypsinogen* (both from the pancreas) and all other pancreatic zymogens to active forms. The result of these digestions are oligopeptides and dipeptides which are cleaved by mucosal enzymes, e.g., carboxypeptidases. Several intestinal active transport systems exist. Absorbed amino acids go to the liver via the venous portal system. There are about 8-10 essential amino acids which have to be supplied in the diet (some are isoleucine, leucine, phenylalanine, histidine). Protein provides about 4 kcals/gm.

### 2.13.1.3   ORIGINS AND FUNCTIONS OF SOME DIGESTIVE ENZYMES

| Enzyme | Origin | Function |
|---|---|---|
| Amylase | Salivary glands, pancreas | Starch breakdown |
| Pepsin (a protease) | Stomach | Protein breakdown |
| Trypsin (a protease) | Pancreas | Further breakdown of protein |
| Lipase | Pancreas | Fat breakdown |
| Peptidase | Intestinal epithelium | Breakdown of short polypeptides |
| Maltase | Intestinal epithelium | Maltose breakdown |

### 2.13.2   Questions to Review the Digestive System

(1)   Which type of tooth, in the normal adult with a full set of teeth, has the *incorrect* maximum number in parenthesis?

(a) incisors (4)
(b) canines (4)
(c) premolars (8)
(d) molars (12)

(2)   All are functions of saliva *except*:

(a) digestion of starch
(b) digestion of protein
(c) lubrication of food
(d) protection against bacteria

(3)   Select the incorrect association:

(a) stomach—grinds and liquefies food
(b) pancreas—digestive enzymes
(c) small intestine—absorption of fluid and food
(d) colon (large intestine)—absorption of food

(4)   Select the *incorrect* association:

(a) chymotrypsin—protein
(b) trypsin—carbohydrates
(c) amylase—carbohydrates
(d) lipases—fats

(5)   The correct sequence of structures in the gut is

(a) stomach, esophagus, small intestine, large intestine
(b) esophagus, stomach, large intestine, small intestine
(c) esophagus, stomach, small intestine, large intestine
(d) esophagus, small intestine, stomach, large intestine

(6)   Which of the following is not a function of the liver?

(a) synthesis of insulin
(b) synthesis of carbohydrates, proteins, fats
(c) detoxifies drugs
(d) synthesis of bile

(7)    Most nutrients are absorbed in the:

    (a) esophagus
    (b) stomach
    (c) small intestine
    (d) large intestine

(8)    Digestion of carbohydrates occurs *mostly* by enzymes from the:

    (a) pancreas
    (b) liver
    (c) stomach
    (d) salivary glands

(9)    All of the following carbohydrates can be digested by humans except:

    (a) starch
    (b) sucrose
    (c) cellulose
    (d) maltose

(10)    Monosaccharides cross the intestinal wall mainly by:

    (a) active transport
    (b) diffusion
    (c) facilitated transport
    (d) both (a) and (c)

(11)    Select the *incorrect* statement concerning bile salts:

    (a) break down (digest) lipids
    (b) emulsify and solubilize lipids
    (c) synthesized in the liver
    (d) stored in the gall bladder

(12)    The products of triglyceride hydrolysis by lipases in the intestine may include:

    (a) fatty acids
    (b) monoglycerides
    (c) diglycerides
    (d) all of these

(13)    Which is the main long-term energy storage substance in animals?

    (a) carbohydrates
    (b) fats
    (c) proteins
    (d) nucleic acids

(14)    All of the following enzymes are important in the digestion of proteins except:

    (a) amylase
    (b) pepsin
    (c) trypsin
    (d) chymotrypsin

(15)    The enzyme responsible for the activation of trypsinogen in the intestine is:

    (a) pepsin
    (b) enterokinase
    (c) chymotrypsin
    (d) carboxypeptidase

(16)    Swallowing is:

    (a) voluntary
    (b) involuntary
    (c) both

(17)   Secretion of bicarbonate and fluid from the pancreas is stimulated by:

(a) secretin
(b) cholecystokinin
(c) enterokinase
(d) gastrin

(18)   Acid secretion from the stomach may be stimulated by:

(a) gastrin
(b) vagus nerve
(c) neither
(d) both

(19)   Select the enzyme not made in the pancreas:

(a) trypsin
(b) lipase
(c) amylase
(d) pepsin

(20)   Vitamin $B_{12}$ is absorbed in the:

(a) ileum
(b) jejunum
(c) duodenum
(d) stomach

(21)   Iron is absorbed in the:

(a) stomach
(b) jejunum
(c) ileum
(d) duodenum

(22)   The absorptive area of the small intestine is increased by structures called:

(a) crypts
(b) villi
(c) microvilli
(d) both (b) and (c)

(23)   The liver does *not* play a role in the metabolism of:

(a) fats
(b) carbohydrates
(c) proteins
(d) it plays a role in the metabolism of all of these

(24)   The digestion of starch by amylase produces:

(a) galactose
(b) glucose
(c) maltose
(d) both (b) and (c)

(25)   The digestion of small peptides and disaccharides occurs

(a) in the stomach lumen;
(b) in the lumen of the bowel;
(c) on the mucosal cell surface;
(d) inside the mucosal cell.

(26) Certain lipids, in contrast to other nutrients, leaving the intestine enter the:

  (a) portal system
  (b) lymphatics
  (c) arteries
  (d) no different from other nutrients

(27) Chylomicrons primarily contain:

  (a) carbohydrates
  (b) lipids
  (c) proteins
  (d) nucleic acids

## 2.13.3 Answers to Questions in Section 2.13.2

( 1) a  ( 2) b  ( 3) d  ( 4) b  ( 5) c  ( 6) a  ( 7) c  ( 8) a  ( 9) c  (10) d  (11) a
(12) d  (13) b  (14) a  (15) b  (16) c  (17) a  (18) d  (19) d  (20) a  (21) d  (22) d
(23) d  (24) d  (25) c  (26) b  (27) b

## 2.13.4 Discussion of Answers to Questions in Section 2.13.2

All answers are adequately discussed in the Section.

## 2.13.5 Vocabulary Checklist for the Digestive System

| | | |
|---|---|---|
| _____ incisor | _____ ileum | _____ saliva |
| _____ small intestine | _____ liver | _____ pepsin |
| _____ pyloric sphincter | _____ sucrase | _____ appendix |
| _____ premolar | _____ amylase | _____ enterokinase |
| _____ feces | _____ starch | _____ gastrin |
| _____ cholecystokinin-pancreozymin | _____ chylomicrons | _____ villi |
| _____ stomach | _____ chymotrypsin | _____ bile salts |
| _____ large intestine (colon) | _____ peristalsis | _____ duodenum |
| _____ zymogens | _____ canine | _____ crypts |
| _____ trypsin | _____ jejunum | _____ mucosal cells |
| _____ mucus | _____ secretin | _____ gluconeogenesis |
| _____ cecum | _____ molar | _____ maltase |
| _____ bile | _____ sigmoid colon | _____ lactase |
| _____ chyme | _____ rectum | _____ triglycerides |
| _____ microvilli | _____ pancreas | _____ salivary gland |

## 2.13.6 Concepts, Principles, etc. Checklist for the Digestive System

_____ types and purposes of teeth
_____ process of swallowing
_____ role of stomach, intestines in digestion and absorption
_____ role of pancreas in digestion
_____ functions of the liver
_____ location of absorption of the key nutrients
_____ digestion of key nutrients
_____ digestive enzymes

## 2.14    SKELETAL SYSTEM

### 2.14.1    Review of the Skeletal System

Bone is composed of a crystal part (mostly *hydroxyapatite* which is a complex of $Ca^{+2}$ and $PO_4^{-3}$, but also $Na^+$, $K^+$, $Mg^{+2}$ and other anions) and an organic part (mostly the fibrous protein, *collagen*). Collagen, whose fibrils are arranged end to end, serves as the focus for the deposition of the crystals. This is the basic composition of all types of bone.

Bone can be formed without a cartilaginous model (*intramembranous bones* such as skull bones) or can be formed from a cartilaginous model (*endochondral bone* formation, such as long bones). The cartilage is first removed and then the bone is laid down in its place. Bone does not come from the cartilage. *Osteoblasts* make the inorganic matrix which crystallizes around the collagen. Osteoblasts become *osteocytes* (mature bone cells) when bone formation is complete. Bone is in a dynamic state with bone formation (osteoblasts) and bone destruction (osteoclasts) occurring simultaneously and continously. *Haversian systems* (Fig. 2.30) are present in mature bone. They consist of central nutrient blood vessels and nerves which connect by *canaliculi* to osteocytes located in *lacunae* arranged circumferentially around the central canal.

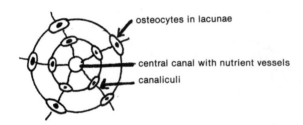

*Fig. 2.30—Haversian Canal System*

When bone is laid down it may be spongy or compact. *Spongy bone* (Fig. 2.31) has many air pockets, like a sponge, with the bone present as spicules. *Compact bone* (Fig. 2.32) is densely packed bone with no air spaces. It is very strong bone and is found where great strength is required as in the cortex of long bones:

*Fig. 2.31—Spongy Bone*              *Fig. 2.32—Compact Bone*

Bones in the human are of two types, flat bones and long bones. *Flat bones* (Fig. 2.33) include the skull bones, ribs and vertebrae, contain red marrow (much blood cell production), are found where little movement is required, and perform protective functions in general. *Long bones* (Fig. 2.34) include the bones of the hands, feet, arms and legs, contain yellow marrow, are involved in locomotion and motion primarily.

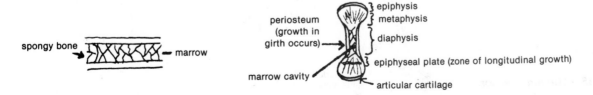

*Fig. 2.33—Flat Bone*              *Fig. 2.34—Long Bone*

Joints allow for motion between bones. The contacting and mobile surfaces between bones are covered by *cartilage*. *Ligaments* help hold bones together at the joint—that is, they are attached bone to bone. *Tendons* connect muscles to bones—they also help hold bones together at joints.

*Parathyroid hormone* (PTH) causes $Ca^{+2}$ (and phosphate) to be removed from the bony matrix, thus causing demineralization of bone. The $Ca^{+2}$ appears in the serum. The bone matrix serves as a storage depot for many cations ($Ca^{+2}$, $K^+$, $Mg^{+2}$, $Na^+$) and serves to buffer (help control the levels of) these in the blood (as well as an $H^+$ buffer). PTH is stimulated by low serum calcium. *Calcitonin* is secreted from special cells in the thyroid gland. It is stimulated by high serum calcium and causes $Ca^{+2}$, etc., to be deposited in bone. A schematized drawing of some of the bones of the human body is in Fig. 2.35.

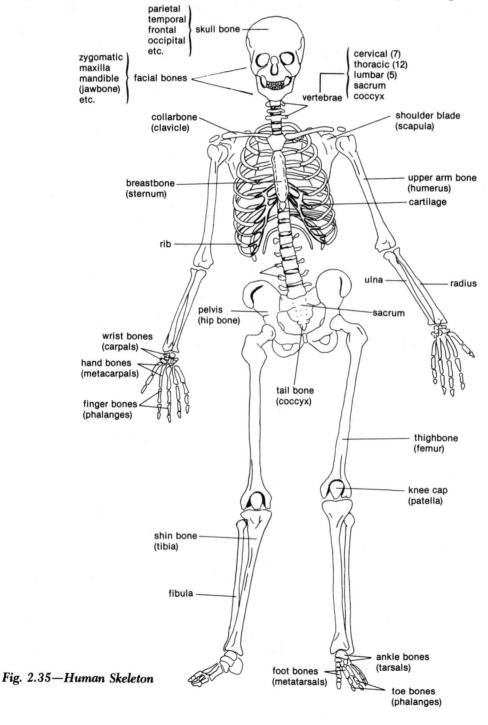

*Fig. 2.35—Human Skeleton*

## 2.14.2    Questions to Review the Skeletal Sysem

(1)    All bone is formed

(a) from a cartilage model
(b) without a cartilage model
(c) either (a) or (b)
(d) neither (a) nor (b)

(2)    Parathyroid Hormone:

(a) demineralization of bone
(b) mineralization of bone
(c) increases basal metabolic rate
(d) Graves' disease results when in excess

(3)    Which cell makes bone?

(a) osteoblast
(b) osteocyte
(c) osteoclast
(d) all of these

(4)    Haversian canals:

(a) markings seen on Mars
(b) nutrient systems of bone
(c) found in the inner ear
(d) communication between the left and right cerebral hemispheres

(5)    Components of a *mature* Haversian canal system would include all except:

(a) osteoblasts
(b) lacunae
(c) canaliculi
(d) blood vessels

(6)    Components of the human axial skeleton include all except:

(a) sternum
(b) vertebral column
(c) hips
(d) skull

(7)    Components of the appendicular human skeleton include all except:

(a) shoulder girdle
(b) arm bones
(c) ribs
(d) leg bones

(8)    The humerus, radius and ulna are found in the:

(a) vertebral column
(b) shoulder girdle
(c) arm
(d) leg

(9)    All are parts of the vertebral column except:

(a) cervical
(b) thoracic
(c) caudal
(d) lumbar

(10) The parietal and occipital bones are found in the:

    (a) vertebral column
    (b) skull
    (c) hip girdle
    (d) foot

(11) The bones of the wrist are called:

    (a) carpals
    (b) metacarpals
    (c) tarsals
    (d) metatarsals

(12) The hip bone connects the _____ to the _____.

    (a) femur, sternum
    (b) humerus, sacrum
    (c) femur, sacrum
    (d) humerus, sternum

(13) Phalanges are found in the:

    (a) fingers
    (b) toes
    (c) both
    (d) neither

(14) Bone is composed of _____ and _____.

    (a) calcium; phosphate
    (b) globular proteins; ions
    (c) collagen; hydroxyapatite
    (d) none of the above

(15) _____ serves as the focus of the deposition of the crystal matrix.

    (a) collagen
    (b) osteocytes
    (c) hydroxyapatite
    (d) cartilage

(16) The hormone that mobilizes $Ca^{+2}$ from bone:

    (a) thyroxin
    (b) parathyroid hormone
    (c) calcitonin
    (d) Vit D

## 2.14.3    Answers to Questions in Section 2.14.2

( 1) c  ( 2) a  ( 3) a  ( 4) b  ( 5) a  ( 6) c  ( 7) c  ( 8) c  ( 9) c  (10) b  (11) a
(12) c  (13) c  (14) c  (15) a  (16) b

## 2.14.4    Discussion of Answers to Questions in Section 2.14.2

All questions are adequately discussed in the Section.

**Vocabulary Checklist for the Skeletal System**

_____ hydroxyapatite
_____ intramembranous
_____ osteoblasts
_____ osteoclasts
_____ canaliculi
_____ spongy bone
_____ flat bones
_____ parathyroid hormone

_____ collagen
_____ endochondral
_____ osteocytes
_____ Haversian systems
_____ lacunae
_____ compact bone
_____ long bones
_____ calcitonin


**2.14.6     Concepts, Principles, etc. Checklist for the Skeletal System**

_____ composition of bone
_____ formation of bone
_____ types of bone (histologically, grossly)


**2.15     MUSCLES**

**2.15.1     Review of Muscles**

The three types of muscles are smooth, striated (skeletal), and cardiac. _Smooth muscle_ is composed of distinct spindle shaped cells with central nuclei and no visible markings. They are innervated by the autonomic nervous system and are largely involuntary. Smooth muscles can contract slowly and maintain contractions for long periods of time. This feature is useful for their function in organs where they are found. These include the gut (for peristalsis and churning of food), in blood vessels (for regulation of blood pressure), and in many ducts (e.g., the ureter for peristalsis).

_Cardiac muscle_ is composed of distinct cells separated by condensed cell membranes called intercalated discs. Heart cells are connected by gap junctions (specialized cell membrane regions) to speed impulse conduction. Cardiac muscle appears striated. The muscle fibers are highly branched—this probably adds to their strength. Innervation is by the autonomic nervous system but beats are originated by specialized muscle cells (see section 2.9.1.1).

_Skeletal muscle_ are a _syncytium_ (many cells fused together with loss of intervening membranes and retention of nuclei) and appear striated. Skeletal muscles are innervated by the somatic nervous system and are voluntary. The control of voluntary movements originates in a portion of the _cerebral cortex_ (surface of cerebrum) and are coordinated by impulses from the _cerebellum_. Skeletal muscles contract rapidly but tire easily. A simple _twitch_ of a muscle involves the following steps: (1) impulse from a nerve stimulates the muscle, (2) a brief latent period, (3) then the phase of contraction, and (4) a phase of relaxation. If the muscle is stimulated during the relaxation phase it can be made to contract again. If these stimuli are in rapid succession the contractions can be made to _summate_ to a sustained contraction called _tetanus_.

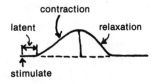

_Fig. 2.36—Phases of Contraction_

Muscle *tone* differs from tetanus in that groups of muscle fibers of a muscle alternatingly contract and relax. This allows form and position (at rest) to be maintained.

Skeletal muscle uses $O_2$ (oxygen) in aerobic metabolism (Sec. 2.2.1) when it is available. In the absence of $O_2$, the production of energy requires that there be a final electron acceptor. This electron acceptor becomes pyruvate which is converted to lactate (Fig. 2.37).

$$H_3C-\overset{\overset{O}{||}}{C}-\overset{\overset{O}{||}}{C}-O^{\ominus} \quad \xrightarrow{H:^{\ominus} \; H+} \quad H_3C-\overset{\overset{O-H}{|}}{\underset{H}{C}}-\overset{\overset{O}{||}}{C}-O^{\ominus}$$

pyruvate                                          lactate

e.g., NADH could transfer an $H:^-$ and $H^+$ is picked up from solution.

*Fig. 2.37—Formation of Lactate*

The amount of lactate formed becomes a measure of the lack of $O_2$ (the usual electron acceptor). This is a partial measure of the oxygen debt that muscles incur during exercise when their rate of $O_2$ demand exceeds that supplied. After exercise, the lactate is converted back to pyruvate, and the electrons are passed to $O_2$ as $O_2$ is supplied to the muscles and the oxygen debt is repaid. *In summary*, during exercise the energy metabolism of muscle switches from aerobic to anaerobic and an oxygen debt is incurred which is repaid when the exercise ends.

The skeletal muscles act across joints to move body parts. Each muscle has an *origin* and an *insertion*. In general, the origin is stationary, and when the muscle contracts, the insertion (and the bone it is attached to) moves toward the origin (Fig. 2.38).

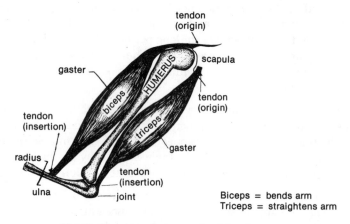

Biceps = bends arm
Triceps = straightens arm

*Fig. 2.38—Attachments of a Muscle*

Muscles work in pairs (or in more complex arrangements). For a muscle that moves a joint in one direction there is an *antagonistic muscle* that will move the joint in the opposite direction (i.e., undo that motion). There are also *synergistic muscles* that aid in the motion caused by a given muscle. At the elbow, the triceps (extension) and biceps (flexion) are examples of antagonistic muscles. At the shoulder, the deltoid (raises arm) and supraspinatous (raises arm) are examples of synergistic muscles. Complex neural pathways insure coordination of the muscle groups. A *flexor* decreases the angle of a joint. An *extensor* increases the angle of a joint. An *abductor* moves a limb away from the midline. An *adductor* moves a limb toward the midline.

The functioning unit of the muscle is the *myofibril* (muscle fibers are composed of myofibrils). Myofibrils are composed of linearly arranged sarcomeres. A *sarcomere* is limited by regions that anchor the *actin* (thin filaments) called the *Z-lines*. *Myosin* (thick filaments) alternate with the actin and are not anchored. Bands are labeled as shown in Fig. 2.39.

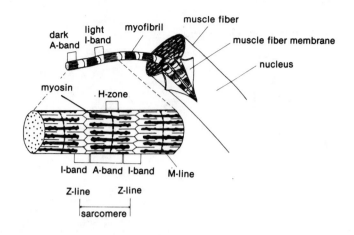

**Fig. 2.39—Components of a Sarcomere**

When the muscle contracts, the Z-lines move together, the I and H bands decrease in size, and the A-band remains the same size. The *actin complex* is composed of actin, tropomyosin and troponin. *Actin* has sites which bind to heavy meromyosin when contraction occurs. *Tropomyosin* is an $\alpha$-helical protein wound around the actin (which is two intertwined $\alpha$-helical chains) and blocks the myosin binding site. *Troponin* is a regulator protein bound to tropomyosin and has a site for binding $Ca^{+2}$ and a site that inhibits myosin's binding to actin. When there is no $Ca^{+2}$ present, the troponin and tropomyosin prevent myosin binding and, hence, contraction. When $Ca^{+2}$ is present, the $Ca^{+2}$ binds to troponin causing a conformational change which in turn causes tropomyosin to shift, uncovering the actin binding region for myosin, and contraction proceeds. *Myosin* is composed of *light meromyosin* (the tail) and *heavy meromyosin* (the head). The head binds to actin and contains an ATPase to break the bonds to actin. *Contraction* is caused by the heads of myosin alternatingly binding and releasing actin in a rachet-like fashion. The *sarcolemma* (cell membrane of muscle) sends a system of membranes (T-tubules) into the muscle. When an impulse from a nerve reaches the sarcolemma, this is transmitted down the *T-tubules* which release $Ca^{+2}$ into the sarcoplasm (muscle cell interior) for contraction. The *sarcoplasmic reticulum* (specialized smooth endoplasmic reticulum) abuts upon the T-tubules; its role is to remove the $Ca^{+2}$ from the sarcoplasm.

## 2.15.1.1   OXYGEN DEBT AND VOLUNTARY MUSCLE CONTROL

As discussed above, during intense physical activity oxidative metabolism cannot supply all the ATP that muscles require. As soon as intense muscular activity ceases, aerobic processes must provide ATP for the resynthesis of creative phosphate. These aerobic activities account for the deep, rapid breathing that continues after muscular activity has ceased. The elevated rate of respiration provides the oxygen required to produce ATP for the resynthesis of creative phosphate and to convert lactic acid back to glucose and glycogen.

When skeletal muscles are not used, the muscle fibers diminish in size. Regular exercise, on the other hand, can produce increases in muscle size, endurance, and strength. Endurance exercises, such as running, produce cardiovascular and pulmonary changes, causing the muscles to be better supplied with materials such as oxygen and carbohydrates. Cramps are involuntary muscle contractions that are painful. Their precise cause is unknown—possibly a low oxygen supply causes them.

## 2.15.2    Questions to Review Muscles

(1)    All of the following are muscle proteins except:

   (a) actin
   (b) myosin
   (c) fibrinogen
   (d) troponin

(2)    One of the histologic muscle types has striated fibers and is involuntary. It is:

   (a) smooth muscle
   (b) skeletal muscle
   (c) cardiac muscle
   (d) none

(3)    Select the muscle type composed of distinct cells:

   (a) smooth
   (b) skeletal
   (c) cardiac
   (d) both (a) and (c)

(4)    Intercalated discs are found in which type of muscle?

   (a) skeletal
   (b) cardiac
   (c) smooth
   (d) all

(5)    Which type of muscle is a syncytium?

   (a) skeletal
   (b) cardiac
   (c) smooth
   (d) all

(6)    All are true concerning smooth muscle except:

   (a) composed of distinct spindle cells
   (b) largely involuntary
   (c) have intercalated discs
   (d) found in the gut

(7)    All are true concerning cardiac muscle except:

   (a) it is a syncytium
   (b) it is striated
   (c) it is involuntary
   (d) gap junctions speed conduction

(8)    All are true concerning skeletal muscle except:

   (a) they are a syncytium
   (b) they are involuntary
   (c) they are responsible for locomotion
   (d) they contract rapidly but tire readily

(9)    Select the incorrect statement concerning muscles:

   (a) ligaments attach bone to bone
   (b) flexors decrease the angle at a joint
   (c) adductors move a limb away from the midline
   (d) tendons attach muscle to bone

(10) The A-band of striated muscle represents:

(a) myosin only
(b) actin only
(c) both (a) and (b)
(d) neither (a) nor (b)

(11) The Z-line as seen in striated muscle anchors:

(a) both actin and myosin
(b) neither actin nor myosin
(c) actin
(d) myosin

(12) During muscle contraction, all of the following occur except:

(a) Z-lines move together
(b) A-band decreases in size
(c) I-band decreases in size
(d) H-band decreases in size

(13) Which of the following ions is of most importance in the mechanical contraction of muscle?

(a) $Na^{+1}$
(b) $Ca^{+2}$
(c) $K^{+1}$
(d) $Cl^{-1}$

(14) Muscle tone depends upon

(a) continual low level contraction of all fibers in the muscles
(b) summation of twitches to a plateau
(c) presence of short fibers that constantly appear contracted
(d) alternating contractions of different fiber groups in a muscle

(15) During exercise

(a) muscles depend on the Kreb's Cycle for energy
(b) $O_2$ becomes the electron acceptor
(c) lactate levels decrease
(d) energy metabolism changes from aerobic to anaerobic

(16) Troponin

(a) binds $Ca^{+2}$
(b) binds to tropomyosin
(c) inhibits myosin's binding to actin
(d) all of the above

(17) The phase of contraction of a muscle occurs when

(a) tropomyosin binds and releases actin
(b) myosin alternately binds and releases actin
(c) actin alternately binds and releases myosin
(d) none of the above

## 2.15.3    Answers to Questions in Section 2.15.2

( 1) c   ( 2) c   ( 3) d   ( 4) b   ( 5) a   ( 6) c   ( 7) a   ( 8) b   ( 9) c   (10) c   (11) c
(12) b   (13) b   (14) d   (15) d   (16) d   (17) b

## 2.15.4 Discussion of Answers to Questions in Section 2.15.2

All questions are adequately discussed in the Section except,

*Question #10* (Answer: c) Technically, the band is visible as such because of the myosin, but within the limits of the band actin is also present.


## 2.15.5 Vocabulary Checklist for Muscles

———— smooth muscle
———— cardiac muscle
———— origin
———— insertion
———— sarcomere
———— synergistic
———— tetanus
———— myosin
———— flexor
———— pyruvate
———— troponin
———— abductor
———— adductor
———— myofibril

———— A-band
———— Z-line
———— skeletal muscle
———— actin
———— antagonistic
———— muscle tone
———— tropomyosin
———— extensor
———— lactate
———— sarcolemma
———— sarcoplasmic reticulum
———— T-tubules
———— I-band


## 2.15.6 Concepts, Principles, etc. Checklist for Muscles

———— types of muscle and differences between them
———— locus of control of voluntary muscles
———— difference between tone and tetanus
———— concept of oxygen debt
———— muscles as movers of bones
———— antagonistic and synergistic muscles
———— molecular mechanism of muscle contraction


## 2.16 NERVOUS SYSTEM

### 2.16.1 Review of the Nervous System

#### 2.16.1.1 THE CENTRAL AND PERIPHERAL NERVOUS SYSTEMS; NERVE CONDUCTION

*Histologically,* the nervous system is composed of neurons and glial cells. Neurons conduct impulses, and *glial cells* provide some sort of supportive function. There are many kinds of neurons and glial cells—only a typical neuron will be discussed. A *neuron* has a cell body or soma that is characterized by having *Nissl bodies* (ribosomes), one or more short branched projections off the body called *dendrites*, and, usually, one long projection called an *axon*. Although impulses can travel in either direction in a dendrite or an axon, dendrites usually convey impulses toward the soma, and axons usually convey impulses away from the soma. This directionality is achieved by the presence of *synapses* between adjacent neurons or a neuron and an effector (muscle or gland). Synapses typically include an axon ending with *transmitter substance*, a synaptic cleft, and a dendrite or muscle or gland with receptors for the transmitter substance.

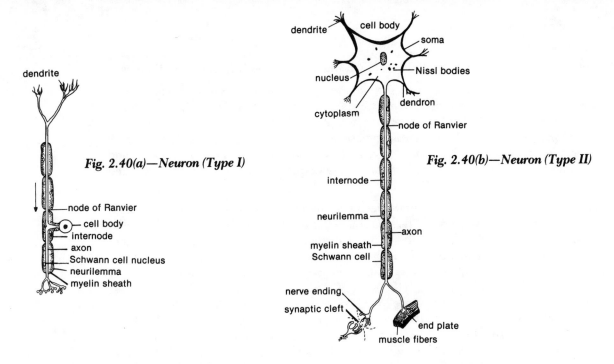

dendrite

*Fig. 2.40(a)—Neuron (Type I)*

node of Ranvier
cell body
internode
axon
Schwann cell nucleus
neurilemma
myelin sheath

dendrite — cell body
soma
nucleus — Nissl bodies
cytoplasm — dendron
node of Ranvier

*Fig. 2.40(b)—Neuron (Type II)*

internode
neurilemma
axon
myelin sheath
Schwann cell

nerve ending
synaptic cleft
end plate
muscle fibers

There are three special types of neurons: sensory, motor, and association. *Sensory neurons* transfer impulses from the various sense organs to the spinal cord or brain, e.g., picking up a hot frying pan with your hand. *Association neurons* transfer and connect the messages between the sensory neurons and the motor neurons. They are located in the brain and spinal cord. Association neurons transfer impulses similar to a switching station at a telephone exchange. In case of the hot frying pan, the impulse travels from the spinal cord to motor neurons, with the help of association neurons. *Motor neurons* transfer impulses to various muscles and glands. These impulses cause stimuli in the body. For the hot frying pan, the impulse travels along motor neurons to muscles in the arm. This causes the muscles in the arm to contract. This results in your hand dropping the frying pan. After you drop the frying pan, the brain receives this impulse, causing pain.

An impulse causes the axon to release the chemical transmitter; this diffuses across the cleft to the receptors and induces an impulse there which is then transmitted. An *impulse or action potential* is set up in a neuron when the *potential difference* (voltage) across its membrane reaches a *threshold potential*. The *resting potential* of a neuron is determined by the balance of $Na^+$ (most outside) and $K^+$ (most inside) on each side of the cell membrane—the outside is positive relative to the inside. An impulse or transmitter substance can disturb the ionic balance in such a way that $Na^+$ moves inside and $K^+$ moves outside (only $Na^+$ moves in the early phase of the action potential). This causes the cell potential to move toward the threshold potential. Once the threshold potential is reached, the action potential is initiated and this moves down the neuron to the axon end, releases transmitter and the process continues as such.

A *Na-K ATPase* maintains the concentration across the nerve membrane by active transport of the ions. *Myelin sheaths* (condensed cell membranes) around axons increase the speed of conduction (saltatory conduction). Details in Fig. 2.41.

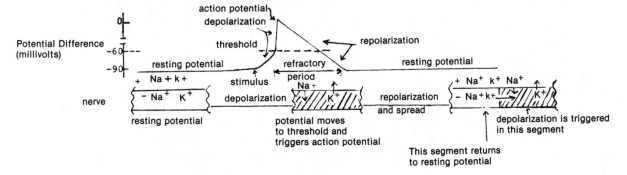

*Fig. 2.41—Various Potentials of a Nerve*

The *refractory period* is that time during which the nerve cannot respond to a stimulus.

*Anatomically*, the nervous system is divided into the *central nervous system (CNS)*, consisting of the brain and spinal cord, and the *peripheral nervous system (PNS)*, consisting of the cranial nerves (CN) and peripheral nerves (PN). The PNS may be divided into the *autonomic nervous system (ANS)* and the *somatic nervous system (SNS)*. The ANS and SNS also have components in the CNS. The ANS is divided into the *sympathetic* and *parasympathetic* branches. The SNS contains the *sensory* (*afferent*—toward the CNS) and *motor* (*efferent*—away from the CNS) nerves.

Hindbrain (rhombencephalon), midbrain (mesencephalon), and forebrain (prosencephalon) are the gross divisions of the *brain*. The *hindbrain* consists of the *myelencephalon (medulla)* and *metencephalon (pons)*. The midbrain is not further divided. The forebrain consists of the *diencephalon* (hypothalamus and thalamus) and the *telencephalon* (the *cerebral hemispheres*). The *cerebellum* is a derivative of the metencephalon. Respiratory and circulatory regulation, coughing, and vomiting reflexes, are functions of the medulla. Note that these are functions basic to life. The cerebellum is concerned with muscle coordination. No general functions are localized in the midbrain or pons; they serve important relay functions. The hypothalamus is the important regulator of the internal environment (controls hormones of the pituitary via releasing factors, thirst and hunger centers, water balance, temperature regulation) and also behavior (sexual, aggressive). The thalamus is the relay center for nearly all sensory input. The cerebrum (especially the cerebral cortex, i.e., surface) is the integrating and interpretation center for all sensory input and voluntary motor activity. In addition, memory, learning, emotions, etc., are also located here (Fig. 2.42).

The *spinal cord (SC)* has an interior of *gray matter* (neuron cell bodies) surrounded by *white matter* (myelinated axons). Serving as a path between the brain and the periphery (senses and muscles or glands) is the primary function of the SC. *Descending tracts* (from the brain to the SC) and *ascending tracts* (from SC to brain) are in the *white matter*. *Sensory nerves* enter dorsally and *motor nerves* exit ventrally. Several *reflexes* are at the SC level, e.g., the knee jerk (Fig. 2.43).

The *sympathetic system* (SS) peripherally consists of a chain of ganglia (neuron cell bodies outside the CNS) called the sympathetic chain which is parallel to and adjacent to the spinal cord. From these, nerves travel to many organs and tissues and may affect them all simultaneously (i.e., in a diffuse manner). In general, the SS moves the organism away from homeostasis as in the "fight or flight" phenomenon. Sympathetic discharges, e.g., cause the heart rate to increase, digestive process to stop, circulation to the skin to decrease, and blood flow to the heart and muscles to increase. The ganglia of the *parasympathetic system (PS)* are located near the end-organ, and it can exert specific effects directed at one organ or tissue. The PS tends to maintain homeostasis and, in general, opposes actions of the SS. Actions of the PS include slowing of the heart rate and increasing the digestive processes. The *Vagus nerve* (cranial nerve X) is a very important parasympathetic nerve to the heart and abdominal viscera. *Acetylcholine* is the postganglionic (after the synapses in the ganglia discussed above) transmitter in the PS. *Norepinephrine* is the postganglionic transmitter for the SS. The PS originates from the cranio-sacral CNS, and the SS originates from the thoraco-lumbar CNS.

There are 31 *spinal nerves (SN)*. They are classified according to the level of their connection with the spinal cord—8 cervical, 12 thoracic, 5 lumbar, 5 sacral, 1 coccygeal. Each nerve contains motor and sensory components.

There are 12 *cranial nerves (CN)*. *Olfactory* (I) for smell. *Ocular* (II) for vision. *Oculomotor* (III), *Trochlear* (IV) and *Abducens* (VI) for eye movements. *Trigeminal* (V) for sensory perception (pain, temperature, touch, pressure) over the face and head and for mastication (chewing). The *Facial* (VII) for taste and facial expression. The *Vestibulocochlear* (VIII) for balance and hearing. The *Glossopharyngeal* (IX) for taste and swallowing. The *Vagus* (X) for voice, swallowing, digestive functions (secretions, peristalsis), and slowing heart rate. The *Spinal Accessory* (XI) helps rotate head and move shoulders. The *Hypoglossal* (XII) for tongue movement.

The brain and spinal cord are covered by *meninges*. These are, from the outside in: the *dura mater* (tough fibrous layer), the *arachnoid* (vascular and nutrient layer), and the *pia mater* (fragile layer directly attached to nervous tissue).

Summary of the above information is in Fig. 2.44.

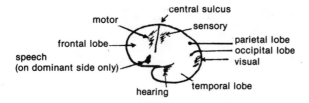

Lateral View of the Brain

*Fig. 2.42—The Cerebral Cortex*

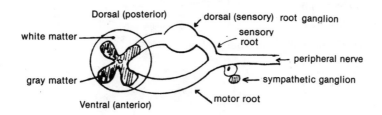

*Fig. 2.43—The Spinal Cord*

Divisions of the Nervous System

| Nervous System | | | | | | | | | |
|---|---|---|---|---|---|---|---|---|---|
| CNS | | | | | | | | PNS | |
| Brain | | | | | | | SC | ANS | SNS |
| Hindbrain | | | Midbrain | Forebrain | | | ///// | PS | SS |
| Myelen-cephalon | Metencephalon | | " | Diencephalon | | Telencephalon | | | |
| Medulla | Pons | Cere-bellum | " | Thal-amus | Hypo-thalamus | Cerebral Hemispheres | | | |

*Fig. 2.44—Summary of CNS Organization*

The simplest functional organization of the nervous system is the *reflex arc*. The basic structure consists of a sensory neuron which detects a stimulus and transmits it to the spinal cord where a motor neuron is stimulated that transmits the impulse to an effector (gland or muscle), which causes the organism to respond (Fig. 2.45).

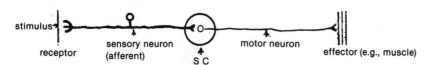

*Fig. 2.45—Reflex Arc*

Not all neurons stimulate other neurons. Some inhibit other neurons. This adds another level of functional complexity. In the example above the afferent neuron could have also stimulated an *interneuron* (in the spinal cord) which could have inhibited the motor neuron of the antagonist of the muscle that contracted:

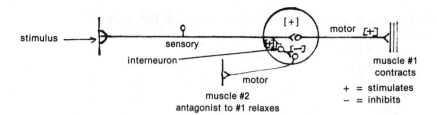

This can be magnified many times thereby affording numerous possibilities for antagonistic or synergistic actions in the nervous system.

### 2.16.2    Questions to Review the Nervous System

(1)    Select the incorrect statement concerning the spinal cord:

(a) gray matter is central
(b) white matter is peripheral
(c) sensory nerves enter ventrally
(d) motor nerves exit ventrally

(2)    Which is(are) not part of the central nervous system?

(a) thalamus
(b) hypothalamus
(c) spinal cord
(d) cranial nerves

(3)    Glial cells are found in the:

(a) muscular system
(b) endocrine system
(c) nervous system
(d) skeletal system

(4)    All are specifically associated with a neuron except:

(a) lack of a nucleus
(b) Nissl bodies
(c) dendrite
(d) axon

(5)    What entity of neurons allow for one-way conduction of impulses in the nervous system?

(a) axons
(b) dendrites
(c) synapses
(d) somas

(6)    Which of the following can conduct impulses away from the neuron cell body or toward it?

(a) axon
(b) dendrite
(c) both
(d) neither

(7)    When the potential difference across a nerve membrane equals the threshold, what results?

(a) an action potential
(b) synthesis of transmitter substances
(c) destruction of transmitter substances
(d) nothing until the resting potential is exceeded

(8)    What ion(s) determine the resting potential of a nerve cell?

(a) sodium
(b) potassium
(c) calcium
(d) both (a) and (b)

(9)    The concentrations of ions across the cell membrane is maintained by:

(a) diffusion
(b) active transport
(c) osmosis
(d) facilitated transport

(10)   Myelin sheaths are found:

(a) surrounding tendons
(b) covering the brain
(c) covering muscles
(d) around axons of neurons

(11)   During the early phase of the action potential

(a) only $Na^+$ moves
(b) only $K^+$ moves
(c) $Na^+$ moves into the cell and $K^+$ moves out
(d) $Na^+$ moves out of the cell and $K^+$ moves in

(12)   The refractory period occurs

(a) before threshold is exceeded
(b) before the action potential
(c) after the action potential
(d) roughly during the action potential

(13)   The peripheral nervous system includes:

(a) spinal nerves
(b) cranial nerves
(c) spinal cord
(d) both (a) and (b)

(14)   The autonomic nervous system includes:

(a) sympathetic system
(b) parasympathetic system
(c) somatic nervous system
(d) both (a) and (b)

(15)   The hindbrain contains:

(a) thalamus
(b) medulla
(c) cerebrum
(d) spinal cord

(16)   All are associated with the forebrain except:

(a) diencephalon
(b) telencephalon
(c) myelencephalon
(d) hypothalamus

(17)   All are functions of the medulla except:

(a) voluntary movements
(b) respiratory regulation
(c) circulatory regulation
(d) cough reflex

(18) The cerebellum:

(a) regulates respiration
(b) is the site of memory
(c) coordinates motor activity
(d) is the site of behavior

(19) Select the *incorrect* statement concerning the sympathetic nervous system:

(a) sympathetic ganglia are near the spinal cord
(b) causes the heart rate to increase
(c) increases blood flow in certain tissues
(d) moves the organism toward homeostasis

(20) Select the *incorrect* statement concerning the parasympathetic system:

(a) ganglia are located near the end-organ
(b) increases the heart rate
(c) maintains homeostasis
(d) increases digestive actions

(21) Vagus Nerve:

(a) parasympathetic
(b) supplies gut and the heart
(c) a cranial nerve
(d) all are correct

(22) Select the correct sequence of the meninges from outside inward: (A = arachnoid, D = dura, P = pia)

(a) A, D, P
(b) D, P, A
(c) P, A, D
(d) D, A, P

## 2.16.3  Answers to Questions in Section 2.16.2

( 1) c  ( 2) d  ( 3) c  ( 4) a  ( 5) c  ( 6) c  ( 7) a  ( 8) d  ( 9) b  (10) d  (11) a
(12) d  (13) d  (14) d  (15) b  (16) c  (17) a  (18) c  (19) d  (20) b  (21) d  (22) d

## 2.16.4  Discussion of Answers to Questions in Section 2.16.2

All questions are adequately discussed in the Section.

## 2.16.5  Vocabulary Checklist for the Nervous System

| | | |
|---|---|---|
| _____ glial cell | _____ trochlear (IV) | _____ parasympathetics |
| _____ sympathetics | _____ hypothalamus | _____ sensory nerves |
| _____ efferent | _____ myelin sheath | _____ axon |
| _____ Nissl body | _____ abducens (VI) | _____ acetylcholine |
| _____ vagus nerve (X) | _____ cerebral hemispheres | _____ hindbrain |
| _____ motor nerves | _____ central nervous system | _____ soma |
| _____ dendrite | _____ vestibulocochlear (VIII) | _____ spinal nerves |
| _____ norepinephrine | _____ brain | _____ medulla |
| _____ myelencephalon | _____ autonomic nervous system | _____ transmitters |
| _____ synapse | _____ spinal accessory (XI) | _____ olfactory (I) |
| _____ cranial nerves | _____ gray matter | _____ pons |
| _____ metencephalon | _____ dura mater | _____ threshold potential |
| _____ action potential | _____ pia mater | _____ oculomotor (III) |
| _____ ocular (II) | _____ reflex arc | _____ thalamus |
| _____ diencephalon | _____ afferent | _____ Na-K ATPase |
| _____ resting potential | _____ neuron | _____ trigeminal (V) |

_____ telencephalon
_____ refractory period
_____ facial (VII)
_____ spinal cord
_____ peripheral nervous system
_____ glossopharyngeal (IX)

_____ white matter
_____ somatic nervous system
_____ hypoglossal (XII)
_____ arachnoid
_____ meninges
_____ interneuron

## 2.16.6 Concepts, Principles, etc. Checklist for the Nervous System

_____ structure of nerve cell
_____ structure and function of synapse
_____ origin and propagation of the action potential
_____ organization and functions of the central nervous system
_____ organization and functions of the peripheral nervous system
_____ structure and function of the sympathetic system
_____ structure and function of the parasympathetic system
_____ coverings of the brain
_____ structure of a reflex arc
_____ basic idea of antagonism/synergism in the nervous system

## 2.17 ENDOCRINE SYSTEM

### 2.17.1 Review of Endocrine System

*Hormones* are substances released from special secretory tissues, called endocrine glands, *into the blood*. From there they circulate to their target tissue, combine with the target receptor and exert their effect. Hormones are regulators, not catalysts (as enzymes are), of organism homeostasis. The *major glands* are the hypothalamus, pituitary, thyroid, parathyroid, adrenal, pancreas, gut, ovaries, testis, liver, kidney, pineal gland, thymus gland, skin and placenta. *Gut hormones* (gastrin, secretin, cholecystokinin-pancreozymin) are discussed in Section 2.13.1. Ovarian, placental and testicular hormones and FSH, LH and prolactin are discussed in Section 2.18.1.

The *hypothalamus* synthesizes releasing factors (RF), inhibiting factors (IF), vasopressin (antidiuretic hormone—ADH) and oxytocin. *Vasopressin* causes the kidney to retain water. *Oxytocin* causes contraction of certain smooth muscles and plays a role in uterine contractions of labor and milk ejection in lactation. Oxytocin and vasopressin are stored in the posterior pituitary until released. RFs and IFs act upon the anterior pituitary (AP). RFs cause the corresponding hormones of the AP to be synthesized and released from it. IFs inhibit release of the corresponding hormones. All of the hormones of the hypothalamus are peptides or proteins. Examples are TRF (TSH Releasing Factor) and PIF (Prolactin Inhibiting Factor).

The *anterior pituitary* (AP) synthesizes and releases several trophic (growth stimulating and supporting) hormones among others. Hormones secreted are *thyroid stimulating hormone (TAH), adrenal cortex stimulating hormone (ACTH), follicle stimulating hormone (FSH),* and *luteinizing hormone (LH)* which are all trophic hormones to the glands indicated by their names. The AP also secretes growth hormone (GH) and prolactin (also called lactogenic hormone). GH functions via somatomedin (produced in the liver) to stimulate the growth of many tissues in the body. Oversecretion of GH results in *Giantism* (if before adolescence) or *acromegaly* (if as an adult). All of the AP hormones are proteins or glycoproteins. *MSH* (melanocyte stimulating hormone) is secreted by the intermediate lobe of the pituitary gland.

The *thyroid gland* produces thyroxin and calcitonin. *Thyroxin*, which is a modified tyrosine with iodine attached, works by increasing the rate of metabolism. *Calcitonin* decreases the calcium in the blood by causing it to move into the bones.

The *adrenal gland* is composed of a cortex and medulla. The *cortex* is stimulated by ACTH to synthesize *glucocorticoids* (the primary one being *cortisol*) which perform many functions including regulation of blood sugar (increases it) and fighting stress (e.g., infections). *Mineralocorticoids* (primary one is *aldosterone*) are also synthesized by the cortex but usually as a result of stimulation by angiotensin II (see below). Aldosterone causes the kidney to retain sodium (and hence water) and secrete potassium. The *medulla* synthesizes *epinephrine* which is a sympathetic stimulant (see Section 2.15.1.1). The cortical hormones are steroids. The medullary hormones are modified tyrosines.

*Parathyroid glands* (located on the thyroid gland, but not part of it) secrete parathyroid hormone (PTH, a protein) which regulates calcium and phosphorus metabolism. Calcium and phosphate are resorbed from bone under the influence of PTH.

The *pancreas* secretes insulin (from $\beta$-cells) and glucagon (from $\alpha$-cells) among other hormones and substances. *Insulin* acts to lower blood glucose by causing cells to take up glucose, it also causes amino acid and fatty acid uptake. *Glucagon* works to increase blood glucose by stimulating *glycogenolysis* (glycogen breakdown) and *gluconeogenesis* (synthesis of glucose from amino acids) by the liver. Insulin and glucagon are both proteins. Diabetes mellitus is due to a deficiency of insulin.

*Vitamin D* is taken in as a nutrient, then goes through a series of activation steps. First, it is activated by ultraviolet light in the skin, then it is hydroxylated successively in the liver and kidney. Its main role is to increase absorption of calcium by the gut through the stimulation of the synthesis of a calcium binding protein. Vitamin D is a steroid.

The *kidney* secretes renin, erythropoietin, and helps in the synthesis of active Vitamin D (above). *Renin* is an enzyme molecule that splits a small peptide called angiotensin I off the *renin substrate* (produced in the liver). Angiotensin I is further split by enzymes in the lung or blood to yield *angiotensin II* which is a potent constrictor of blood vessels and also stimulates synthesis and release of aldosterone from the adrenal. *Erythropoietin* is a protein hormone which stimulates the bone marrow to synthesize more red blood cells.

The *pineal gland* probably produces a host of hormones, but the best known is melatonin which is a modified tryptophan. The pineal gland suppresses pituitary, gonadal (ovary and testis), adrenal and thyroid function. These effects may be mediated via the hypothalamus.

*Thymosin* is produced by the *thymus gland* and plays a role in the immunologic system.

Hormones regulate themselves by means of a process called *feedback inhibition*. A gland produces a hormone and this hormone, or a product, feeds back at some level to shut off its synthesis. This is illustrated in Fig. 2.46. Note the following points:

(1) *Long Loop*—the specific hormone feeds back on the hypothalamus to inhibit release of the RF. This then prevents release of the trophic hormone which prevents the synthesis of the specific hormone. As this decreases, its inhibition on the hypothalamus decreases and more of the RF is released which causes more trophic hormone to be released, etc. This cycle can continue as such or be modified positively or negatively by factors outside of the axis (hypothalamus-pituitary-gland) shown.

(2) & (3) *Short Loops*—Mechanisms as above, but the hormones feed back on the gland that stimulated their synthesis (i.e., the pituitary) instead of a point farther removed (i.e., the hypothalamus).

For a given hormone all combinations of the above may exist.

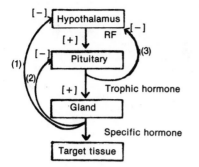

(−) = inhibition of that gland
(+) = stimulation of that gland

Fig. 2.46—Feedback Loops

Hormones *exert their actions* in many ways (some still unknown). Some protein hormones seem to act via cAMP by combining with specific receptors on the target cell membrane. Some steroids exert their effect by combining with receptors in the target cell cytoplasm (they diffuse through the lipid cell membrane). They then move into the nucleus to interact with DNA to cause synthesis of mRNA, which makes specific proteins (usually enzymes).

## 2.17.1.1   MAJOR HORMONES OF ENDOCRINE GLANDS

| Gland | Hormone | Function |
|-------|---------|----------|
| Pituitary | a) Growth<br>b) Gonadotropic<br>c) ACTH<br><br>d) Prolactin<br><br>e) TSH | a) regulates growth of bones<br>b) development of sex organs and sex hormones<br>c) stimulates secretion of adrenal cortex hormones, e.g., glucocorticoids<br>d) stimulates secretion of milk by the mammary glands<br>e) stimulates activity of the thyroid gland |
| Hypothalamus | a) Oxytocin<br><br>b) ADH | a) regulates blood pressure and stimulates uterine smooth muscles<br>b) controls water absorption in the kidneys |
| Thyroid | a) Thyroxine<br>b) Calcitonin | a) increases metabolism<br>b) releases calcium from bones, lowers blood calcium and phosphates |
| Parathyroid | PTH | a) increases release of calcium from bone<br>b) decreases plasma phosphate levels |
| Adrenal Cortex | Corticoids | multiple metabolism, blood cell production, reabsorption of $Na^+$, excretion of $K^+$ |
| Medulla | Adrenaline (Epinephrine and Norepinephrine) | increases heart rate, stimulates the nervous system, causes sweating, cardiac muscle contraction |
| Pancreas | a) Glucagon<br>b) Insulin | a) helps breakdown of glycogen<br>b) controls sugar storage in liver, causes hypoglycemia |
| Ovaries | a) Estrogen<br>b) Progesterone | a) enhances female sex characteristics<br>b) growth of uterine lining |
| Testes | Testosterone | enhances male sex characteristics |

| Symbol Key: | | |
|---|---|---|
| ACTH | = | Adrenocorticotropin |
| TSH | = | Thyrotropin |
| ADH | = | Antidiuretic Hormone |
| PTH | = | Parathyroid Hormone |

### 2.17.2    Questions to Review the Endocrine System

(1)    Insulin:

    (a) secreted by the pancreas
    (b) a protein
    (c) involved in the metabolism of glucose, amino acids, fats
    (d) all of the above

(2)    Vitamin D:

    (a) is actually a hormone after modification in the body
    (b) increases absorption of calcium from the gut
    (c) requires metabolic changes in the skin, liver, and kidney to function
    (d) all of the above

(3)    Select the *incorrectly* paired hormone and disease or deranged process associated with an excess/deficiency of it:

    (a) growth hormone—acromegaly
    (b) insulin—diabetes mellitus
    (c) cortisol—abnormal calcium/phosphate metabolism
    (d) thyroxin—altered metabolic rate

(4)    All of the following hormones are correctly paired with one of its major functions except:

    (a) thyroxin—increases metabolic rate
    (b) glucocorticoids—increases blood sugar levels
    (c) aldersterone—role in "fight or flight" sympathetic response
    (d) parathyroid hormone—regulation of calcium/phosphorous metabolism

(5)    Select the endocrine gland that is *incorrectly* paired with its hormone product:

    (a) adrenal cortex—cortisol
    (b) adrenal medulla—aldosterone
    (c) adrenal medulla—epinephrine
    (d) adrenal cortex—mineralocorticoids

(6)    Select the hormone *incorrectly* paired with its target tissue:

    (a) TSH—thyroid glands
    (b) ACTH—anterior pituitary
    (c) LH—ovary or testis
    (d) MSH—melanocytes

(7)    Which hormones are synthesized by the hypothalamus?

    (a) releasing factors
    (b) vasopressin
    (c) oxytocin
    (d) all of the above

(8)    Hormones synthesized and released by the anterior pituitary is(are)

    (a) Thyroid Stimulating Hormone (TSH)
    (b) Follicle Stimulating Hormone (FSH)
    (c) Growth Hormone
    (d) all of the above

(9)    Which of the following tissues secrete hormones?

    (a) pancreas
    (b) ovaries
    (c) gastrointestinal tract
    (d) all of the above

(10)    All of the following are general characteristics of hormones except

(a) hormones are secreted into the blood
(b) hormones are regulators not initiators of homeostatic processes
(c) hormones are all proteins
(d) hormones do not function like enzymes

(11)    All of the following are general characteristics of hormones except

(a) hormones regulate themselves by feedback inhibition
(b) hormones may be proteins, peptides, steroids, or modified amino acids
(c) some protein hormones act via cAMP
(d) most steroid hormones act via cAMP

(12)    Melatonin is produced by the:

(a) pineal gland
(b) skin
(c) liver
(d) pituitary gland

(13)    Thymosin is concerned with:

(a) metabolic rate
(b) immunologic competence
(c) calcium/phosphate
(d) none of the above

(14)    Calcitonin:

(a) decreases serum calcium
(b) has no effect on serum calcium
(c) is made in the parathyroid gland
(d) is a steroid

(15)    All of the following are true about glucagon except:

(a) causes glycogenolysis
(b) is a steroid
(c) causes gluconeogenesis
(d) make in the pancreas

(16)    In the hypothalamic-pituitary-adrenal axis, if the long feedback loop holds then

(a) ACTH inhibits the production of ACTH-RF by the hypothalamus
(b) cortisol inhibits the production of ACTH by the pituitary
(c) cortisol inhibits the ACTH-RF produced by the hypothalamus
(d) none of the above

## 2.17.3    Answers to Questions in Section 2.17.2

( 1) d   ( 2) d   ( 3) c   ( 4) c   ( 5) b   ( 6) b   ( 7) d   ( 8) d   ( 9) d   (10) c   (11) d
(12) a   (13) b   (14) a   (15) b   (16) c

## 2.17.4    Discussion of Answers to Questions in Section 2.17.2

All questions are adequately discussed in the Section except:

*Question #16* (Answer: c) In the long feedback loop, the specific hormone (cortisol) of the gland (adrenal) feeds back past the pituitary to the hypothalamus.

### 2.17.5 Vocabulary Checklist for the Endocrine System

_____ hormone
_____ thyroid gland
_____ hypothalamus
_____ thyroxin
_____ releasing factors
_____ calcitonin
_____ inhibiting factors
_____ adrenal gland
_____ vasopressin
_____ adrenal cortex
_____ oxytocin
_____ adrenal medulla
_____ pituitary
_____ glucocorticoids
_____ TSH
_____ cortisol
_____ gluconeogenesis

_____ Vitamin D
_____ renin
_____ angiotensin I
_____ erythropoietin
_____ melatonin
_____ thymosin
_____ short loop
_____ feedback inhibition
_____ ACTH
_____ mineralocorticoids
_____ FSH
_____ aldosterone
_____ LH
_____ epinephrine
_____ growth hormone
_____ parathyroid gland
_____ prolactin

_____ PTH
_____ giantism
_____ pancreas
_____ acromegaly
_____ insulin
_____ MSH
_____ glucagon
_____ glycogenolysis
_____ kidney
_____ renin substrate
_____ angiotensin II
_____ pineal gland
_____ thymus gland
_____ long loop
_____ trophic hormone

### 2.17.6 Concepts, Principles, etc. Checklist for the Endocrine System

_____ characteristics of hormones
_____ the different endocrine glands and hormones
_____ role of the hypothalamus and pituitary gland
_____ concept of feedback inhibition
_____ general mechanisms of action of hormones

## 2.18 REPRODUCTIVE SYSTEM

### 2.18.1 Review of the Reproductive System

### 2.18.1.1 FEMALE AND MALE ANATOMY

<u>Female anatomy</u> The *labia* are composed of the *major folds* or *labia major,* and the *minor folds* or *labia minora.* The *clitoris* (located between the minor folds ventrally) is very sensitive. The *vagina,* the passage from the external genital opening, terminates in the *cervix* (part of the uterus), which has an *os* (opening) to the uterine cavity (where the fertilized egg implants). The *placenta* derives from the uterus and the developing embryo. Connected to the uterus are the *Fallopian tubes* that lead to the *ovaries* (but are not connected to them).

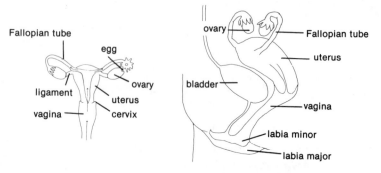

*Fig. 2.47—Female Reproductive System*

The female gonads, the ovaries, lie within the abdominal cavity. They produce female hormones. They also produce the female gametes. Each female gamete is called an egg, or ovum. An ovum is huge compared to a sperm. Ova (plural of ovum) are produced by meiosis. Even before a female is born, egg-producing cells in the ovary have developed into primary oocytes. At birth, all the primary oocytes for a life-time are present. Primary oocytes are diploid.

**Male anatomy** The *testicles* are located outside the body because spermatogenesis requires a temperature lower than body temperature. The *scrotum* is the sack that contains the testicles. Sperm travels from the testis to the *epididymis* (where sperm maturation is completed) to the *vas deferens* to the *ejaculatory duct* to the *penile urethra* to the exterior. The *seminal vesicles* and *prostate gland* contribute fluid to the ejaculate (which averages 1-2cc). The *penis* consists of a *glans penis* (very sensitive) and a shaft (consisting of cavernous tissue for blood engorgement). *Penile erection* (mostly parasympathetic stimulation) results from veins of the penis clamping down and, hence, holding blood in the penis. Ejaculation is a reflex mediated by the sympathetic nervous system. Males continue to produce sperm from puberty onwards.

The sperm is produced by the process of meiosis, which results in haploid gametes. Gametes have only half the number of chromosomes contained in the body cells. Human body cells contain 46 chromosomes. Gametes contain only 23 chromosomes. It may be noted that before a male is born, the testes develop within the abdominal cavity.

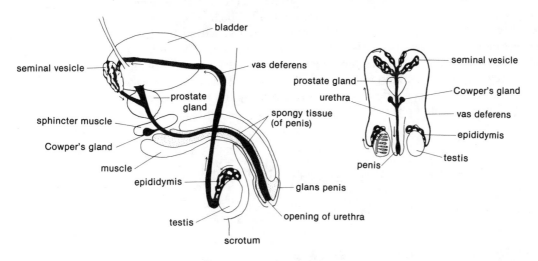

*Fig. 2.48—Male Reproductive System*

## 2.18.1.2   GAMETOGENESIS

**Gametogenesis in Females** (Fig. 2.49) The ovary consists of *oogonia* (2n) which divide and differentiate (before birth) into *primary (first degree) oocytes* (2n) which become surrounded by *follicular cells* (from the mesenchymal stroma), and together constitute the *primordial follicle*. The primary oocytes are arrested in the prophase of the first meiotic division, and they may remain as such from birth to menopause. There are about 5 million oogonia, but only 1 million primary oocytes at birth and about 40,000 at puberty—the remainder degenerate (become *atretic follicles*). Beginning at puberty, a group of primordial follicles begin differentiation to *Graffian follicles*, and the first degree oocyte (2n) becomes the secondary (second degree) oocyte (1n). The second degree oocyte is surrounded by the *zona pellucida* (a gel-like substance), this is surrounded by follicular cells, and these are surrounded by *thecal cells* (which secrete estrogens). Next, *ovulation* occurs by expelling the secondary oocyte and zona pellucida plus some follicular cells (*corona radiata* together) into the *Fallopian tubes*. If fertilization occurs in the Fallopian tubes (the usual location), the secondary oocyte completes meiosis to become an ovum (1n) and fuses with the sperm—if it is not fertilized, it degenerates. The follicular and thecal cells left behind become the *corpus luteum* which is the main source of progesterone which maintains pregnancy. The other follicles that began to develop degenerate because only one follicle completes development and is ovulated from one ovary during each cycle. *Polar bodies* result from the division of the primary oocyte, the secondary oocyte, and possibly the first polar body. Polar bodies have nuclear material but no cytoplasm. Hence, each primary oocyte (2n) produces only one gamete.

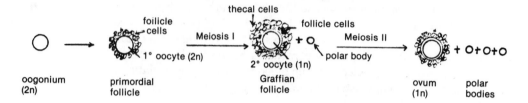

*Fig. 2.49—Gametogenesis in Females*

**Gametogenesis in Males** (Fig. 2.50) The first step is a differentiation of *spermatogonia* (2n) into *primary spermatocytes* (2n) into *secondary spermatocytes* (1n) into *spermatids* (1n) by meiosis. The second step is called *spermiogenesis* in which spermatids (1n) are transformed into *sperm* (1n). A sperm consists of a head, a middle part and a tail. The head contains an *acrosome* (contains digestive enzymes to penetrate egg, probably derived from the Golgi apparatus) and *nuclear material (DNA)* surrounded by very little cytoplasm. The midpiece contains mitochondria for power. The tail has the structure of a centriole and provides locomotion. *Leydig cells* (produce testosterone) and *Sertoli cells* (support sperm development) are also in the testis. Sperm deposited in the vagina by the penis reach the cervix within 90 seconds and migrate up the Fallopian tubes to fertilize the ovum there.

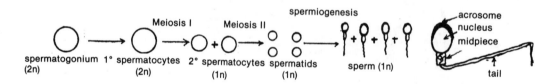

*Fig. 2.50—Gametogenesis in Males*

### 2.18.1.3    MEIOSIS

**Meiosis** (Fig. 2.51) Meiosis has two phases. The first, a *reductional division* is different from mitosis (Section 2.5.1.3). *Prophase I*—the DNA coils to become the chromosome, and there is *exact pairing (synapsis)* of the pairs of homologous chromosomes allowing crossing-over to occur. The nuclear membrane disintegrates, and the centrioles migrate to opposite poles of the nucleus. *Metaphase I*—the two members of the *homologous pair align* along the equatorial plane. The disposition of the maternal and paternal members of the pair toward either pole is random. The spindle fibers attach to the centromere of only one member of each homologous pair. *Anaphase I*—chromosomes of each homologous pair *separate* and move toward opposite poles, the *centromeres do not divide*. *Telophase I*—cytokinesis occurs. In spermatocytes the distribution of the cytoplasm is equitable giving two cells of equal size. In oocytes, the division is unequal giving one secondary oocyte and one polar body. *Interphase I*—a short period in which chromosomes may uncoil somewhat and the nuclear membrane may be partially reconstituted. The daughter cells now contain the haploid number of chromosomes each composed of two daughter chromatids. *Prophase II*, *metaphase II* and *anaphase II* are all like the corresponding mitosis phases. *Telophase II* is like mitosis but has haploid cells.

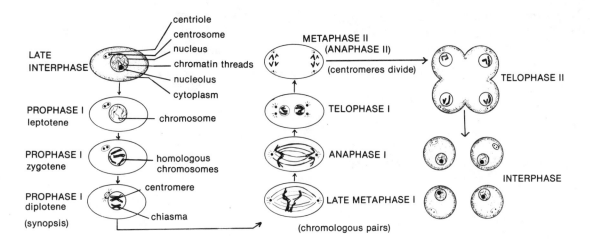

*Fig. 2.51—Meiosis*

## 2.18.1.4    THE MENSTRUAL PERIOD

The female period is typically 28 days and consists of a menstrual flow (mensus), a *follicular phase (ovary)/proliferative phase (uterus)*, ovulation, and a *luteal phase (ovary)/secretory phase (uterus)* in that order. The first day of mensus is conveniently taken as the first day of the cycle. Shedding of the uterine lining occurs during the menstrual flow. Development of the follicle under the stimulation of *FSH* (Follicle Stimulating Hormone) and proliferation of the cells of the uterine lining under the stimulation of *estrogen* (from the ovary) occurs in the follicular/proliferative phase. A rapid increase of estrogen triggers a surge of *LH* (Luteinizing Hormone) at midcycle which causes ovulation to occur (at about 14 days *prior to* the first day of mensus). Just before ovulation, there is a slight dip in body temperature which then rises with ovulation—the progesterone is responsible for the temperature rise. During the luteal/secretive phase, the corpus luteum secretes progesterone, which, with estrogen, causes the uterus to secrete different substances. If fertilization and implantation occur, the corpus luteum continues to secrete progesterone under the stimulation of *HCG* (Human Chorionic Gonadotropin) from the placenta. If implantation does not occur, the corpus luteum degenerates and there is no progesterone to support the uterus, and mensus (shedding of the uterine lining) occurs. Then the cycle repeats itself as FSH and estrogen concentrations rise. Menstrual cycles occur until nearly all the oocytes are depleted—this results in menopause. (Fig. 2.52)

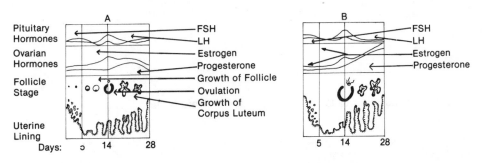

*Fig. 2.52—Menstrual Cycle: (A) Without Pregnancy, (B) With Pregnancy*

## 2.18.2    Questions to Review the Reproductive System

(1)    The testicles are located outside the body because

(a) that is the normal embryologic location
(b) there is direct connection from the epididymis to the penile urethra
(c) there is a need for automatic peripheral nerves
(d) spermatogenesis requires a temperature lower than body temperature

(2)    Sperm travels through all of the following structures except:

(a) ureter
(b) urethra
(c) vas deferens
(d) epididymis

(3)    What structure is directly attached to the ovary?

(a) vagina
(b) uterus
(c) Fallopian tubes
(d) none of the above

(4)    The placenta of humans is composed of tissue derived from the

(a) uterus and developing embryo
(b) uterus only
(c) developing embryo only
(d) none of the above

(5)    The menstrual period (total cycle) is typically closest to:

(a) 2 weeks
(b) 4 weeks
(c) 2 months
(d) 1 year

(6)    The sequence of stages of the menstrual cycle (in reference to the ovary) following the menstrual flow is: (F = follicular phase, L = luteal phase, O = ovulation)

(a) F, O, L
(b) L, O, F
(c) O, F, L
(d) F, L, O

(7)    Ovulation usually occurs

(a) 1-3 days after menses (blood flow)
(b) 14 days before menses
(c) 1-3 days before menses
(d) during menses

(8)    The corpus luteum secretes:

(a) progesterone
(b) LH
(c) FSH
(d) HCG

(9)    The organ in the female analogous to the glans penis in the male is the:

(a) vagina
(b) labia minora
(c) labia majora
(d) clitoris

(10) Which hormone below is found primarily during the first half (follicular/proliferative phase) of the menstrual cycle?

(a) FSH
(b) progesterone
(c) prolactin
(d) HCG

(11) Synapsis and crossing over of chromosomes occur in which phase of meiosis?

(a) Interphase I
(b) Prophase I
(c) Prophase II
(d) Metaphase I

(12) When do the centromeres divide in meiosis?

(a) Anaphase I
(b) Anaphase II
(c) Telophase I
(d) Telophase II

(13) Which substance is not secreted by the ovary or uterus in a pregnant female?

(a) FSH
(b) HCG
(c) progesterone
(d) estrogen

(14) In males, gametes are formed in the:

(a) vas deferens
(b) Leydig cells
(c) epididymis
(d) seminiferous tubules

(15) Polar bodies:

(a) the poles of magnets
(b) result from gametogenesis in the male
(c) result from gametogenesis in the female
(d) dipoles

(16) Fertilization of the ovum by the sperm usually occurs in the:

(a) ovary
(b) Fallopian tubes
(c) uterus
(d) vagina

(17) Select the incorrect association:

(a) oogonia—1n
(b) primary oocyte—2n
(c) secondary oocyte—1n
(d) ova—1n

(18) Corpus luteum:

(a) mature ovum
(b) no hormones
(c) before ovulation
(d) after ovulation

(19)   Tissue/cells not found in the testis:

   (a) seminiferous tubules
   (b) Leydig cells
   (c) spermatogonia
   (d) seminal vesicles

(20)   The primary oocyte remains arrested in what phase of meiosis from birth to puberty:

   (a) Prophase I
   (b) Prophase II
   (c) Metaphase I
   (d) Metaphase II

(21)   Which of the following contains *no* developing ovum?

   (a) Graffian follicle
   (b) primordial follicle
   (c) corpus luteum
   (d) none of the above

(22)   Select the incorrect association:

   (a) spermatogonia—2n
   (b) primary spermatocytes—2n
   (c) secondary spermatocytes—1n
   (d) spermatozoa—2n

(23)   Which is not associated with the male reproductive system?

   (a) Epididymis
   (b) Leydig cells
   (c) Thecal cells
   (d) Sertoli cells

(24)   The number of mature gametes resulting from meiosis of the primary oocyte in the female:

   (a) 1
   (b) 2
   (c) 3
   (d) 4

(25)   The number of mature gametes resulting from meiosis in the male:

   (a) 1
   (b) 2
   (c) 3
   (d) 4

(26)   The key difference(s) in Anaphase I of meiosis and anaphase of mitosis is:

   (a) crossing over occurs in Anaphase I of meiosis
   (b) centromeres divide in Anaphase I of meiosis
   (c) homologous chromosomes move to opposite poles in Anaphase I of meiosis
   (d) all of the above

## 2.18.3    Answers to Questions in Section 2.18.2

( 1) d   ( 2) a   ( 3) d   ( 4) a   ( 5) b   ( 6) a   ( 7) b   ( 8) a   ( 9) d   (10) a   (11) b
(12) b   (13) a   (14) d   (15) c   (16) b   (17) a   (18) d   (19) d   (20) a   (21) c   (22) d
(23) c   (24) a   (25) d   (26) c

### 2.18.4 Discussion of Answers to Questions in Section 2.18.2

All questions adequately discussed in the Section.

### 2.18.5 Vocabulary Checklist for the Reproductive System

_____ scrotum
_____ spermatogonia
_____ testicles
_____ secondary spermatocytes
_____ epididymis
_____ vas deferens
_____ spermiogenesis
_____ penile urethra
_____ spermatids
_____ seminal vesicles
_____ sperm
_____ prostate gland
_____ acrosome
_____ penis
_____ menses
_____ Sertoli cells
_____ ejaculation
_____ oogonia
_____ labia minora
_____ primary oocytes
_____ Anaphase I
_____ ovulation
_____ Telophase I
_____ secretory phase
_____ Interphase I
_____ FSH
_____ Telophase II
_____ estrogens
_____ luteal phase
_____ vagina

_____ cervix
_____ zona pellucida
_____ os
_____ thecal cells
_____ placenta
_____ ovary
_____ ovulation
_____ Fallopian tubes
_____ corona radiata
_____ meiosis
_____ corpus luteum
_____ reductional division
_____ polar bodies
_____ Leydig cells
_____ glans penis
_____ follicular phase
_____ Prophase I
_____ proliferative phase
_____ Metaphase I
_____ labia majora
_____ follicular cells
_____ clitoris
_____ primordial follicle
_____ LH
_____ atretic follicle
_____ progesterone
_____ Graffian follicle
_____ HCG
_____ penile erection

### 2.18.6 Concepts, Principles, etc. Checklist for the Reproductive System

_____ male anatomy, female anatomy; relationships and differences between them
_____ meiosis and how it differs from mitosis and differences in males and females
_____ gametogenesis in males
_____ gametogenesis in females
_____ the menstrual period

## 2.19 BEHAVIOR

### 2.19.1 Review of Behavior

General behavioral responses, the effect of neurological changes upon behavior, and behavioral relationships in populations will be discussed. _Motivation_ is considered to be the driving force of all behavior, innate and learned. It is believed that the internal state of the individual determines this motivation. A simple example being hunger causing an animal to search out food. The hypothalamus is probably a major control center. Much needs to be learned concerning motivation.

## 2.19.1.1  BASIC BEHAVIORAL RESPONSES

Behavioral responses may be divided broadly into those considered innate versus those considered learned. *Innate* implies a predominant inherited component that is only slightly modifiable by external factors. *Learned* implies a behavior that is largely modifiable by external factors, but it still depends, to some extent, upon inherited characteristics. Note that inheritance tends to set the limits of possible behavior, and the environment (external) determines the realization of behavior within those limits. In general, the limits set by inheritance increase as the evolutionary scale is ascended, and this implies that environmental factors may also play a greater role within those widened limits.

Innate types of behavior are reflexes, taxis, instincts, and bioryhthms. *Reflexes* may be considered as the basic unit of behavior, even though they may be difficult to discern or not be present in advanced behaviors. The simplest reflex involves a stimulus perceived by a sensor, and the conduction of the stimulus to an effector which gives the response, e.g., the knee jerk reflex. There are more complex reflexes. Reflexes are, in general, rigid and automatic and essentially not modifiable by external factors. *Taxis* is a simple orienting movement usually in some relation to a stimulus, but not necessarily so. It may involve one or more reflexes. An example is the preference of a paramecium to be in a region of higher acidity (but not very high) than one of lower acidity. *Instinct* is generally considered to be rigid and stereotyped behavior little affected by learning. There is a strong inherited component, but the correct environmental opportunity must be present for it to express itself. For example, bird songs may be considered instinctive, but if a baby bird is not exposed to the song of its species during a given time period, it may not be able to sing. The inherited component allows the capacity for a specific type of song, but the correct environmental situation must be present. Note there is little room for "learning" because other species of birds cannot "teach" the baby birds their songs. *Biorhythms* exist not only for behaviors but for physiological functions as well. They tend to depend upon, or at least correlate with, environmental cycles such as day length (or night length), precipitation, and temperature. Daily cycles (24 hrs.) are called *Circadian Rhythms*. Many hormones are secreted in Circadian cycles, i.e., a peak secretion followed by a minimum secretion within a 24-hour period. Mating patterns of many animals follow seasonal cycles. The mechanisms of these cycles are not known, but the internal metabolism of the animal is suspected to play a role. Also, most of these cycles can be modified by environmental factors. For example, a 24-hour cycle can be changed to a 22-hour cycle.

*Learning* is the process whereby behavior is changed in an enduring (not necessarily permanent) manner by experiences and the environment. Changes in behavior due to learning must be distinguished from behavioral changes due to maturation (e.g., babies cannot physically walk until a certain age). Also the ability to learn can vary with a setting, may depend on a critical period during which "teaching" must occur, and may be delayed from the time of the "teaching." Note that all forms of learning are dependent upon adequate motivation. Types of learning include habituation, conditioning, trial and error, imprinting, and insight learning or reasoning as its ultimate extension.

*Habituation* is the gradual decline in the responses to insignificant stimuli due to the lack of positive reinforcement. *Conditioning* may be viewed as the establishment of active reflex neural pathways (by facilitation) which were present but not used. Conditioning is more complex than the usual reflex. *Pavlov conditioning* is the classic example of conditioning. If there exists a natural stimulus (called the unconditioned stimulus—US) which elicits a natural response (R), then if an artificial stimulus (called the conditioned stimulus—CS) is paired with the US, eventually the CS alone will elicit the R. This is because the animal comes to interpret the CS and US as interchangeable in eliciting the given R. But if the CS is continually given without the US, the CS will eventually cease to elicit the R—this is called *extinction.* To summarize:

| | |
|---|---|
| already existing | US → R |
| experimentally add | CS, US → R |
| eventually | CS → R |

The intensity, duration, character, and timing relative to US of the CS are all important in eliciting the R. *Trial and error* learning is just what the words imply, and it is a very common method of learning. Similar to trial and error learning (some consider them to be the same) is *operant conditioning.* In this there is a response (R) for which there is no clear preceding stimulus. But following the response there is a *reinforcement (RI). A positive reinforcement (PRI),* also called a reward (such as food), increases the likelihood of future similar responses. A *negative reinforcement (NRI),* also called punishment (such as electric shock), decreases the likelihood of future responses. Note that the termination of NRI increases the likelihood of future responses. To summarize for operant conditioning:

| **present** | | **future** | |
|---|---|---|---|
| Response (R) leads to | then | if more rewards (PRI), | |
| Reinforcement (RI) | | then more responses (R) | [↑PRI → ↑R] |
| [R → RI] | | if less rewards (PRI), | |
| | | then less responses (R) | [↓PRI → ↓R] |
| | | if more punishment (NRI), | |
| | | then less responses (R) | [↑NRI → ↓R] |
| | | if less punishment (NRI), | |
| | | then more responses (R) | [↓NRI → ↑R] |

*Imprinting* is a form of learning that occurs within a very short critical period, is difficult to reverse, and is not affected by reward or punishment. An example is baby geese who learn that the first object they see is the parent and follow it. *Insight learning* merges with *reasoning* and will be considered together. This involves the application of prior learning and knowledge to totally new situations. This is different from *generalization* from a learning experience in which similar but not identical stimuli may lead to the same response.

An evolutionary scheme of potential behavior patterns and the evolutionary scale is shown in Fig. 2.53.

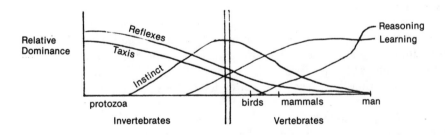

**Fig. 2.53—Behavior Patterns in Evolution**

## 2.19.1.2 EFFECT OF EVOLUTION OF NEUROLOGICAL STRUCTURES UPON BEHAVIOR

*Irritability,* the ability to respond to stimuli, is a universal property of protoplasm. *Conduction* of the stimulus and *response* to it exist as well. These are the basic units of the neurological mechanism of behavior. As evolution progressed, specific cells called neurons became specialized for receiving stimuli (in special sense organs), conducting stimuli as nerve impulses, coordination and integration of stimuli (as in the CNS—see Section 2.16.1), and in conducting impulses to effectors to cause responses. The general changes in the nervous system as evolution progressed are: (1) increased centralization into a CNS, (2) an increase in the complexity for pathways within the CNS, (3) an increase in segregation within the CNS of cells performing different functions, (4) an increase in the concentration of integration and coordinating functions in the brain, (5) an increase in one-way conduction paths such as sensory and motor nerves (see Section 2.16.1), and (6) an increase in the number and complexity of sense organs. All of these changes allowed for the reception of an increased variety, complexity and number of stimuli, an increase in interpretation of these, and an increase in the number of possible responses. All of these added up to more complex behaviors.

The *brain* proceeded to evolve from the three basic divisions—hindbrain, midbrain, forebrain—to the complex structure found in humans (see Section 2.16.1). The medulla of the hindbrain became a control center for autonomic and some somatic functions. The cerebellum of the hindbrain developed rapidly to coordinate muscular movements. Initially, the optic lobes off the midbrain were the dominant *control center*, but this eventually gave way to the thalamus which gave way to the cerebrum. In fish, the cerebrum was primarily an olfactory (smell) center. But in amphibians a *neocortex* (gray matter of neuron bodies) began to grow over the surface of the cerebrum. Two paths emerged in the reptiles. One group with a continued growth of the neocortex led to mammals. The other group with no neocortex, but a dominance of the internal part of the cerebrum, led to birds. Initially, the neocortex of mammals was concerned with sensory and motor functions. But in humans, these covered less of the neocortex, and associational areas came to dominate. The neocortex and especially the associational areas of man led to more complex behaviors characterized by more complex types of learning and reasoning, while in birds, where there was no neocortex (or very little), more innate behaviors (e.g., instinct) and simpler learning modes (e.g., imprinting) remained dominant.

## 2.19.1.3   BEHAVIORAL MODES IN POPULATIONS

Organisms interact with members of the same species (intraspecific) and with members of different species (interspecific). *Intraspecific interactions* are characterized by the fact that members of the same species exhibit antagonism or competition as well as cooperation with each other. Types of relationships established include territoriality, hierarchies, societies, and competition. *Territoriality* is the establishment of a specific area by each member, usually the male of a species, for its own use. Members tend to avoid each others' territories. Areas are delimited in various ways such as behavorial demonstrations, fecal droppings, scents, etc. These territories serve the purposes of spacing members of a species, decreasing competition and antagonism, increasing social stability, and controlling the size of the breeding population. Dominant members of a species usually get the better territories, and, hence, usually survive better because they have access to better food, mates, and living conditions. If members of a species are organized into a group, dominance patterns become apparent in the form of *hierarchies*. Hierarchies are established usually during the first encounter between members of a species. This occurs by behavioral demonstrations of aggression usually, and, if necessary, by outright fighting. Various types of hierarchies exist such as despotism (one individual dominant over others without ranking of other members), straight chains (each individual is dominant over those below it in a sequential manner), closed loops (where no one individual is dominant over all other individuals), and other more complex patterns. *Societies* are highly structured groups where there are clearly defined social roles and divisions of labor. In general, insect societies are dominated by a single female, a division of labor based on biological differences, and behavioral patterns tend to be instinctive with little room for modification. In general, human societies consist of an aggregation of individuals and family groups, the division of labor is not based upon biological differences or castes, there is a considerable choice of roles, and behavioral patterns are based on learning and are highly modifiable. *Competition* between members of a species can be intense because they require the same types of resources. Wide fluctuations in numbers occur when imbalances between numbers of a species and resources exist.

*Interspecific interactions* include symbiosis (commensalism, mutualism, and parasitism), predation, and competition. *Symbiosis* means the living together of different organisms. *Commensualism* is when one species benefits and the other is not affected by the relationship. *Mutualism* is when both species benefit from the relationship. *Parasitism* is when one species benefits and the other is harmed by the relationship. Parasitism merges with commensualism on one end and predation on the other. It differs from predation because the parasite is usually tied to the host, whereas a predator lives independently of its prey. Also, a parasite is specific for its host and is specialized (which usually means loss of all unnecessary organs and functions). The best adapted parasites do not kill their hosts. *Predators* are free-living from their prey, have less specificity for prey (i.e., they can prey on a variety of organisms), and can greatly affect the numbers of their prey. The prey usually increase and the predators then increase after a lag period. As the predators increase, the number of prey decrease and fewer predators are supported and they decrease. This allows prey to increase and the cycle recurs. Predators are, in general, beneficial to prey species because prey are prevented from outgrowing and, hence, ruining their needed resources. Interspecific *competition* is considered in the context of *niches* which include every factor (food, physical environment, other species, etc.) that affects the life of an organism. The *habitat* is just the physical environment. The guiding concept is the *Competitive Exclusion Principle* which states that two different species cannot occupy the same niche for long. One of several options must occur because resources become limited: (1) extinction of one of the species, (2) the range of one or both of the species is restricted, and (3) evolution of one or both species which results in greater differentiation.

### 2.19.1.4 COMMUNICATION BETWEEN INDIVIDUALS

*Communication* is the process of affecting behavior of individuals to assure survival and/or reproduction of the species through a variety of signals transmitted between its members. Communicative signals also permit structural complexity within groups of organisms, and may affect the development of species outside the usual mechanisms of evolution. Signals received by the senses (smell, taste, vision, and hearing), individually or in combination, are the basis of communication.

*Pheromones* are chemicals produced by cells and transmitted via air, water, objects, etc., to a second individual. They may be effective over long distances. They are extremely potent in small amounts. Pheromone communication is the most common type and is found from single organisms to mammals, including plants. A *releasor pheromone* causes a behavioral response in the receiving organism. It plays a role in reproduction, territorial determinations, recognition of individuals, trail marking, etc. A *primer pheromone* causes a physiological change (often via hormonal changes) in the receiving organism that may be permanent. An example is the suppression of additional queens in a variety of insects.

*Visual* communications involves colors, shapes, visual cues, etc. Humans, birds, butterflies, e.g., utilize this method heavily. It is more restricted than pheromones. It is also used for territory delineations and especially sexual/reproductive functions. *Auditory* communication is valuable in situations in which vision is restricted (night, water, dense foliage, etc.). It is fairly common and effective. Its uses are similar to visual communication.

## 2.19.2   Questions to Review Behavior

(1)   Motivation

   (a) is not dependent upon the internal physiological state
   (b) is not required for innate behavior
   (c) is required for learned behavior
   (d) all of the above

(2)   Which region of the brain is thought to be most associated with motivation?

   (a) hypothalamus
   (b) thalamus
   (c) cerebrum
   (d) medulla

(3)   Innate behavior differs from learned behavior by the former being

   (a) highly modifiable by external factors
   (b) slightly modifiable by external factors
   (c) totally unaffected by external factors

(4)   Select the correct statement:

   (a) innate behavior depends on inherited factors only
   (b) learned behavior depends on environmental factors only
   (c) both types of behavior depend on both inherited and environmental factors
   (d) both (a) and (b)

(5)   The wider the behavioral limits set by inherited factors

   (a) the greater the role exerted by environmental factors
   (b) the lesser the role exerted by environmental factors
   (c) has no effect on the role exerted by environmental factors

(6)   All are innate types of behavior except:

   (a) reflexes
   (b) taxis
   (c) instincts
   (d) imprinting

(7)   The most basic of the following units is the:

   (a) reflex
   (b) taxis
   (c) instinct
   (d) imprinting

(8)   An instinct:

   (a) is little affected by learning
   (b) always is expressed as a behavior
   (c) has a strong inherited component that requires no environmental opportunity
   (d) all of the above

(9)   A Circadian Rhythm

   (a) has a cycle of about 4 months as the seasons
   (b) exists only for behavioral cycles
   (c) is not affected by environmental factors
   (d) none of the above

(10) All of the following are types of learning except:

(a) habituation
(b) maturation
(c) conditioning
(d) imprinting

(11) Facilitation may be involved in

(a) habituation
(b) conditioning
(c) imprinting
(d) reflexes

(12) In Pavlovian conditioning,

(a) the unconditioned stimulus cannot elicit the response until it has been paired with the conditioned stimulus
(b) the response is created by experiment
(c) the conditioned stimulus is a natural (already existing in nature) stimulus
(d) extinction may occur if the conditioned stimulus is continually given without the unconditioned stimulus

(13) Operant conditioning is similar to:

(a) trial and error learning
(b) Pavlovian conditioning
(c) imprinting
(d) habituation

(14) In operant conditioning,

(a) a decrease in negative reinforcement increases the likelihood of future responses
(b) positive reinforcement precedes the response
(c) a stimulus precedes the response
(d) all of the above

(15) All of the following are correct about imprinting except:

(a) it is a form of learning
(b) rewards can increase its likelihood of occurrence
(c) must occur within a very short critical period
(d) it is not the same as instinct

(16) All of the following are correct about reasoning except:

(a) it is similar to generalization
(b) it is similar to insight learning
(c) it requires application of prior experiences to totally new situations
(d) it is unrelated to motivation

(17) All of the following modes of behavior are dominant among invertebrates except:

(a) learning
(b) instinct
(c) reflexes
(d) taxis

(18) Modes of behavior dominant in humans include all except:

(a) reasoning
(b) learning
(c) reflexes
(d) all of these are dominant

(19)　All of the following occurred in the evolution of the nervous system except:

(a) increased centralization into a central nervous system
(b) increased complexity of pathways in the central nervous system
(c) increased segregation in the periphery of neurons performing specific functions
(d) increased number and complexity of sense organs

(20)　The earliest control center in the brain was probably the:

(a) cerebellum
(b) midbrain
(c) thalamus
(d) cerebrum

(21)　In early vertebrates (fish, amphibians) the cerebrum was primarily concerned with:

(a) smell
(b) vision
(c) all sensory modalities
(d) integration of information

(22)　The development of what structure was important in separating behavioral potentials of birds and mammals?

(a) midbrain
(b) thalmus
(c) neocortex
(d) cerebellum

(23)　The neocortex of man differs from that of other mammals by having a dominance of which area(s)?

(a) sensory
(b) association
(c) autonomic
(d) motor

(24)　Types of intraspecific competition include all except:

(a) territoriality
(b) mutualism
(c) hierarchies
(d) societies

(25)　Function(s) of territoriality are(is):

(a) spacing members of a species
(b) decreasing competition among members of a species
(c) increasing social stability of a species
(d) all of the above

(26)　In hierarchies

(a) there is always one dominant individual
(b) social stability is usually decreased
(c) dominance by an individual is usually established in the first encounter
(d) all of the above

(27)　Human societies are characterized by all except

(a) aggregation of individuals and families
(b) roles based on biological differences
(c) behavioral patterns are greatly modifiable by learning
(d) all of the above are correct

(28) Insect societies are characterized by all except

(a) domination by a single female
(b) division of labor based on biological differences or castes
(c) behavioral patterns based upon instincts
(d) all of the above are correct

(29) Types of interspecific interactions include all except:

(a) hierarchies
(b) parasitism
(c) mutualism
(d) predation

(30) "One species benefits and the other not affected" is called:

(a) mutualism
(b) predation
(c) commensalism
(d) parasitism

(31) "Both species benefitting from a relationship" is called:

(a) mutualism
(b) predation
(c) commensalism
(d) parasitism

(32) "One species benefitting and the other being harmed in a relationship" is called:

(a) mutualism
(b) commensalism
(c) parasitism
(d) none of these

(33) Parasitism, at its extremes, is similar to:

(a) commensalism
(b) predation
(c) neither (a) nor (b)
(d) both (a) and (b)

(34) A parasite differs from a predator by

(a) being specific for its host
(b) being tied (versus living free) to its host
(c) both (a) and (b)
(d) neither (a) nor (b)

(35) Predators in general

(a) increase the number of prey in an area
(b) decrease the number of prey in an area
(c) have no effect on the number of prey

(36) "Two different species cannot occupy the same niche for long" is a statement of the:

(a) Hardy-Weinberg Law
(b) Darwin's Natural Selection Theory
(c) Competitive Exclusion Principle
(d) none of the above

(37) Which of the following may occur if two different species occupy the same niche?

(a) extinction of one of the species
(b) range restriction of one of the species
(c) evolution of one of the species
(d) all of the above may occur

(38) If a bright light is placed near a planarian, it will move toward the light. This will occur repeatedly as the light is moved. This is an example of:

(a) taxis
(b) reflex
(c) habituation
(d) conditioning

(39) A sound is produced that startles a pigeon. The sound is repeated a second time but has less of an effect on the pigeon. By the tenth time the pigeon is not affected by the sound. This process is best characterized as:

(a) Pavlov Conditioning
(b) habituation
(c) Operant Conditioning
(d) insight learning

*For Questions 40, 41, and 42*

Ducklings will run and hide if a hawk flies overhead. Actually, it is the pattern of the hawk's shape and motion that is detected by the ducklings. This effect can be created in a lab setting by a moving hawk-shaped cardboard. A bell is rung when the cardboard is presented to the ducklings who continue to seek shelter. Eventually, the bell is rung but without the cardboard hawk, and the ducklings still seek shelter.

(40) This is an example of:

(a) trial and error learning
(b) imprinting
(c) Pavolian conditioning
(d) operant conditioning

(41) The bell is called the:

(a) conditioned stimulus
(b) unconditioned stimulus
(c) positive reinforcement
(d) negative reinforcement

(42) If the bell continues to be rung without the presence of the cardboard hawk, a process called _____ will occur:

(a) forgetting
(b) insight learning
(c) extinction
(d) facilitation

(43) Some citizens decided that the wolf population in a fairly isolated but fertile valley had grown too large and was destroying too many deer. To save the deer, they decided to destroy all the wolves, the only natural predators of the deer in the valley. The succeeded in removing all of the wolves. Over a representative period of time, which graph probably shows the growth of the deer? (a) = initial level of deer before wolf eradication; ↑ = elimination of all wolves.

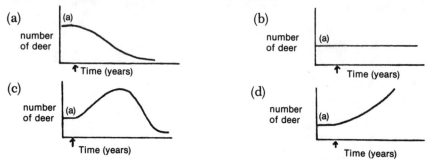

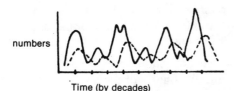

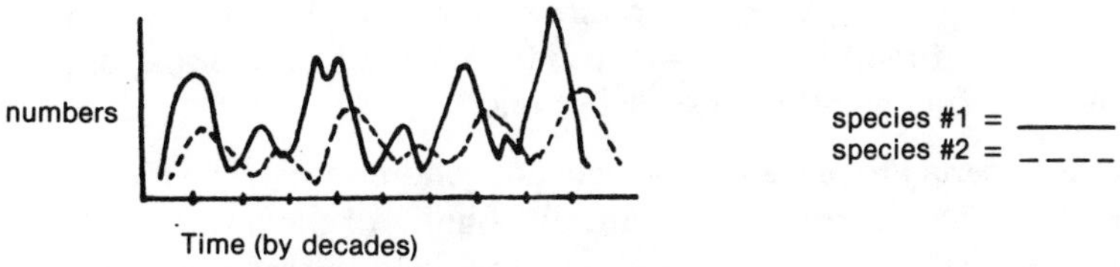

species #1 = _____
species #2 = _ _ _ _

Time (by decades)

(44) The above graph probably represents what type of relationship between these species?

(a) commensualism
(b) mutualism
(c) parasitism
(d) predation

(45) Cows do not have digestive enzymes to digest cellulose. Cellulose is a very important component of a cow's diet. The cellulose is digested by bacteria in the cow's stomach. These bacteria can use some of the cellulose products for their own purposes. This relationship is called:

(a) commensualism
(b) mutualism
(c) parasitism
(d) competition

(46) Bacterial species #1 and bacterial species #2 are very similar in their requirements for life. The "diet" of both consists primarily of small organic molecules. The following experiments are done as shown in the graphs below:

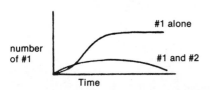 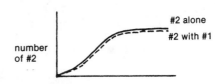

The bacteria alone or in combination are placed in identical culture media.

This experiment may be considered to be an example of:

(a) commensualism
(b) the Competitive Exclusion Principle
(c) parasitism
(d) predation

## 2.19.3    Answers to Questions in Section 2.19.2

( 1) c   ( 2) a   ( 3) b   ( 4) c   ( 5) a   ( 6) d   ( 7) a   ( 8) a   ( 9) d   (10) b   (11) b
(12) d   (13) a   (14) a   (15) b   (16) a   (17) a   (18) c   (19) c   (20) b   (21) a   (22) c
(23) b   (24) b   (25) d   (26) c   (27) b   (28) d   (29) a   (30) c   (31) a   (32) c   (33) d
(34) c   (35) b   (36) c   (37) d   (38) a   (39) b   (40) c   (41) a   (42) c   (43) c   (44) d
(45) b   (46) b

## 2.19.4    Discussion of Answers to Questions in Section 2.19.2

*Questions #1 to #37* Adequately discussed in Section.

*Question #38* (Answer: a) The motion is an orienting motion and simply a rigid stereotyped response (as a reflex). There is no evidence of habituation (decreased response to the stimulus) nor that the organism was conditioned. Taxis is the best of the possible answers.

*Question #39* (Answer: b) The response of the pigeon decreases with repeated application of the sound which was presented without reinforcement—this is the meaning of habituation. There is no evidence in the question for the other answer options.

*Question #40* (Answer: c) All the criteria are present for Pavlovian conditioning. The hiding is a natural response found in ducklings elicited by the natural stimulus of the hawk (or its stand-in). The bell is the conditioned stimulus which eventually can elicit the response after being paired with the unconditioned stimulus (the hawk). But upon repeated presentations of the bell without the hawk the response is elicited less and less—this is the extinction phenomenon.

*Questions #41, #42* See discussion of #40 above.

*Question #43* (Answer: c) As soon as the wolves are removed the deer population will begin to increase because the wolves were the major limiting factor of the deer. So the deer population will increase. But the resources of the valley are limited and the deer population will reach a brief plateau as the carrying capacity of the valley is reached. Then, because the valley is relatively isolated and the deer can't move on, they will tend to destroy foliage faster than it can be replenished and the carrying capacity will decrease; hence, the deer population will decrease. This is as in graph (c).

*Question #44* (Answer: d) Species #2 tends to lag behind species #1 as to peaks and valleys. Also, as species #2 increases, species #1 decreases; as #1 increases, #2 increases. And, species #2 is always less abundant than species #1. Of the relationships given, the predator (#2)/prey(#1) relationship would best explain the graph. As the prey (#1) increase, more predators can be supported and they increase. But when the predator:prey ratio reaches a critical point, more prey are destroyed than are created so they decrease. The decrease in prey causes the predators to decrease because fewer can be supported. Thus the numbers fluctuate.

*Question #45* (Answer: b) The cow benefits by having the cellulose digested for it. The bacteria benefit by being provided with an abundant supply of cellulose. This is the definition of mutualism.

*Question #46* (Answer: b) These two species occupy the same niche as alluded to in the question; they are, therefore, in competition with each other. The experiments show that, when put with #2, species #1 is decreased in number (goes toward extinction) as is predicted by the Competitive Exclusion Principle. Parasitism, predation and commensualism are most likely all excluded by the fact that both organisms survive well when grown alone. Also, it is noted that the diet of both is small organic molecules.

## 2.19.5    Vocabulary Checklist for Behavior

| | |
|---|---|
| _____ motivation | _____ unconditioned stimulus |
| _____ instinct | _____ reflexes |
| _____ maturation | _____ biorhythms |
| _____ extinction | _____ habituation |
| _____ punishment | _____ reward |
| _____ generalization | _____ imprinting |
| _____ territoriality | _____ neocortex |
| _____ societies | _____ hierarchies |
| _____ commensualism | _____ symbiosis |
| _____ parasitism | _____ mutualism |
| _____ competition | _____ predation |
| _____ insight learning | _____ niche |
| _____ Circadian Rhythms | _____ taxis |
| _____ Pavlov conditioning | _____ conditioning |
| _____ conditioned stimulus | _____ reasoning |

_____ operant conditioning
_____ habitat
_____ trial and error learning
_____ negative reinforcement

_____ Competitive Exclusion Principle
_____ positive reinforcement
_____ pheromones

## 2.19.6    Concepts, Principles, etc. Checklist for Behavior

_____ innate behavorial responses
_____ learned behavioral responses
_____ distinction between innate and learned behavior
_____ evolution of innate and learned behaviors
_____ evolution of the nervous system
_____ behavioral consequences of evolution of the nervous system
_____ intraspecific interactions
_____ interspecific interactions
_____ visual communication
_____ auditory communication

## 2.20    GENETICS

### 2.20.1    Review of Genetics

Each organism has a set of chromosomes. *Chromosomes* of eukaryotes are a complex of DNA, *histone* (basic protein), and non-histone protein. The normal complement of chromosomes is called *diploid (2n)* as occurs in somatic cells. Gametes (male and female) are *haploid (1n)*. Gametes combine to form the diploid cell. The complement of chromosomes may be divided into *autosomes* and *sex chromosomes* (having to do with sex determination). Humans have 22 pairs of autosomes and 1 pair of sex chromosomes (X, Y) for a total of 46. The female is XX, and the male is XY. Either the whole set of chromosomes can be in some multiple of n which is called *polyploidy*, e.g., 4n = *tetraploidy*, or one or more chromosomes may be missing or in excess, which is called *aneuploidy*, e.g., *monosomy* (only one of a chromosome type is present) or trisomy (three of a chromosome type is present). Down's Syndrome (Mongolism) is caused by trisomy 21 (i.e., there are three of the chromosomes numbered 21 instead of two).

On each chromosome there is a sequence of *genes*. For this section, a gene is a specific trait. Hence, each *locus* (or position) on a chromosome is for a specific trait. In the diploid (2n) cell, there is a pair of *homologous chromosomes* (which pair in meiosis). Homologous chromosomes are similar by having the same sequence of trait loci (except the pair X and Y, see below); hence they are the same size. For any given general trait (e.g., eye color), there are many alternative genes (e.g., blue, brown) for its determination. The alternative genes for a general trait constitute a set of *alleles* for that trait. Since there is only one locus (usually) for a simple trait on a chromosome, there can be only one allele of that trait per homologous chromosome. Then, for any given trait, there is a maximum of two alleles per diploid cell (one on each homologous chromosome). But the total number of different alleles for a given trait can be greater than two (e.g., there are many different alleles for types of hemoglobin—normal adult, fetal, sickle, hemoglobin C, hemoglobin Milwaukee, etc.). For an individual, the specific alleles present is called the genotype. If the alleles for a given trait on each homologous chromosome are identical, the genotype is called *homozygous*. If the alleles for a given trait on each homologous chromosome are different, the genotype is called *heterozygous*. The term genotype can refer to the alleles of a specific trait or the total genetic makeup (all of the alleles) of an individual. Each of the alleles (genes) of a given trait will attempt to express itself via its protein product. If one allele of a pair expresses itself over another (e.g., eye color with brown over blue), that allele is said to be *dominant* and the other *recessive*. (Note that these terms go together like oxidation-reduction in chemistry.) If both alleles express themselves, they are called *codominant*. The expression (what is seen as the trait of the individual) of the genotype is called the *phenotype*. Note that different genotypes can give rise to the same phenotype, but a given genotype will not usually give rise to different phenotypes.

Gametes (haploid) are formed during meiosis by the separation of homologous chromosomes (diploid state). This results in the separation of each of the alleles into a different gamete. This is *Mendel's First Law of Segregation* (of alleles of the same trait). Different traits (i.e., loci) may be on the same chromosome or on different chromosomes. If the traits are on different chromosomes, the alleles of these different traits should separate independently of each other into gametes. This is *Mendel's Second Law of Independent Assortment* (of alleles of different traits). But if different traits are on the same chromosome, they may be far apart or close together. Traits far apart on the same chromosome separate into gametes as if they were on separate chromosomes. This is possible because of *crossing-over* (reciprocal exchange of parts of homologous chromosomes) during *synapsis* in the first meiotic prophase. The farther apart two different traits are on a chromosome, the easier it is for cross-over to occur. Alleles of traits which are close together do not separate frequently by the mechanism of crossing-over into different gametes because they tend to remain on the same chromosome. So they cannot independently (of each other) assort, do not follow Mendel's Second Law, and are called *linked traits* (or genes). (Fig. 2.54) *Recombination* is the process of separating alleles of linked traits into different gametes, i.e., onto different homologous chromosomes. *Linkage (recombination)* studies and cytogenetics (study of markings, e.g., band on chromosomes) are used to map chromosomes as to the loci of traits. Another of Mendel's great contributions to genetics was his recognition that genes are *particulate* (i.e., not indivisible or blendable). Mendel's mechanisms of assortment and segregation and the later discovered ideas of recombination illustrate mechanisms of *genetic variability* which can be viewed as the passage to offspring, via gametes, of different combinations of alleles than existed in the parent. Another set of mechanisms responsible for genetic variability is *mutations*. A mutation may be considered a stable heritable change in genetic material (DNA). Mutations that may occur at the level of the chromosome (see Fig. 2.55) are:

(1) *inversion*—sequence of genes on the chromosomes is reversed
(2) *translocations*—a part of one chromosome attaches to another
(3) *deletion*—a part of the chromosome is missing
(4) *duplication*—part of the chromosome is repeated.

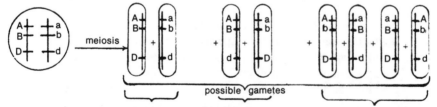

possible gametes

| | | | |
|---|---|---|---|
| Diploid (2n) cell showing a pair of homologous chromosomes with loci for three different traits with alleles A,a and B,b and D,d. Traits A,a and B,b are linked. Traits A,a and D,d and traits B,b and D,d are not linked. | Mendel's 1st Law, each allele of a given trait (A vs. a, B vs. b, and D vs. d) segregate independently of each other. | Mendel's 2nd Law, consider A,a vs. D,d. These alleles of different traits assort independently of each other (also for B,b vs. D,d). Not true for A,a vs. B,b because these are linked. | Recombination of the linked genes A,a vs. B,b. A,a and B,b do not assort independently of each other because they are so close together. One would normally expect A & B or a & b to be together in gametes. But by crossing over, Ab and aB also are possible but at frequencies less than expected. |

*Fig. 2.54—Mendel's Law; Crossing-over; Recombination; Gamete Formation*

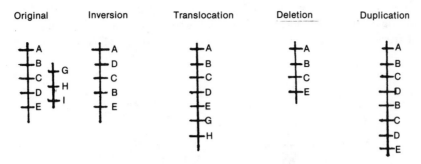

*Fig. 2.55—Chromosomal Mutations*

In the sex chromosomes, the X is larger than the Y (i.e., has more loci for traits), and hence, traits on the X may not appear on the Y. Traits of this type are called *sex-linked traits.* Examples in humans are hemophilia, color blindness, and glucose-6-phosphate dehydrogenase deficiency. The X and Y chromosomes are homologous because they can pair (synapse) in meiosis. Sex-linked traits are unique in their inheritance because the male (with only one X chromosome) can express (phenotypes) recessive alleles because there is only one allele present. The female requires both recessive alleles to be present for expression of the recessive trait. Also note that transmission to the male occurs usually only from the mother. Whereas if the daughter is diseased, both mother and father must have passed on the allele. In passing, *Barr bodies* are inactivated "excess" X chromosomes (only one X remains active). This phenomenon is referred to as the *Lyon* or *Lyon-Russel* hypothesis. The above concepts are illustrated in Fig. 2.56.

Given a trait with alleles A = dominant, a = recessive and phenotypes A and a.

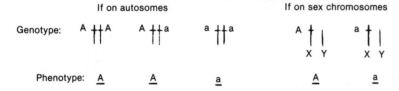

Note that the *a* allele can only be expressed when it is present on both chromosomes (i.e., it is homozygous).

Note that *a* (the allele) is alone and is expressed.

*Fig. 2.56—Autosomal and Sex Chromosomes: Phenotype Expressions*

*Cytoplasmic inheritance* is the determination of genetic traits by constituents of the cytoplasm rather than the nucleus. This inheritance does not follow Mendelian Laws. The mother (most of the cytoplasm of the zygote comes from the ovum) plays the major role in this type of inheritance. Chloroplasts (contain DNA), mitochondria (contain DNA), centrioles, and basal bodies of flagella and cilia are examples of structures that replicate without input from the nucleus.

*Pedigrees* are convenient diagrams for showing phenotypic appearance of traits in a family. The basic nomenclature is given in Fig. 2.57.

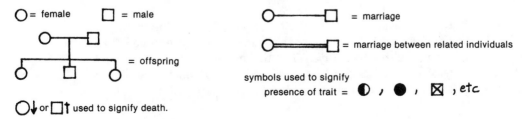

*Fig. 2.57—Pedigree Terminology*

A dominant autosomal or sex-linked trait, with complete *penetrance* (i.e., the trait appears in all with the allele), will have a pedigree that shows both sexes affected, many individuals affected, passage of trait from affected parent to children even if heterozygous. (Fig. 2.58).

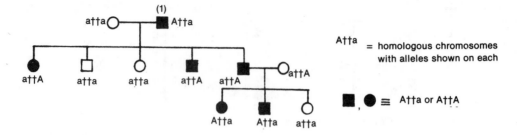

Atta = homologous chromosomes with alleles shown on each

■, ● ≡ Atta or A†tA

Case (1) is probably heterozygous for the trait because if homozygous then all offspring would be affected.

*Fig. 2.58—Dominant Pedigree*

An autosomal recessive trait will also show both sexes affected, but fewer individuals will be affected and passage may be from an unaffected parent (because heterozygous) to an affected offspring (Fig. 2.59).

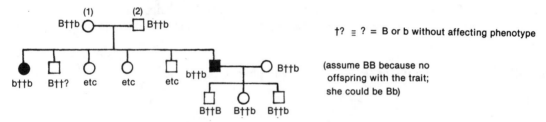

†? ≡ ? = B or b without affecting phenotype

(assume BB because no offspring with the trait; she could be Bb)

Both parents are heterozygous for the recessive allele.

*Fig. 2.59—Recessive Pedigree*

A sex-linked recessive trait usually shows only males affected and passage of the trait from an unaffected mother to a son. A daughter can get the trait only if the father has it and the mother is, at least, heterozygous. (Fig. 2.60).

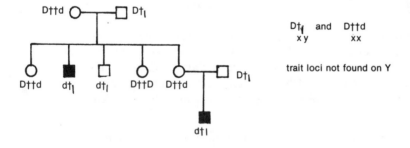

Dt† and D††d
x y      x x

trait loci not found on Y

*Fig. 2.60—Sex-Linked Pedigree*

*Punnet squares* are useful ways of determining the genotypes possible from the mating of two individuals with known genotypes. First the possible gametes are determined (Fig. 2.61), then these are combined in all possible ways. Then by knowing dominant-recessive relationships, the frequency of phenotypes can be ascertained. The Punnet square gives expected ratios only. Fig. 2.62 and Fig. 2.63 are examples.

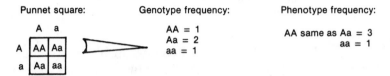

Genotype (Diploid): (1) AaBb  (2) AaBB  (3) AABbDd  (4) AaBbDd

Possible Gametes: (Haploid)  AB,Ab,aB,ab   AB,aB   ABD,ABd,AbD,Abd   ABD,ABd,AbD,Abd,aBD,aBd,abD,abd

*Fig. 2.61—Gamete Formation by Example*

Punnet square:          Genotype frequency:          Phenotype frequency:

|   | A | a |
|---|---|---|
| A | AA | Aa |
| a | Aa | aa |

AA = 1
Aa = 2
aa = 1

AA same as Aa = 3
aa = 1

*Fig. 2.62—Punnet Square With One Trait*

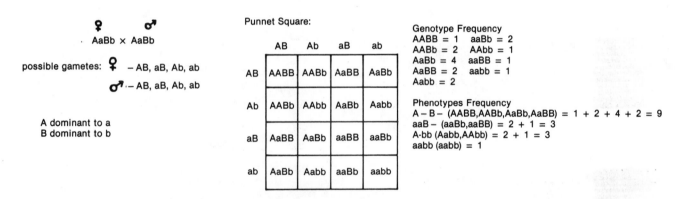

*Fig. 2.63—Punnet Square With Two Traits*

*Simple gene mapping* is done utilizing recombinant techniques. This is done with viral and bacterial DNAs. The map is a linear, one-dimensional structure. The map units indirectly represent the percent recombination between various traits (genetic loci). The traits must be measurable in some manner (e.g., nutrient utilization, products produced, temperature dependence, etc.). The combination of traits in the offspring, as compared with the parents, helps determine the recombinant frequencies (percentages) that help determine the gene map. An example of a two-factor (trait) cross:

| Parents | | Offspring | |
|---|---|---|---|
| a |  $a^+$ | a | |
| $\times$ | | $b^+$ | — 35% |
| $b^+$  b | | $a^+$ | |
| | | b | — 35% |

— the original genotypes are in
  the highest frequency.

a
b — 15%

— the larger percentage of
  recombinants, the farther apart

$a^+$
$b^+$ — 15%

  the traits are on the map and
  the less tightly linked the traits are.

— the trait loci (a *or* $a^+$ and b *or* $b^+$) are linked (see below).

A series of two-factor crosses may be used to sequence the gene loci. The maximal possible frequency of any recombinant is 50%. If the frequency of recombination between the loci is near 50%, then there is no linkage. The smaller the recombination frequency between two loci, the stronger the linkage (i.e., the closer together the traits). Triple factor (i.e., three traits at three loci) are used to order gene loci. The (original) parental genotypes will appear in the highest frequency, single recombinants next, and double recombinants in the lowest frequency. The probability of the central locus recombining with both outside loci (double recombination) is equal to the products of the probability of it combining with each individually (single recombination).

Example: **Parents**

x   x$^+$
y   y$^+$
z   z$^+$

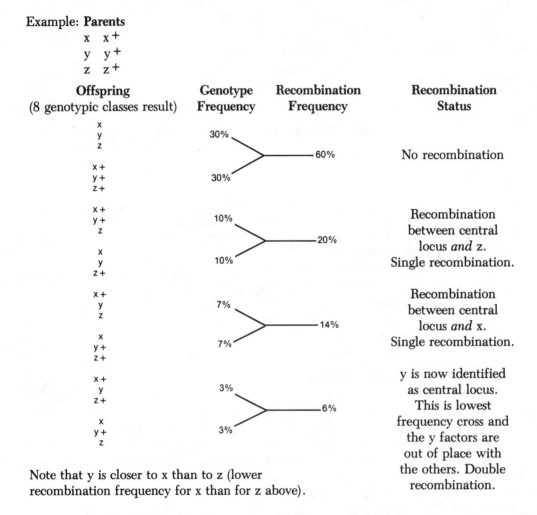

| Offspring (8 genotypic classes result) | Genotype Frequency | Recombination Frequency | Recombination Status |
|---|---|---|---|
| x<br>y<br>z | 30% | 60% | No recombination |
| x+<br>y+<br>z+ | 30% | | |
| x+<br>y+<br>z | 10% | 20% | Recombination between central locus *and* z. Single recombination. |
| x<br>y<br>z+ | 10% | | |
| x+<br>y<br>z | 7% | 14% | Recombination between central locus *and* x. Single recombination. |
| x<br>y+<br>z+ | 7% | | |
| x+<br>y<br>z+ | 3% | 6% | y is now identified as central locus. This is lowest frequency cross and the y factors are out of place with the others. Double recombination. |
| x<br>y+<br>z | 3% | | |

Note that y is closer to x than to z (lower recombination frequency for x than for z above).

There are factors that modify the percentage distributions of the offspring and may affect the analysis. Besides the probability factor (i.e., each cross will not lead to exact ratios just as in Mendelian crosses), conditional lethal mutations may occur and cause some genotypes not to survive, and therefore, not to be counted.

## 2.20.1.1   USE OF THE HARDY-WEINBERG PRINCIPLE

The Hardy-Weinberg principle states that under certain random mating conditions, gene frequencies will remain constant from generation to generation. This principle is useful in population genetics. Gene frequencies may be expressed as a decimal or as a percent. Under the Hardy-Weinberg principle, the gene frequency of dominant and recessive alleles remains the same from generation to generation. In other words, the sum of all the allele frequencies for a gene within a population is equal to 1.0, or 100%. Each genotype is made of two alleles. The chance of getting a particular genotype is the product of the probabilities of the two alleles.

The Hardy-Weinberg equation states, $p^2 + 2pq + q^2 = 1$.

    p = frequency of dominant allele
    q = frequency of recessive allele

As a simple example, consider a population of dogs, 16 percent are white. The gene for white is recessive. In order to find the frequency of the dominant gene (dominant = W, recessive = w), apply Hardy-Weinberg principle as shown:

WW = homozygous dominant
2Ww = heterozygous dominant
ww = homozygous recessive

$$(p + q)(p + q) = 1$$
$$p^2 + 2pq + q^2 = 1$$
$$p + q = 1$$

In the population of dogs provided, 16% are white (these are the homozygous recessive dogs). Hence, $q^2 = 0.16$, $q = 0.4$, $p = 1-0.4 = 0.6$. The frequency of the dominant gene W = p = 0.6.

In order to determine the frequency of heterozygosity for whiteness/non-whiteness for the dog population, determine $2pq = 2(0.6)(0.4) = 0.48$.

Finally, p = 0.6 = 60%
        q = 0.4 = 40%
      2pq = 0.48 = 48%
      $p^2 = (0.6)^2 = 0.36 = 36\%$
      $q^2 = (0.4)^2 = 0.16 = 16\%$
$p^2 = 2pq + q^2 = 36\% + 48\% + 16\% = 100\%$

The above examples should be studied and applied to various population genetics problems.


### 2.20.2    Questions to Review Genetics

(1)    Which of the following is correct for gene mapping?

(a) only three-factor crosses may be used to sequence gene loci
(b) the recombination frequencies are always representative of the recombination rates of the gene loci
(c) the recombination frequency is equal to the map units
(d) viral DNAs are used for gene mapping

(2)    Cytoplasmic inheritance:

(a) does not follow Mendelian Laws
(b) the maternal cytoplasm plays the dominant role
(c) replication of mitochondria is an example
(d) all of the above

(3)    Homozygous refers to

(a) similar types of chromosomes
(b) having similar functions on an evolutionary basis
(c) particles in a solution not being separable microscopically
(d) identical alleles for a given trait

(4)    Which statement is *incorrect* concerning X and Y chromosomes?

(a) X is larger than Y
(b) they are not homologous
(c) XY is a genotypic male
(d) traits appearing on X but not on Y are called sex-linked traits

(5)     Select the *incorrect* statement:

(a) genotype is the alleles for a given trait in an individual
(b) phenotype is the expression of the genotype
(c) a given genotype will give rise to different phenotypes
(d) different genotypes may give rise to the same phenotype

(6)     Crossing-over of chromosomes

(a) involves reciprocal exchanges of homologous chromosomes
(b) occurs in Metaphase I of meiosis
(c) is more frequent between traits located close together
(d) prevents independent assortment of traits on the same chromosome

(7)     Genetic recombination

(a) occurs by exchange of chromosomes between gametes
(b) is the exchange of similar alleles between gametes
(c) is the mixing of alleles of different traits on homologous chromosomes by crossing-over
(d) is not used to make chromosome maps

(8)     An allele for a trait:

(a) is a gene
(b) can be different on homologous chromosomes in a given cell
(c) both (a) and (b)
(d) neither (a) nor (b)

(9)     Barr bodies:

(a) the densities associated with desmosomes
(b) crystals of enzymes seen in lysosomes
(c) inactivated X-chromosomes seen in certain cells
(d) synonym for polar bodies resulting during oogenesis

(10)    Which of the following is an example of aneuploidy?

(a) 4n
(b) trisomy 21
(c) XO (no Y chromosome)
(d) both (b) and (c)

(11)    Select the *incorrect* statement about the number and type of chromosomes in the normal human male:

(a) there are 44 autosomal chromosomes
(b) there are 46 chromosomes total
(c) there are two X chromosomes
(d) there is one Y chromosome

(12)    In the typical somatic cell, the number of chromosomes is symbolized as:

(a) 1n
(b) 2n
(c) 3n
(d) 4n

(13)    Chromosomes (eucaryotes) are composed of all except:

(a) histones
(b) non-histone protein
(c) DNA
(d) RNA

(14) Select the *incorrect* statement:

(a) a recessive allele is only expressed when it is homozygous
(b) a dominant allele can be expressed when heterozygous
(c) a codominant allele may express itself completely or partially when homozygous or heterozygous, respectively
(d) dominant alleles may not be expressed

(15) Mendel's First Law:

(a) alleles of the same trait segregate (separate on homologous chromosomes) in the formation of gametes
(b) alleles of different traits separate independently of each other in the formation of gametes
(c) genes are particulate in nature
(d) genes are indivisible (i.e., cannot be subdivided and yet produce a given trait)

(16) Select the *incorrect* statement regarding homologous chromosomes:

(a) except for X and Y, they are the same size
(b) they have identical sequences of genes
(c) they synapse in meiosis
(d) except for X and Y, they have the same sequence of loci as traits

(17) Sex-linked traits:

(a) are found more in females than in males
(b) are found on the X and Y chromosomes
(c) allow recessive alleles to be expressed when one such allele is present in the male
(d) males have a 50% chance of receiving sex-linked alleles from the father

(18) If the genotype for a trait is Aa (A dominant to a), possible gametes are:

(a) Aa only
(b) AA and aa
(c) A,a
(d) Aa,A, and a

(19) Given the following pedigree, select the correct explanation assuming that the pedigree is representative of the inheritance patterns (blackened symbols mean trait is present):

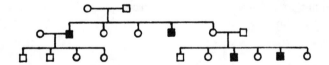

(a) autosomal dominant
(b) autosomal recessive
(c) sex-linked dominant
(d) sex-linked recessive

(20) Given the following representative pedigree, select the most likely pattern of inheritance (blackened symbols mean the trait is present):

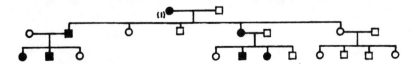

(a) autosomal dominant
(b) autosomal recessive
(c) sex-linked dominant
(d) sex-linked recessive

(21) Given the following representative pedigree, what is the *most likely* pattern of inheritance (blackened symbols mean trait is present)?

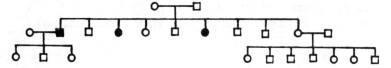

(a) autosomal dominant
(b) autosomal recessive
(c) sex-linked recessive
(d) mutation

(22) If brown eyes (B) is dominant to blue eyes (b), the parents have what genotype for eye color (open symbol: brown eyes; blackened symbol: blue eyes)?

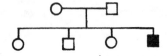

(a) father Bb, mother BB
(b) father BB, mother Bb
(c) father Bb, mother Bb
(d) cannot be determinned from information given

(23) Suppose gray (G) is dominant to white (g) coat color for rats. Given the following representative pedigree, what are the most likely genotypes of the parents (open symbol: white; blackened symbol: gray)?

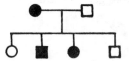

(a) father GG, mother gg
(b) father Gg, mother Gg
(c) father gg, mother Gg
(d) cannot be determined from the information given

(24) Suppose round peas (R) are dominant to wrinkled peas (r) and green peas (G) are dominant to yellow peas (g). The following cross is made:

$$RrGg \times RrGg$$

What are the expected phenotypes and their frequencies in the offspring (assume the traits are not linked)?

(a) 3 round, green: 1 wrinkled, yellow
(b) 2 round, green: 1 round, yellow: 1 wrinkled, green
(c) 9 round green: 3 wrinkled, green: 3 round, yellow: 1 wrinkled, yellow
(d) all round, green

(25) If red (R) is dominant to white (r) and parents with genotypes RR(male) and rr(female) are crossed, what are the colors and their expected frequencies in the offspring?

(a) 1 red: 3 white
(b) 1 red: 1 white
(c) 3 red: 1 white
(d) all red

(26) If the offspring from Question #25 are crossed with each other, what are the colors and their frequencies in the offspring from this second cross?

(a) 1 red: 2 pink: 1 white
(b) 3 red: 1 white
(c) 1 red: 1 white
(d) all red

(27) If the genotype for two traits is AaBB, the possible gametes are:

(a) Aa,BB
(b) AB,aB
(c) A,a,B,B
(d) Ab,ab,AB,aB

(28) Mendel's Second Law:

(a) alleles of the same trait segregate (separate on homologous chromosomes) in the formation of gametes
(b) alleles of different traits separate independently of each other in the formation of gametes
(c) genes are particulate in nature
(d) genes are indivisible

(29) Suppose the only alleles that determine blood type are A and B, and that they are codominant. If parents, both with Type AB, have children, what are the ratios of the childrens' expected blood types? Type A = AA, Type B = BB, Type AB = AB (genotypes of each type).

(a) 1 Type A: 2 Type AB: 1 Type B
(b) 1 Type A: 1 Type B
(c) 3 Type AB: 1 Type A: 1 Type B
(d) all Type AB

(30) The following three-factor cross is done. Which answer is correct?

| Parent Genotypes: | Offspring Genotypes | Percentage of Total |
|---|---|---|
| r      r+ <br> s+     s <br> t      t+ | r <br> s+ <br> t | 26% |
|  | r+ <br> s <br> t+ | 26% |
|  | r <br> s+ <br> t | 16% |
|  | r+ <br> s <br> t | 16% |
|  | r+ <br> s+ <br> t+ | 6% |
|  | r <br> s <br> t | 6% |
|  | r+ <br> s+ <br> t | 2% |
|  | r <br> s <br> t+ | 2% |

*Question #30 Answer Choices:*

   (a) the genotypes representing the double recombination are r s t and r+ s+ t+
   (b) the s locus is farthest from the central locus
   (c) the map distance between the three loci is 16 units
   (d) the r locus is the central locus

## 2.20.3    Answers to Questions in Section 2.20.2

( 1) d  ( 2) d  ( 3) d  ( 4) b  ( 5) c  ( 6) a  ( 7) c  ( 8) c  ( 9) c  (10) d  (11) c
(12) b  (13) d  (14) a  (15) a  (16) b  (17) c  (18) c  (19) d  (20) a  (21) b  (22) c
(23) c  (24) c  (25) d  (26) b  (27) b  (28) b  (29) a  (30) d

## 2.20.4    Discussion of Answers to Questions in Section 2.20.2

*Questions #1 to #9, #15, #28* — Adequately discussed in Section.

*Question #10* (Answer: d) Aneuploidy is the deletion (Y is lost in XO) or addition (an extra #21 is added in trisomy 21) of one or more individual chromosomes. Polyploidy means a multiplication of the whole set of chromosomes as in 4n.

*Question #11* (Answer: c) The normal male has 44 autosomes, one X and one Y chromosome. The normal female has 44 autosomes and two X chromosomes.

*Question #12* (Answer: b) 2n = diploid. Gametes are haploid (1n). Occasionally, somatic cells will be triploid (3n) or tetraploid (4n).

*Question #13* (Answer: d) RNA is made using the DNA of chromosomes as a template; it is not an integral part of a chromosome.

*Question #14* (Answer: a) Recessive alleles may be expressed when sex-linked. Dominant alleles may not have penetrance.

*Question #16* (Answer: b) A gene is a specific sequence of nucleotides which codes for a specific protein which may be expressed as a phenotypic variation (blue, brown) of a given trait (eye color). Homologous chromosomes do not usually have an identical sequence of genes; they do have a set sequence of loci for the alleles (contrasting genes) for a given trait.

*Question #17* (Answer: c) This is possible because only the X chromosome carries the trait and the Y is the homologous chromosome in the male. Hence: a

$$\overset{\mathsf{a}}{\underset{\mathsf{X}}{|}} \qquad \underset{\mathsf{Y}}{|}$$

The allele, a, will express itself because it is the only allele present for the trait.

*Question #18* (Answer: c) The genotype Aa produces the gametes with A and a separately by Mendel's First Law of Segregation of alleles of the same trait. Note that A and a are on different but homologous chromosomes.

*Question #19* (Answer: d) Note that the trait appears only in males, can be carried by females, and the males apparently inherit it only from their mothers.

*Question #20* (Answer: a) There is no sex preference and no skipped generations. It (the trait) is only passed from those parents expressing the disease, and many individuals are affected. All of this is characteristic of a highly penetrated autosomal dominant allele. The initial mother (1) is heterozygous for the allele; because if she were homozygous, every one of her children would have the trait.

*Question #21* (Answer: b) There is no sex preference, and since the initial father did not have the disease, it would be improbable that his daughters would have it if it was sex-linked recessive. A mutation is unlikely (but possible) because three offspring have the trait, few people are affected, and the trait is not passed by affected individuals. Autosomal recessive is the most likely, and the initial parents must have been heterozygous for the recessive allele.

*Question #22* (Answer: c) Since both parents have brown eyes, their genotype must be at least B – for each. Since one child has blue eyes (bb), one b allele must have come from each parent. Therefore, each parent must be Bb.

*Question #23* (Answer: c) The father must be gg because he is white. The mother is gray and she is, at least, G – . Since the pedigree is representative, white offspring do appear. Since each white offspring must get one g from the father, they must also get a g from the mother—otherwise there would be no white offspring. Therefore, the mother must be Gg.

*Question #24* (Answer: c) Use the Punnet square to get genotypic frequencies (gametes are RG, Rg, rG, rg for each parent):

|      | RG   | Rg   | rG   | rg   |
|------|------|------|------|------|
| RG   | RRGG | RRGg | RrGG | RrGg |
| Rg   | RRGg | RRgg | RrGg | Rrgg |
| rG   | RrGG | RrGg | rrGG | rrGg |
| rg   | RrGg | Rrgg | rrGg | rrgg |

Then, based on the dominance-recessive relationships given, the phenotypes and their ratios are:

> all R-G- are round, green (RRGG-1, RRGg-2, RrGG-2, RrGg-4) = 9
> all rrG- are wrinkled, green (rrGG-1, rrGg-2) = 3
> all R-gg are wrinkled, yellow (RRgg-1, Rrgg-2) = 3
> rrgg is wrinkled, yellow (rrgg-1) = 1

*Question #25* (Answer: d) Since the gametes will be r (female) and R (male) only, all offspring will be Rr or red. See Question #26.

*Question #26* (Answer: b) Using the genotype Rr derived in Question #25, determine the genotypes of the new offspring by using a new Punnet Square (gametes are R,r for both parents):

♀

Rr = red

♂

|   | r  | r  |
|---|----|----|
| R | Rr | Rr |
| R | Rr | Rr |

for #25

|   | R  | r  |
|---|----|----|
| R | RR | Rr |
| r | Rr | rr |

for #26

Then using the dominance-recessive relationship given, the phenotypes and their ratios are determined:

> R- is red (RR-1, Rr-2) = 3
> rr is white (rr) = 1.

*Question #27* (Answer: b) Each gamete will contain one allele of each trait in all possible combinations with each other. Then each gamete can have an A or a, and it must have a B. This gives AB, aB.

*Question #29* (Answer: a) Use the Punnet Square to determine the genotypes (gametes of each parent are A,B):

|   | A  | B  |
|---|----|----|
| A | AA | AB |
| B | AB | BB |

Using the informtion relating phenotypes to genotypes given in the question:

$$\text{Type A} \quad (AA = 1) \ = \ 1$$
$$\text{Type B} \quad (BB = 1) \ = \ 1$$
$$\text{Type AB} \ (AB = 2) \ = \ 2$$

*Question #30* (Answer: d) The lowest frequency recombinant is  r+  s+  t  and  r  s  t+ . The locus out of line with the parents is the r locus. Then, r must be the central locus. The t is farther from r (32% recombination frequency) than the s (12% recombination frequency). Map units are not recombination frequency units.

## 2.20.5    Vocabulary Checklist for Genetics

_____ chromosome
_____ diploid
_____ polyploidy
_____ tetraploidy
_____ monosomy
_____ heterozygous
_____ penetrance
_____ alleles
_____ cytoplasmic inheritance
_____ dominant
_____ crossing-over
_____ trisomy
_____ histone
_____ autosomes
_____ translocation
_____ aneuploidy
_____ pedigrees
_____ homozygous

_____ genes
_____ homologous chromosomes
_____ codominant
_____ recessive
_____ sex-linked
_____ linked traits
_____ mutation
_____ sex chromosomes
_____ duplication
_____ Barr bodies
_____ recombination
_____ Punnet square
_____ inversion
_____ deletion
_____ phenotype
_____ genotype
_____ Lyon Hypothesis

## 2.20.6    Concepts, Principles, etc. Checklist for Genetics

_____ chemical composition of chromosomes
_____ the set of human chromosomes and variations
_____ organization of chromosomes (genes, alleles, etc.)
_____ Mendel's Laws
_____ mechanisms of genetic variability
_____ sex-linked traits
_____ cytoplasmic inheritance
_____ use of pedigrees
_____ use of Punnet squares
_____ two-factor cross
_____ three-factor cross
_____ recombination frequency
_____ map units
_____ linkage
_____ ordering of gene loci

## 2.21 EVOLUTION AND ADAPTATION

### 2.21.1 Review of Evolution and Adaptation

#### 2.21.1.1 THE MECHANISM OF EVOLUTION

*Evolution* is the study of the changes that occur in organisms, how the changes occur, and the results of the changes. These changes may be minor and lead to better adaptation to an environment, or they may be major and lead to a totally different species. Changes come about when organisms are *"selected"* on the basis of *phenotypic differences* to survive. These phenotypic differences must be based upon underlying *genetic differences*, as found in the germ cells, to lead to evolutionary change. The survival of selected organisms leads to *changes in the gene frequencies and gene combinations* in the population, which in turn leads to *changes in phenotypic characteristics* and, hence, evolution.

Mutations (see Section 2.20.1) are the ultimate source of all new genes in the population, and as such, they are the raw material for all evolutionary changes. Genes mutate forward to new genes and backward to the old gene. The *mutation pressure* is the net change of these two processes. Genes arising by mutation tend to be recessive, and since they are rarely homozygous, they tend to be carried silently, i.e., not expressed, in the population for long periods of time. Stable alleles are those with low mutation rates and they tend to increase in frequency. This contrasts with unstable alleles which have high mutation rates and tend to decrease in frequency. This process results in a slow shift in gene frequencies in the population. It seems reasonable that mutation alone could cause evolutionary change. The major reason that mutation per se does *not* cause evolutionary change is that *mutation is random* and, consequently, usually is in a direction away from the organism's evolutionary trend. So mutation alone has a slow and non-directional effect on evolution with the exception of polyploidy (Section 2.20.1). *Polyploidy* is the doubling (e.g., 2n → 4n), of the set of chromosomes usually by nondisjunction during meiosis. What results is an organism with a larger set of chromosomes which result in phenotypic differences in them. Also, note that mutations in somatic cells have no effect on evolution because they are not passed on to the offspring.

Mutations produce a small but important change in the gene frequencies of the *gene pool* (Section 2.20.1) of a population. These gene frequencies determine the genotypic ratios which determine the distribution of phenotypes in the population. *Genotypic ratios* (i.e., numbers and types of genotypes) can be determined from the gene frequencies and the Punnet square method as shown in Fig. 2.64.

allele B = 0.8, allele b = 0.2 as frequencies in the population

Punnet Square to determine genotypes:

|  | B (0.8) | b (0.2) |
|---|---|---|
| B (0.8) | BB (0.64) | Bb (0.16) |
| b (0.2) | Bb (0.16) | bb (0.04) |

genotypic frequencies BB = 0.64, Bb = 2(0.16) = 0.32, bb = 0.04.

*Fig. 2.64—Genotypic Frequencies*

The *Hardy-Weinberg Law* states that under certain conditions the above gene frequencies and genotypic frequencies remain constant from generation to generation in sexually reproducing populations. This means no evolution would occur under *these conditions* which are: (1) large populations, (2) no mutations or the existence of mutation equilibrium, (3) no immigration or emigration of the population, and (4) random reproduction. The reason large populations (#1) are required is that gene frequencies undergo random fluctuations called *genetic drift*. In a small population, these random changes may cause an increase in certain alleles which leads to homozygosity. This effect is small in large populations (e.g., greater than 10,000 breeding individuals). As noted above, mutations always occur so #2 does not hold. Immigration or emigration leads to loss or gain of certain alleles which change gene frequencies. Reproduction includes all the steps from mate selection through mating and development of the embyro to growth of the young to reproductive maturity. All of these steps, and all in between, must be random for gene frequencies to remain constant (#4). But in all populations, non-random reproduction exists, and this non-random reproduction is called *natural selection* as first set forth by *Darwin*. The reason reproduction is non-random is because phenotypes vary, and different phenotypes result in differences in reproductive capabilities. Natural selection does change gene frequencies by causing new combinations of genes which result in new phenotypes. Additionally, recombination and gene mutation, if left alone, can destroy favorable gene combinations and substitute unfavorable combinations for them. Natural selection also serves a conservative function by eliminating these unfavorable combinations. Note that natural selection can act on gene frequencies only when the genetic variation is expressed as phenotypic variation, and that phenotypic variation can lead to changes in gene frequencies only when it reflects underlying genetic variation.

Phenotypic differences are in a distribution in any population. The distribution is often an approximation of the bell shaped curve.

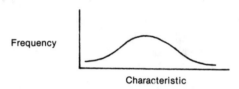

An example is the distribution of height in humans. *Environmental factors* (meteorologic, geographic, physical, or biologic) also vary greatly. It is a small step to infer that certain characteristics are better suited for certain environments. Or, to look at it differently, environments may select organisms with certain phenotypic characteristics that are most likely to survive in them. As above, if these phenotypic characteristics reflect genetic differences then a change in gene frequencies and evolution can occur. Environmental factors and reproductive factors (i.e., natural selection) interact with each other.

*In summary*, mutations provide the raw material for evolution. But it is the *selection pressure* for certain phenotypes exerted by natural selection and environmental factors that determines the course of evolution.

## 2.21.1.2    CONSEQUENCES OF EVOLUTION

The consequences of evolution are seen in the changes that may occur in a given species. These changes can be minor and reflected as *clines*. Clines are gradual variations in a species due to geographic (environmental) variations such as altitude or latitude. *Subspecies (races)* result when an abrupt environmental change is associated with an abrupt change in characteristics. Finally, the evolutionary changes may be so great as to result in a totally new species—a process called speciation.

A *species* is viewed as a set of genetically distinct organisms that share a common gene pool (i.e., gene flow is possible between them) and are reproductively isolated from all other such groups. The first step in *speciation* is usually *geographic isolation* of two populations of the same species. A *barrier* (e.g., rivers, oceans, canyons, mountains, etc.) prevent the populations from coming together to mate. The two separate populations will tend to differ because: (1) gene frequencies usually differ, (2) each population experiences different mutations, (3) the different environments will exert different selection pressures, and (4) if small, genetic drift can cause differences. The second factor in speciation then comes into play; it is *reproductive isolation*. The two populations will begin to differ such that gene flow between them is no longer possible even if they are brought together. This is brought about by *intrinsic reproductive isolating mechanisms* which act at all the steps of reproduction discussed earlier. These are: (1) *ecogeographic isolation* (organisms can no longer survive in each other's environment), (2) *habitat isolation* (organisms may occupy only certain, but different, habitats within the same range), (3) *seasonal isolation* (the breeding periods may be at different times of the year), (4) *behavioral isolation* (mating rituals differ), (5) *mechanical isolation* (nonfitting of genitals), (6) *gametic isolation* (fertilization cannot occur), (7) *hybrid unviability* (the offspring cannot reproduce), and (9) *developmental isolation* (fertilization can occur, but the embryo dies). So, by geographic isolation followed by reproductive isolation, the mechanisms of evolution lead to new species.

General *patterns* of evolution are *divergent* (moving from one species to different species, the usual pattern), *convergent* (moving from separate to common species), or *parallel* (two species resulting from one but evolving in a parallel fashion). *Adaptive radiation* is the gradual divergent differentiation of a species, usually as a response to environmental variations. *Homologous* structures are those that arose from a common structure even though functions may be different. *Analogous* structures have common functions but arose from different structures.

## 2.21.1.3 TAXONOMY

A hierarchical classification that exists for organisms was due primarily to *Linnaeus*. Organisms are grouped at each level on the basis of similarities. As the hierarchy is ascended (shown below), the similarities become more general. A well-known mnemonic is given with the hierarchy:

| | |
|---|---|
| Kings | Kingdom |
| Play | Phyllum |
| Chess | Class |
| On | Order |
| Fine | Family |
| Grain | Genus |
| Sand | Species |

All organisms are given a two-component Latin name. The first is the genus (capitalized), and the second is the species (not capitalized), e.g., *Homo sapiens*.

## 2.21.1.4 MAJOR ADAPTIVE EVOLUTIONARY CHANGES IN VERTEBRATES

*Chordates* are distinguished by (1) a dorsal, hollow nerve cord, (2) gill slits in the throat region, and (3) a notochord. Chordates are divided into invertebrate chordates (tunicates, acorn worms, cephalochordates or amphioxus) and vertebrates. *Vertebrates* have a vertebral column, closed circulatory system (enabling large growth), a better developed nervous system and improved sensory apparatus. *Fish* include the Agnatha (jawless, e.g., lampreys), Chondrichthyes (e.g., sharks, all cartilage except inner ears) and Osteichthyes (bony fish). The pectoral fins, pelvic fins and lateral line system are important for balance. Lobe fin fish (or crossopterygians, e.g., latimeria) invaded land, had lungs, had stubby fins (bones into fins—was a crucial step for land invasion) and gave rise to the amphibians. *Amphibians* (frogs, toads, salamanders) are still tied to water because their eggs are easily dessicated. *Reptiles* (snakes, turtles, lizards, crocodiles and alligators) arose from amphibians. Total land life was possible because of the amniotic egg which wouldn't dessicate and which had a sufficient food supply. Reptiles are also advanced beyond amphibians by (1) internal fertilization by copulation, (2) ventricle of heart is partly divided to separate oxygenated and unoxygenated blood, (3) ribs aid in respiration, and (4) the brain has small cerebral hemispheres. The pterosaurs (extinct) gave rise to the birds. *Aves* (birds) can fly because of special feathers (modified reptile scales, large quills for flying surface, fanlike tail feathers for stabilization, contour and down feathers for insulation), light skeleton and a special breastbone for flight muscles, warm-blooded, efficient respiration with the four-chambered heart, advanced sight and muscular coordination by the brain. *Mammals* arose from a different type of reptile than did the birds. Key distinguishing features of mammals are: (1) internal development of young and nutrition by mammary glands, (2) jaw is strengthened and teeth are differentiated, (3) a diaphragm is present to separate thorax and abdomen and is used in breathing, (4) legs are swung underneath the body, and (5) the brain is greatly enlarged.

## 2.21.1.5   POPULATION GROWTH

Although many factors affect the ultimate growth of a population (species), four factors can be used to describe the growth rate (R). These are the birth rate (B), the death rate (D), the carrying capacity (C), and the number of individuals in the population (N). B is the rate of live births per unit population (e.g., 5/1000 means 5 live births per 1000 individuals). D is similarly defined. Both are dependent on the age of the population and the reproductive capacity of the population. Very old or young populations will have high D. C represents the number of individuals the environment is able to support. C is independent of the R of the population, but over time the total N can affect its value (e.g., by using up the food supply). The maximum growth rate may vary as the C of particular environments varies. The equation linking these four factors is:

$$R = (B - D) \times \left(\frac{C - N}{C}\right) \times N.$$

Note that B − D is the intrinsic growth rate (IGR) of the population. The key points to remember are:

(1) R is directly proportional to IGR;
(2) R is directly proportional to N;
(3) when N is small, the term C-N/C is about one and growth is exponential;
(4) when N approaches and equals C, the term C-N/C is zero and the population is in zero growth (mild fluctuations may occur);
(5) the C-N/C factor results in the logistic (S shaped) growth curve for populations.

Growth curves are:

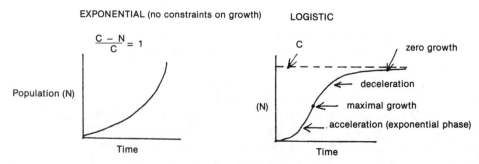

Note the maximal growth rate occurs in approximately the center of the curve (logistic). The maximal growth rate of the exponential growth curve is not reached as it is always increasing (and is never realized except for very short periods and then the logistic curve will intervene). The point of maximal growth is also the point of optimal yield of a population. This means to get the greatest number of individuals (including more mature) out of a population, the population size (N) should be kept near this point. It is always near the center of the logistic growth curve.

Age distributions of populations are important in understanding and predicting changes in population growth. Age distribution curves may be done in many different graphic representations. One example is (with different distributions):

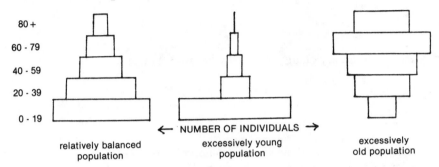

Survivorship of the population may also be graphically represented as:

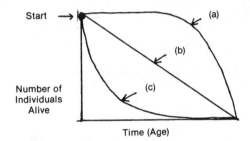

(a) individuals live to older ages, many younger & older
(b) death rates same at all ages, equal representation of all ages
(c) younger die at high rates, few older in population

The factors limiting population growth may be divided into density dependent (DD) and density independent (DI) effects. DD effects (as population grows, these are more important) include space, food, diseases, predation, and other competitive factors. DI effects include weather, natural disasters, and aging. The limitations on population growth can be overcome by emigration (relocation to alleviate DD effects), migration (relocating annually to maximize environments), evolution of different characteristics, or undergoing population cycles (increases and decreases in population size on a regular basis by mechanisms unknown, e.g., the lemmings). If unsuccessful, the population may become extinct.

## 2.21.2   Questions to Review Evolution and Adaptation

(1)   Select the correct statement:

   (a) Phenotypic differences alone serve as a basis for evolution.
   (b) Phenotypic differences serve as a basis for evolution when they reflect somatic cell genetic differences.
   (c) Phenotypic differences serve as a basis for evolution when they reflect germ cell genetic differences.
   (d) None of the above.

(2)     The ultimate source of all new genes in a population is due to:

(a) mitosis
(b) mating
(c) meiosis
(d) mutation

(3)     Mutations tend to be:

(a) recessive
(b) dominant
(c) codominant

(4)     Mutations do not affect evolutionary change primarily because they are:

(a) expressed
(b) recessive
(c) too rare
(d) random

(5)     "Under certain conditions the gene frequencies and genotypic frequencies remain constant from generation to generation in sexually reproducing populations" was put forth by:

(a) Dalton
(b) Hardy-Weinberg
(c) Mendel
(d) Mendeleev

(6)     All of the following are conditions under which evolution would *not* occur except:

(a) large populations
(b) nonrandom reproduction
(c) no mutations
(d) no immigration or emigration

(7)     Genetic drift may lead to evolution in populations that are:

(a) any size
(b) large
(c) small

(8)     Which is *not* considered as part of the evolutionary concept of the reproductive process?

(a) mate selection and mating behavior
(b) embryo development
(c) growth of young to reproductive maturity
(d) all of the above are part of the reproductive process

(9)     Darwin's idea of natural selection is the same as:

(a) polyploidy
(b) mutation pressure
(c) genetic drift
(d) nonrandom reproducion

(10)    Natural selection results in:

(a) increased favorable gene combinations
(b) decreased unfavorable gene combinations
(c) both
(d) neither

(11) Selection pressure depends on:

(a) nonrandom reproduction
(b) environmental factors
(c) both
(d) neither

(12) The first step in the formation of a new species is:

(a) reproductive isolation
(b) geographic isolation
(c) both occur together

(13) Populations that are separated by geographic barriers will tend to differ because

(a) gene frequencies usually differ between them
(b) mutations vary between populations
(c) there are different environmental pressures
(d) all of the above

(14) Structures that have different functions but arose from a common structure are called:

(a) convergent
(b) divergent
(c) analogous
(d) homologous

(15) Assuming all other factors are constant, which situation will not result in an increase in the population growth rate?

(a) increase in the total individuals in the population near the carrying capacity
(b) decrease in the death rate
(c) increase in the birth rate
(d) increase in the intrinsic growth rate

(16) Important features in the development of mammals are:

(1) internal development of young
(2) jaw is strengthened and teeth differentiated
(3) diaphragm
(4) legs underneath body
(5) brain greatly enlarged

(a) 1, 3, 5
(b) 1, 3, 4, 5
(c) 1, 2, 3, 5
(d) all of the above

(17) A factor which would be detrimental to the flight of birds is

(a) light skeleton
(b) advanced sight and muscle coordination
(c) three-chambered heart
(d) large quill feathers or fan-like tail feathers

(18) Reptiles differ from amphibians by all of the following *except:*

(a) amniotic egg
(b) internal fertilization by copulation
(c) complete four-chambered heart
(d) ribs aid in respiration

(19)    The primary reason amphibians are still tied to the water is

   (a) lungs are inadequate
   (b) they are cold blooded
   (c) eggs are easily dessicated
   (d) they need to breathe through moist skin

(20)    A fish manager wants to increase the productivity of a lake. He desires greater catches of fish and larger sized fish. He wants to maintain this over a long period of time. This increase will be accomplished best by:

   (a) increasing the bait (food) available to the fish
   (b) keeping the fish population near the maximal growth rate point
   (c) restricting the number of fish caught for several years
   (d) stocking the lake with reproductive size fish this year

(21)    Which type of heart can separate oxygenated and deoxygenated blood completely?

   (a) two chambers
   (b) three chambers
   (c) four chambers
   (d) all can

(22)    Diaphragms are muscles used in the act of breathing. Which of the following utilizes a diaphragm to breathe?

   (a) amphibians
   (b) reptiles
   (c) birds
   (d) none of the above

(23)    What is the correct hierarchy (from highest to lowest) of the given levels of taxonomy?

   (a) class, order, family, genus
   (b) order, family, genus, class
   (c) family, genus, class, order
   (d) family, class, order, genus

(24)    Organisms are given a two-component scientific name. The first part is the:

   (a) class
   (b) order
   (c) species
   (d) genus


## 2.21.3    Answers to Questions in Section 2.21.2

( 1) c   ( 2) d   ( 3) a   ( 4) d   ( 5) b   ( 6) b   ( 7) c   ( 8) d   ( 9) d   (10) c   (11) c
(12) b   (13) d   (14) d   (15) a   (16) d   (17) c   (18) c   (19) c   (20) b   (21) c   (22) d
(23) a   (24) d


## 2.21.4    Discussion of Answers to Questions in Section 2.21.2

*Questions #1 to #19* Adequately discussed in Section.

*Question #20* (Answer: b) The point of optimal yield is at the maximum growth rate (MGR). If the MGR can be determined and the population kept at this level, the lake will produce the greatest yield.

Increasing the food (that is, the carrying capacity) will not increase the yields per se. If the amount of fish caught is restricted, the lake will approach the carrying capacity and zero growth rate, and the yield will decrease. Adding more fish may overload the carrying capacity, and, of itself, may not increase the yield. Arguments for each choice may be made; the best answer is (b).

*Questions #21 - #24* Adequately discussed in Section.


### 2.21.5 Vocabulary Checklist for Evolution and Adaptation

_____ genotypic ratios
_____ reproductive isolation
_____ divergent evolution
_____ adaptive radiation
_____ genetic drift
_____ homologous
_____ speciation
_____ population growth rate
_____ birth rate
_____ exponential growth

_____ geographic isolation
_____ convergent evolution
_____ parallel evolution
_____ gene pool
_____ analogous
_____ vertebrates
_____ intrinsic growth rate
_____ death rate
_____ logistic growth


### 2.21.6 Concepts, Principles, etc. Checklist for Evolution and Adaptation

_____ role of mutations in evolution
_____ Hardy-Weinberg Law
_____ meaning of reproduction in evolutionary terms
_____ natural selection
_____ role of environment in evolution
_____ mechanism of speciation
_____ optimal yield
_____ taxonomy
_____ carrying capacity of population
_____ major adaptive evolutionary changes in vertebrates
_____ survivorship curves
_____ density dependent effects
_____ density independent effects
_____ maximal growth rate
_____ age distributions


## 2.22 REFERENCES FOR REVIEW OF BIOLOGY

Johnson, Leland G. *Biology*. 1983 or latest ed. (Dubuque, Iowa: Wm. C. Brown, Publishers)

Another excellent text.

Keeton, W. *Biological Science*. 2nd or latest ed. (New York: W. W. Norton & Co., Inc.)

An excellent introductory text on general biology. If any questions arise about material presented in this workbook, this textbook should be consulted first.

Wilson, W. O., et al. *Life on Earth*. Latest ed. (Sinauer Associates, Inc.)

# Chapter 3

# Review

# of

# General Chemistry

## 3.1 ATOMIC STRUCTURE

### 3.1.1 Review of Atomic Structure

*Bohr* used the theories and experimental data of Planck, Einstein and Rutherford to develop his theory of the atom. He thought the angular momentum of the electron was in multiples of h/2$\pi$ (or mvr = nh/2$\pi$), and that electrons circulated in discrete circular orbits stabilized by having the centrifugal force on the electron equal the Coulomb force of attraction between the nucleus and the electron. From these inferences he derived the energy states of the electrons given by:

$$E = -\frac{2\pi^2 m Z^2 e^4}{n^2 h^2} \qquad n = 1,2,3,\ldots\ldots$$

$m$ = mass of electron
$e$ = charge on electron
$Z$ = atomic number (nuclear charge)
$h$ = Planck's Constant

Energy transitions occur between states with energy change equal to h$\upsilon$ which could be calculated from above (h = $|E_f - E_i|$). Note that E $\propto 1/n^2$ and as n gets larger, the energy levels get closer together. Bohr was able to explain some of the hydrogen spectrum lines with his theory. Another key to his theory was that electrons in any one of the energy states do not radiate energy. The major flaws in Bohr's theory were the discrete orbits and the determination of exact momentum of the electron concurrently. *Heisenberg's uncertainty principle* stated that it is impossible to determine simultaneously the position and momentum of an electron as in Bohr's theory. This led to the probabilistic theory of electronic structure as derived by Schroedinger. The quantum theory and its natural quantum numbers resulted. The quantum numbers are:

(1)     n = principle quantum number
        takes values n = 1,2,3,4,5....
        higher n means higher total energy of electron defines *shells* of the atom

        1 = K, 2 = L, 3 = M, 4 = N, etc.

(2)     $l$ = angular momentum quantum number
        higher $l$ means higher angular momentum of electron
        angular momentum is limited by the total energy (n)
        $l$ = 0,1,2....n − 1
        *defines orbitals* of atom (along with n)
        0 = s, 1 = p, 2 = d, 3 = f, etc.

(3)    $m_l$ = magnetic quantum number
orientation of the electron's magnetic field in an external field—limited
by the angular momentum ($l$)
$m_l = l, l-1, \ldots 0, \ldots, -l+1, -l$
(i.e., takes all values between $+l$ and $-l$) determines spatial
orientation of orbitals and, consequently, the *number* of orbitals of
type $l$

(4)    $m_s$ = spin quantum number
does not arise from solution of the Schroedinger equation
the spin of an electron in its axis also generates a magnetic field which
can orient two ways with an external field
values have been chosen as $+\frac{1}{2}$, $-\frac{1}{2}$ for the direction of spin.

Each electron in an atom has a set (n, $l$, $m_l$, $m_s$) of quantum numbers that uniquely defines it. *Pauli's Exclusion Principle* states that no two electrons in the same atom may have the same set of quantum numbers. Only a certain number of electrons is allowed for each quantum number:

n:    a maximum of 2 $n^2$ electrons
for n = 1, get 2 electrons
for n = 2, get 8 electrons
for n = 3, get 18 electrons

$l$:    a maximum of $4l + 2$ electrons
for $l = 0$ (s orbital), get 2 electrons
for $l = 1$ (p orbital), get 6 electrons
for $l = 3$ (f orbital), get 14 electrons

$m_l$: a maximum of two electrons for each $m_l$

An example of how one gets these numbers is shown for n = 3 (maximum numbers of electrons are in parentheses) in Fig. 3.1.

| n | $l$ | $m_l$ | $m_s$ |
|---|---|---|---|
| 3 (18) | 0(2) | 0(2) | +1/2,-1/2 |
| | 1(6) | +1(2) | +1/2,-1/2 |
| | | 0(2) | +1/2,-1/2 |
| | | -1(2) | +1/2,-1/2 |
| | 2(10) | +2(2) | +1/2,-1/2 |
| | | +1(2) | +1/2,-1/2 |
| | | 0(2) | +1/2,-1/2 |
| | | -1(2) | +1/2,-1/2 |
| | | -2(2) | +1/2,-1/2 |

*Fig. 3.1—Example of the Quantum Number Relationships*

Each orbital is symbolized by using the n and $l$ quantum numbers as follows:
1s, 3p, 5f
n↗      ↘$l$.

The *orbitals are filled* in sequence, from the lowest energy to the highest energy. The pattern of orbitals filled is called the *electron configuration*. The sequence is not that expected because some orbitals, especially those with $s(l = 0)$, penetrate (get closer to the nucleus than others) and are consequently lowered in energy more and are filled first. A useful way to remember the sequence is to add the n and $l$ numerical values. The lowest sum is filled first. In the case of a tie, the lowest n value is filled first (remember s = 0, p = 1, d = 2, f = 3). For example: 1s 2s 2p 3s 3p 3d 4s vs. 1s 2s 2p 3s 4s 3d. In the first configuration 3d is written before 4s. Using the rule for 3d, n(= 3) + d(= 2) = 5, whereas for 4s, n(= 4) + s(= 0) = 4; therefore second configuration should be used.

The orbitals are filled by knowing the number of electrons in the atom (if neutral, this is the atomic number), and then filling each orbital sequentially up to its maximum number of electrons. For example:

$$Al = 13: \quad 1s^2\ 2s^2\ 2p^6\ 3s^2\ 3p^1.$$
$$Ca = 20: \quad 1s^2\ 2s^2\ 2p^6\ 3s^2\ 3p^6\ 4s^2.$$

If the atom is charged, the extra electrons (if negative) are added or the lost electrons (if positive) are removed. For example:

$$Al^{+3}\ (AN = 13): 1s^2\ 2s^2\ 2p^6$$
$$O^{-2}\ (AN = 8): \quad 1s^2\ 2s^2\ 2p^6.$$

Fig. 3.2 shows another way to remember the sequence of filling:

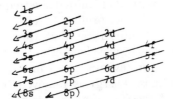

The sequence: 1s 2s 2p 3s 3p 4s 3d 4p 5s, etc.

*Fig. 3.2—A Way of Remembering the Sequence of Filling of Orbitals*

*Hund's rule* describes the way electrons are to be put into each orbital (n, *l*). Electrons go into each orbital of same energy ($m_l$) with parallel spins (same $m_s$) until each orbital is half filled (i.e., all electrons unpaired), then they are paired (put in the same orbital with opposite $m_s$'s) (Fig. 3.3).

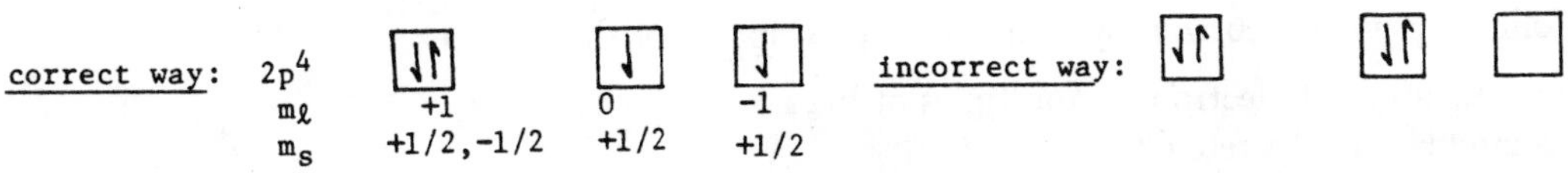

correct way:
| $2p^4$ | $\boxed{\downarrow\uparrow}$ | $\boxed{\downarrow}$ | $\boxed{\downarrow}$ |

incorrect way: $\boxed{\downarrow\uparrow}$ $\boxed{\downarrow\uparrow}$ $\boxed{\phantom{x}}$

| $m_l$ | +1 | 0 | -1 |
| $m_s$ | +1/2, -1/2 | +1/2 | +1/2 |

*Fig. 3.3—Hund's Rule*

*Orbitals* (Fig. 3.4) are determined by the n, *l*, and $m_l$ numbers. The n and *l* are important for determining the energy and shape of the orbital. The $m_l$ determines the orientation (direction in space) of the orbitals. Remember that an orbital describes the probability of an electron being in a region of space; it is not the electron spread out.

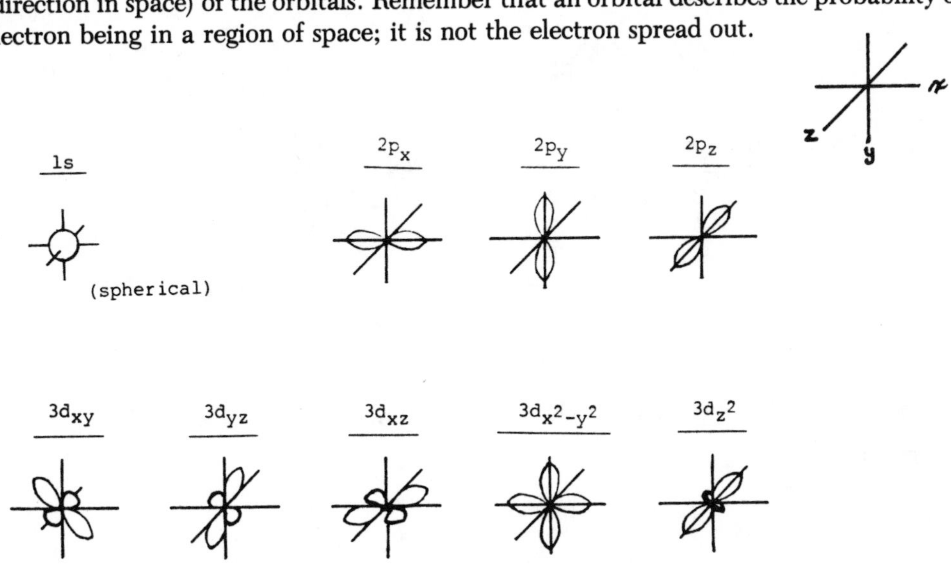

1s
(spherical)

$2p_x$    $2p_y$    $2p_z$

$3d_{xy}$    $3d_{yz}$    $3d_{xz}$    $3d_{x^2-y^2}$    $3d_{z^2}$

*Fig. 3.4—Orbitals*

The *ground state* of the electrons of an atom is when the electrons are in the lowest energy states available to the electrons. For example, the ground state of the aluminum was

$$1s^2 \quad 2s^2 \quad 2p^6 \quad 3s^2 \quad 3p^1.$$

An *excited state* of the atom occurs when one or more electrons occupy orbitals (energy levels) other than the lowest available to the atom. This occurs by "exciting" the electron (by input of some type of energy) to the higher state. For example, for the aluminum:

$$1s^2 \quad 2s^2 \quad 2p^6 \quad 3s^2 \quad 3p^1 \xrightarrow{\text{energy}} 1s^2 \quad 2s^2 \quad 2p^6 \quad 3s^0 \quad 3p^3$$

both 3s electrons are now in the higher energy level 3p.

For the electrons, the higher the n or $l$ quantum numbers, the higher the energies. When electrons shift between the different orbitals, energy is absorbed or emitted as a frequency of light. When energy is emitted (the electron moves from higher orbitals to lower orbitals, i.e., closer to the nucleus in general), a bright band appears at that frequency (or wavelength) in a spectrum (the continuum of all frequencies or wavelengths) — this results in *emission spectra*. When energy is absorbed by the electron (as must occur in the example above), a dark band appears at that frequency because energy is removed from the spectrum. This results in *absorption spectra*. Look at the spectrum as a source of light containing all the frequencies (wavelengths) representing different energies. As this passes through a substance, energy may be added (by emission from atoms) and certain frequencies become more intense (brighter) or energy may be removed (by absorption by atoms) and certain frequencies become less intense (less bright).

### 3.1.2    Questions to Review Atomic Structure

(1)    All of the following were theorized by Bohr in his description of the atom except:

(a) angular momentum of electrons in multiples of $h/2\pi$
(b) electrons circulate in discrete circular orbits
(c) energy of each electron is inversely proportional to $n^2$
(d) electrons radiate energy continuously in a given orbit

(2)    The statement, "it is impossible to determine simultaneously the position and momentum of an electron," is attributable to:

(a) Heisenberg
(b) Einstein
(c) Planck
(d) Schroedinger

(3)    The following shape represents what type of orbital?

(a) p
(b) s
(c) d
(d) f

(4)    The letters s,p,d and f are used to represent which quantum numbers?

(a) angular momentum ($l$)
(b) principal (n)
(c) magnetic ($m_l$)
(d) spin ($m_s$)

(5)     The magnetic quantum number (QN) has its values limited *directly* by the value of:

(a) principal QN
(b) angular momentum QN
(c) spin QN
(d) none of the above

(6)     Hund's Rule:

(a) Electrons go into orbitals with parallel spins until all the orbitals of the same energy are half filled, then they go into suborbitals with anti-parallel (opposite) spins.
(b) Two electrons in the same atom cannot have the same four quantum numbers.
(c) There is a maximum of two electrons in any orbital.
(d) None of the above.

(7)     Pauli's Exclusion Principle states that:

(a) The position and momentum of an electron cannot be simultaneously determined.
(b) Electrons with the same spin cannot go into the same orbital.
(c) No two electrons in an atom may have the same set of the four quantum numbers.
(d) None of the above.

(8)     When an atom emits energy as light, bands in the spectrum will appear:

(a) brighter
(b) darker
(c) remain the same

(9)     The maximum number of electrons in an orbital with $m_l$ (magnetic quantum number) $= -3$ is:

(a) 6
(b) 4
(c) 3
(d) 2

(10)    The maximum number of electrons in a shell with n (principal quantum number) $= 3$ is:

(a) 6
(b) 8
(c) 18
(d) 32

(11)    The maximum number of electrons in an orbital with $l$ (angular momentum quantum number) $= 3$ is

(a) 6
(b) 10
(c) 14
(d) 18

(12)    An element with atomic number $= 22$ has how many electrons in the 2p orbital?

(a) 6
(b) 4
(c) 3
(d) 1

(13)    The electron configuration of magnesium (Mg) with atomic number 12 is:

(a) $1s^2$  $2s^2$  $2p^6$  $3s^2$
(b) $1s^2$  $2s^2$  $3s^2$  $3p^6$
(c) $1s^2$  $2s^2$  $2p^2$  $3s^2$  $3p^2$  $3d^2$
(d) None of the above

(14) Sodium has an atomic number = 11. The electron configuration of the sodium ion ($Na^{+1}$) is:

(a) $1s^2$ $2s^2$ $2p^6$ $3s^2$
(b) $1s^2$ $2s^2$ $2p^5$ $3s^2$
(c) $1s^2$ $2s^2$ $2p^6$ $3s^1$
(d) $1s^2$ $2s^2$ $2p^6$

*Use the following information for Questions #15–#17*

The atomic number of manganese (Mn) is 25.

(15) The electron configuration of the ground state is:

(a) $1s^2$ $2s^2$ $2p^6$ $3s^2$ $3p^6$ $3d^7$
(b) $1s^2$ $2s^2$ $2p^6$ $3s^2$ $3p^6$ $4s^2$ $4p^5$
(c) $1s^2$ $2s^2$ $2p^6$ $3s^2$ $2d^{10}$ $3p^3$
(d) None of the above

(16) An excited state of the atom may be:

(a) $1s^2$ $2s^2$ $2p^6$ $3s^2$ $3p^6$ $4s^1$ $3d^6$
(b) $1s^2$ $2s^2$ $2p^6$ $3s^2$ $3p^6$ $4s^2$ $3d^5$
(c) $1s^2$ $2s^2$ $2p^6$ $2d^{10}$ $3s^2$ $3p^3$
(d) None of the above

(17) In going from $1s^2$ $2s^2$ $2p^6$ $3s^2$ $3p^6$ $4s^2$ $3d^5$ to $1s^2$ $2s^2$ $2p^6$ $3s^2$ $3p^6$ $4s^1$ $3d^6$, the atom would _____ energy.

(a) absorb
(b) emit
(c) not change energy states

### 3.1.3     Answers to Questions in Section 3.1.2

( 1) d   ( 2) a   ( 3) a   ( 4) a   ( 5) b   ( 6) a   ( 7) c   ( 8) a   ( 9) d   (10) c   (11) c
(12) a   (13) a   (14) d   (15) d   (16) a   (17) a

### 3.1.4     Discussion of Answers to Questions in Section 3.1.2

*Questions #1 to #8:* Adequately discussed in Section.

*Question #9* (Answer: d) All orbitals contain a maximum of two electrons.

*Question #10* (Answer: c) Using the formula given in Section, $2n^2 = 2(3)^2 = 2(9) = 18$. See example in Section for alternative method to determine it.

*Question #11* (Answer: c) Using the formula given in the Section, $4l + 2 = 4(3) + 2 = 12 + 2 = 14$.

*Question #12* (Answer: a) There are 22 electrons (from the AN = 22 and the atom is neutral). The electron configuration is:

$$1s^2 \quad 2s^2 \quad 2p^6 \quad 3s^2 \quad 3p^6 \quad 4s^2 \quad 3d^2$$

It might have been clear that the 2p orbital would have been filled. So, the answer would be a filled p orbital which has *six* electrons.

*Question #13* (Answer: a) There are 12 electrons in the neutral atom because AN = 12. The sequence of filling is:

$$1s \quad 2s \quad 2p \quad 3s \quad 3p \quad 4s \quad 3d$$

The *s* has a maximum of 2 electrons, and the *p* has a maximum of 6 electrons. The electron configuration is:

$$1s^2 \quad 2s^2 \quad 2p^6 \quad 3s^2.$$

*Question #14* (Answer: d) There are 10 electrons in the sodium ion. In the neutral atom there are 11 (from atomic number = 11). Since the ion is a positive one, there must be one less electron available. The electron configuration is then:

$$1s^2 \quad 2s^2 \quad 2p^6.$$

*Question #15* (Answer: d) The ground state is when the electrons are in the lowest energy levels available. The sequence of filling for 25 electrons is:

$$1s^2 \quad 2s^2 \quad 2p^6 \quad 3s^2 \quad 3p^6 \quad 4s^2 \quad 3d^5$$

So, none of the answers given is correct.

*Question #16* (Answer: a) An excited state occurs when electrons in the ground state orbitals are "excited" to higher energy orbitals. In (a), a 4s electron is excited to a 3d electron.

*Question #17* (Answer: a) Here the 4s electron is being excited to become a 3d electron. Since 3d electrons are of higher energy than 4s (due to the penetrance of this orbital and consequent lowering of its energy), it would require energy to move 4s to 3d levels. Therefore, the atom must absorb this energy.

### 3.1.5 Vocabulary Checklist for Atomic Structure

| | |
|---|---|
| _____ Heisenberg's Uncertainty Principle | _____ absorption spectra |
| _____ Bohr | _____ excited states |
| _____ Pauli's Exclusion Principle | _____ emission spectra |
| _____ orbital | _____ n |
| _____ shell | _____ $l$ |
| _____ Hund's rule | _____ $m_l$ |
| _____ ground states | _____ $m_s$ |

### 3.1.6 Concepts, Principles, etc. Checklist for Atomic Structure

_____ Bohr theory of atomic structure
_____ quantum numbers and filling of electron orbitals (electronic structure)
_____ relation of spectra to atomic structure

## 3.2 PERIODIC TABLE

### 3.2.1 Review of the Periodic Table

The periodic table is an orderly arrangement of elements by their atomic numbers based on the quantum theory of the atom. Mendeleev was the first to arrange elements by their atomic numbers. Features of the organization of the chart are (see also Fig. 4.5):

(1) Rows or *periods* represent the principal quantum number (n) and have values from n = 1 to n = 7. Each period is the sequential filling of the orbitals within a shell.

(2) Columns or *groups* represent elements with the same electron configuration in the *outermost shell*. There is the A set of elements called *representative*, and these have the s and/or p orbitals as the outermost. The *nonrepresentative*, or B set, elements have the d or f orbitals as the outermost. The Roman Numerals (I, II, etc.) give the number of electrons in the outermost orbitals. From this, the electron configuration and valence can be determined. For the VI A group, for example, there are six electrons in s and p orbitals. This gives an $s^2p^4$. Remember that the second period atoms prefer the *octet state* and that they will gain or lose electrons to reach it, whichever is easier. The common valence in VI A is − 2 because it is easier to gain 2 electrons to go

to $s^2 p^6$ (octet) than to lose 6 electrons and go to $s^0 p^0$ (which would be the next lower octet) and have a $+6$ valence. Elements in the same group tend to have similar chemical properties.

(3) The different *blocks* represent the angular momentum quantum number ($l$). The number of spaces from left to right in each block is the maximum number of electrons for each quantum number: $s$ has a maximum of 2, $p$ has a maximum of 6, $d$ has a maximum of 10, and $f$ has a maximum of 14.

(4) The magnetic quantum number ($m_l$) and spin quantum number ($m_s$) are not represented on the chart.

(5) Representative elements, transition elements, inner transition elements (actinides, lanthanides), inert gases and other special groups are labeled on the chart (Fig. 3.5).

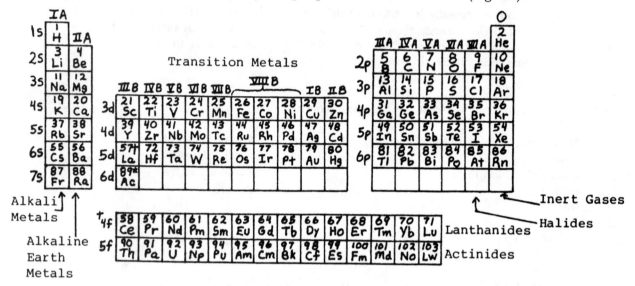

Fig. 3.5-The Periodic Chart

The *periodic properties* are properties of the elements which vary in a more or less regular pattern as a function of the atomic numbers, and, hence, electron configuration. Most can be understood through the following:

(1) As one reads from left to right in a given period, the nuclear pull on the outermost electrons increases. This causes the electrons to be bound tighter and to be closer to the nucleus.

(2) As one reads down a given column, the outermost electrons are bound less tightly because more electrons are between the nucleus and the outermost electrons, and because a shell has been completed and this effectively shields the outer electrons.

Based upon the above discussion, the gross atomic trends of the periodic properties from the chart can be understood. These are:

(1) *Ionization energy (IE)*—The energy (or voltage) required to ionize a gaseous atom, i.e., take the outermost electron away from the atom. The higher the IE, the more difficult it is to remove an electron, and this means the nucleus is holding on tighter. IE increases, generally, from left to right in a period, and it decreases from top to bottom in a group.

(2) *Electron Affinity (EA)*—The energy released when an electron is moved from infinity into the lowest energy vacant orbital in the gaseous atom. The stronger the nuclear attraction for electrons, the higher the EA (absolute value). The EA is subject

to configuration variations (Be $2s^2 <$ Li $2s^1$ but C>B) and repulsion of electrons in the same energy level (F<Cl but Br<Cl). No overall trend is observed.

(3) *Electronegativity (E)* — The relative attraction of the nucleus for the electrons in a chemical bond. Not measured directly, but it can be indirectly obtained from EA, IE and/or bond energies. The E increases from left to right in a period and decreases from top to bottom in a group — this is similar to IE.

(4) *Atomic Radius (AR)* — The distance from the middle of the nucleus to the "outermost limit" of the electrons. The AR is determined by using x-rays on bonded atoms. The AR decreases from left to right in a given period and increases from top to bottom in a given group.

Additional trends of properties can be inferred from the above basic properties. These are:

(1) *Metallic character (MC)* — The key feature of a metal is high mobility of electrons. This requires a low IE and/or a low EA. This means MC decreases from left to right in a period but increases from top to bottom in a group. In the chart, the metals are to the left and bottom, and the non-metals are in the top and right. Between is a region of transition called the semi-metals.

(2) *Oxidation State (OS)* — The OS depends on IE and EA. Low IE elements tend to have positive OS, and high EA elements tend to have negative OS. Metals tend to have positive OS, and non-metals tend to be negative. Determiniation of OS (valence) from the chart is given above. In general, note that the OS of the transition (d orbital) elements tend to be variable but positive. And the OS of the inner transition elements (f-orbitals) tend to be $+3$.

(3) *Chemical Activity (CA)* — This depends on the ease of removing an electron (low IE) or the ease of adding an electron (high EA). Either situation leads to high CA. Hence, CA trends are not usually discussed across a period (because the balance of IE and EA changes), but trends are meaningful for groups. On the left side of the chart, CA increases as you go down the chart in a given group (because IE decreases). On the right side of the chart, CA increases as you go up the chart in a given group (because EA generally increases).

(4) *Acidity Trends* — See Section 3.11.1.

(5) *Hydrogen Bonding (HB)* — HB exists for F, O, N and Cl but would theoretically increase as one ascended a given group.

### 3.2.2 Questions to Review the Periodic Table

(1) The periodic table is based upon:

(a) atomic weights
(b) mass number
(c) neutron number
(d) atomic number

(2) The periods of the periodic table are _____ and represent the _____ quantum number.

(a) horizontal; principal
(b) horizontal; angular momentum
(c) vertical; principal
(d) vertical; angular momentum

(3) Groups of the periodic table:

(a) represent the magnetic quantum number
(b) represent elements with the same outer electron configuration
(c) are horizontal
(d) all of the above are correct

(4) Which of the following quantum numbers is not represented on the periodic chart?

    (a) principal
    (b) angular momentum
    (c) magnetic
    (d) all are

(5) The transition elements have the ____-orbital as the outermost.

    (a) s
    (b) p
    (c) d
    (d) f

(6) Inert gases

    (a) have incomplete shells
    (b) are found in the same period
    (c) are found at the beginning of a period
    (d) are found in the same group

(7) All of the following are correct except:

    (a) The nuclear attraction for the outermost electrons decreases from right to left in a given period.
    (b) In moving down a given column, the outermost electrons are bound less tightly.
    (c) Half-filled or completely filled orbitals have more stability than other incompletely filled orbitals.
    (d) All of the above are correct.

(8) The energy required to ionize a gaseous atom is called the:

    (a) ionization energy
    (b) electron affinity
    (c) electronegativity
    (d) none of the above

(9) The relative attraction of the nucleus for the electrons in a chemical bond is called the:

    (a) ionization energy
    (b) electron affinity
    (c) electronegativity
    (d) none of the above

(10) The energy released when an electron is moved from infinity into the vacant orbital with the lowest energy:

    (a) electron affinity
    (b) electronegativity
    (c) ionization energy
    (d) none of the above

(11) The ionization energy

    (a) generally increases from left to right in a period
    (b) does not change in a period
    (c) increases from top to bottom in a group
    (d) does not change in a group

(12) The electron affinity

    (a) decreases from left to right in a period
    (b) measures the attraction of the atom for electrons
    (c) increases from top to bottom in a group
    (d) variations follow no overall trend

(13) The electronegativity

(a) is measured directly from physical characteristics
(b) does not vary in a group
(c) decreases from left to right in a period
(d) decreases from top to bottom in a group

(14) The atomic radius

(a) is calculated from bond energies
(b) decreases from left to right in a period
(c) decreases from top to bottom in a group
(d) all of the above

(15) Metallic character

(a) depends upon the mass number
(b) decreases from bottom to top in a group
(c) requires a high ionization energy and a high electron affinity
(d) decreases from top to bottom in a group

(16) Oxidation states (OS):

(a) high ionization energy elements have positive OS
(b) metals tend to have negative OS
(c) low electron affinity elements tend to have positive OS
(d) non-metals tend to have negative OS

(17) Chemical activity

(a) increases as ionization energy increases
(b) decreases as electron affinity decreases
(c) in groups on the left side of the chart, chemical activity increases as you read down the chart

(18) Phosphorus (P) is in group VA; the electron configuration of its outermost shell is

(a) $s^2 p^3$
(b) $p^5$
(c) $d^5$
(d) cannot be determined

(19) Bromine (Br) is in group VII A; its most common oxidation state (OS) is probably:

(a) $+1$
(b) $-1$
(c) $-2$
(d) cannot be determined

(20) The electron configuration of selenium is:
$1s^2 2s^2 2p^6 3s^2 3p^6 4s^2 3d^{10} 4p^4$. It is probably in what group?

(a) VI A
(b) IV A
(c) VI B
(d) need more information

(21) The atomic number of chlorine is 17. It is in what group?

(a) VII A
(b) IV A
(c) I A
(d) cannot be determined by trends

(22) Fluorine (F) has an atomic number (AN) = 9 and chlorine (Cl) has an AN = 17. Which has the highest electron affinity?

(a) both are equal
(b) Cl
(c) F
(d) cannot be determined

(23) Sodium (Na) has an atomic number (AN) = 11 and aluminum (Al) has an AN = 13. Which has the highest ionization energy?

(a) both are equal
(b) Na
(c) Al
(d) cannot be determined

(24) Oxygen (O) has an atomic number (AN) = 8 and sulfur (S) has an AN = 16. Which has the greatest electronegativity?

(a) S
(b) O
(c) both are equal
(d) cannot be determined

(25) The atomic number (AN) of magnesium (Mg) is 12, and the AN of sulfur (S) is 16. Which has the largest atomic radius?

(a) Mg
(b) S
(c) both are equal
(d) cannot be determined

(26) Lithium (Li) has an atomic number (AN) = 3 and potassium (K) has an AN = 19. Which has the greater metallic character?

(a) both are equal
(b) Li
(c) K
(d) cannot be determined

(27) Berylium (Be) has an atomic number (AN) = 4, and strontium (Sr) has an AN = 38. Which has the greater chemical activity?

(a) both are equal
(b) Sr
(c) Be
(d) cannot be determined

(28) Magnesium (Mg) has an atomic number (AN) = 12 and Bromine (Br) has an AN = 35. Which has the greater chemical activity?

(a) both are equal
(b) Mg
(c) Br
(d) cannot be determined

### 3.2.3    Answers to Questions in Section 3.2.2

( 1) d  ( 2) a  ( 3) b  ( 4) c  ( 5) c  ( 6) d  ( 7) d  ( 8) a  ( 9) c  (10) a  (11) a
(12) d  (13) d  (14) b  (15) b  (16) d  (17) c  (18) a  (19) b  (20) a  (21) a  (22) d
(23) c  (24) b  (25) a  (26) c  (27) b  (28) d

## 3.2.4 Discussion of Answers to Questions in Section 3.2.2

*Questions #1 to #17:* Adequately discussed in Section.

*Question #18* (Answer: a) The A means the p is a representative element and that its outermost shell contains s and p orbitals. The V means there are 5 electrons, and these give the following electron configuration, $s^2 p^3$.

*Question #19* (Answer: b) Since Br is in group VII A the electron configuration of its outermost shell is $s^2 p^5$. The closest octet is $s^2 p^6$, and this requires an extra electron to give it an OS of $-1$.

*Question #20* (Answer: a) Since the outermost incomplete orbitals are $s$ and $p$ (the d orbital is complete), the selenium is an A element. The $s$ and $p$ contain $2 + 4 = 6$ electrons. This means selenium is group VI A.

*Question #21* (Answer: a) The electron configuration of chlorine is $1s^2 2s^2 2p^6 3s^2 3p^5$. The outermost incomplete orbitals are $s$ and $p$—this makes it A (representative). There are $2 + 5 = 7$ electrons in the $s$ and $p$ orbitals—this makes it a VII. So it is group VII A.

*Question #22* (Answer: d) EA has no overall trend useful for predictions.

*Question #23* (Answer: c) The electron configuration of Na is $1s^2 2s^2 2p^2 3s^1$ and Al is $1s^2 2s^2 2p^6 3s^2 3p^1$. This places them in the same period—highest $n$ number is 3 in each. Ionization energy (IE) increases from left to right on the table. Then Al has a higher IE than Na.

*Question #24* (Answer: b) O has an electron configuration of $1s^2 2s^2 2p^4$, and sulfur has an electron configuration of $1s^2 2s^2 2p^6 3s^2 3p^4$. This places both in group VI A. In a group, the electronegativity decreases from top to bottom. Then O has the greater electronegativity.

*Question #25* (Answer: a) The electron configurations are: $Mg = 1s^2 2s^2 2p^6 3s^2$; $S = 1s^2 2s^2 2p^6 3s^2 3p^4$. They are, therefore, in the same period. The atomic radius decreases from left to right in a period. Then Mg is larger than S.

*Question #26* (Answer: c) The electron configurations are: $Li = 1s^2 2s^1$; $K = 1s^2 2s^2 2p^6 3s^2 3p^6 4s^1$. Therefore, both are in group IA. In a group the metallic character increases from top to bottom. Then K has more metallic character than Li.

*Question #27* (Answer: b) The electron configurations are: $Be = 1s^2 2s^2$; $Sr = 1s^2 2s^2 2p^6 3s^2 3p^6 4s^2 3d^{10} 4p^6 5s^2$. Therefore, they are both in group II A. In a group on the left side, the chemical activity increases from top to bottom. Then Sr is more reactive than Be.

*Question #28* (Answer: d) The electron configurations are: $Mg = 1s^2 2s^2 2p^6 3s^2$; $Br = 1s^2 2s^2 2p^6 3s^2 3p^6 4s^2 3d^{10} 4p^5$. This means they are neither in the same group nor period and cannot be compared by general periodic trends.

## 3.2.5 Vocabulary Checklist for the Periodic Table

_____ periods        _____ periodic properties      _____ electronegativity
_____ groups         _____ oxidation state          _____ atomic radius
_____ representative elements    _____ ionization energy    _____ metallic character
_____ octet state    _____ electron affinity        _____ chemical activity

## 3.2.6 Concepts, Principles, etc. Checklist for the Periodic Table

_____ basis for the periodic table
_____ organization of the table, especially the relation to the quantum numbers
_____ general basis for the variation of the periodic properties
_____ variation of the periodic properties within groups and periods

## 3.3 GAS PHASE

### 3.3.1 Review of the Gas Phase

The metric *pressure* units are mmHg = torr. The English system uses atmospheres (atm). The conversion is 760 torrs = 1 atm. See Section 5.5.1 for temperature scales.

Gases have relatively high translational kinetic energies per molecule as compared with liquids. Gases take the shape of the container they are in, like liquids; but, unlike liquids, they completely fill any container. The *key characteristics* of gases are the pressure (P), the volume (V), the temperature (T), and the quantity (moles = n). Gases are broadly considered as ideal or non-ideal. An *ideal gas* has no intermolecular forces, and the gas molecules occupy no volume (they are points in space). This means the gases should have low density. In general, at high temperatures and low pressures, most gases can be considered to be ideal. A *non-ideal gas* has intermolecular forces, and the molecules do have a finite volume. Laws covering the behavior of ideal gases will be covered first.

*Boyle's Law* states that pressure and volume are inversely related (P ∝ 1/V), i.e, as the pressure increases, the volume decreases and vice versa. *Charles' (Gay-Lussacs) Law* states that the temperature and volume are directly related, i.e., as the temperature increases, the volume increases and vice versa. These laws are combined to give the *Ideal Gas Law* which is:

$$PV = n\,RT$$

P = pressure, V = volume, n = moles, T = absolute temperature
R = Ideal gas constant = 0.0821 $l$ -atm/°K-mole

Another useful way of writing the Ideal Gas Law is,

$$\frac{PV}{T} = \text{constant or,}$$

$$\frac{P_1 V_1}{T_1} = \frac{P_2 V_2}{T_2}$$

Also, note that *22.414 liters of an ideal gas at S.T.P. (Standard Temperature and Pressure—273°K and 1 atmosphere pressure) represent 1 mole of that gas. Avogadro's Principle* is also important for solving problems and states that equal volumes of ideal gases at the same temperature and pressure contain the same number of moles (or molecules). *Dalton's Law* states that the total pressure ($P_t$) of a mixture of gases is equal to the sum partial pressures ($P_i$) of the gases:

$$P_t = P_1 + P_2 + P_3 + \ldots$$

The *partial pressure* ($P_i$) of a gas in a mixture of gases is determined as follows:

$P_i$ = $X_i\,P_t$
$P_t$ = total pressure
$X_i$ = mole fraction of gas in the mixture
$X_i = \dfrac{n_i}{n_1 + n_2 + n_3 + \ldots} = \dfrac{n_i}{\Sigma n_i}$

$n_i$ = moles of a gas
$\Sigma n_i$ = sum of the moles of all gases.

*The Kinetic Theory of Gases* attempts to describe the energy characteristics of gases as a whole by analyzing the motion and mass characteristics (e.g. forces, momentum) of individual molecules. It has its limitations but important results of it are:

(1)    Boyle's Law, Charles' Law, and the Ideal Gas Law are derivable from it;

(2)    P and V can be related to the kinetic energy of molecules,

$PV = 2/3\ NE_k$ (on a molecular scale)

$N$ = # of molecules, $E_k$ = translation energy/molecule

or, $E_k = (3/2)\ RT$ (on a mole scale)

also at a given temperature, all molecules have the same average $E_k$;

(3)     *Graham's Law of Diffusion* can be determined from $E_k$ as follows:

$E_{k_1} = E_{k_2}$ i.e., the average $E_k$s are equal

1, 2 = molecules

also, $\frac{1}{2}m_1v_1^2 = \frac{1}{2}m_2v_2^2$ (see Section 5.4.1)

after solving, get

$v_1/v_2 = \sqrt{m_2}\ /\ \sqrt{m_1} = \sqrt{m_2/m_1}$

$v$ = velocities of diffusion (e.g., mls/min)

$m$ = molecular weights or densities.

(4)     Values for Heat Capacities of Monatomic Gases (see Section 5.5.1).

$C_v = \dfrac{3}{2}\ R$

$C_p = C_v + R$

$C_p/C_v = 1.67$

$R$ = 1.99 cals/mole-°k

One of the simpler equations for nonideal gases is the *van der Waals equation* which takes into account the false assumptions of ideal gases:

$$\left(P + \frac{n^2a}{V^2}\right)(V-nb) = nRT$$

a, b are constants

$n^2a/V^2$ corrects for intermolecular forces

nb corrects for the volume occupied by gas molecules.

Note that if the density is very low, then $V \gg nb$ and $n^2a/V^2 \to O$, and the Ideal Gas Law results. The effect of the intermolecular forces is to decrease the pressure of the gas. The effect of the volume of molecules is to increase the volume occupied by the gas. The terms above bring the pressure and volume back to ideal levels.


### 3.3.2      Questions to Review the Gas Phase

(1)     The variables used to describe gases include all except:

(a) pressure
(b) volume
(c) moles
(d) all of the above

(2)     All of the following are characteristics of ideal gases except:

(a) absence of intermolecular forces
(b) nonideal gases may exhibit ideal behavior at high pressure and low temperatures
(c) the molecules occupy no space
(d) all of the above are correct

(3)     Boyle's Law states that:

(a) volume varies inversely as temperature
(b) volume varies directly as temperature
(c) pressure varies inversely as volume
(d) pressure varies directly as volume

(4) Charles' Law states that

(a) volume varies inversely as temperature
(b) volume varies directly as temperature
(c) pressure varies inversely as volume
(d) pressure varies directly as volume

(5) All are expressions for the Ideal Gas Law except:

(a) $PV = nRT$

(b) $\dfrac{PV}{T} = \text{constant}$

(c) $\dfrac{P_1 V_1}{T_1} = \dfrac{P_2 V_2}{T_2}$

(d) $\left(P + \dfrac{n^2 a}{V^2}\right)(V-nb) = nRT$

(6) One mole of an ideal gas at STP has all of the following characteristics except:

(a) volume = 1 liter
(b) temperature = $273\,°K$
(c) pressure = 1 atmosphere
(d) all of the above are correct

(7) Each gas in a mixture exerts a pressure. The total pressure of all the gases in the container is

(a) less than the sum of the separate pressures of each gas
(b) more than the sum of the separate pressures of each gas
(c) equal to the sum of the separate pressures of each gas
(d) the sum is variable

(8) The correct expression for the partial pressure ($P_A$) of $n_A$ moles of a gas in a mixture of gases with a *total* of $n_T$ moles and a total pressure = $P_T$ is

(a) $P_A = (n_A + n_T)P_T$
(b) $P_A = (n_T - n_A)\,P_T$
(c) $P_A = n_A P_T$
(d) $P_A = (n_A/n_T)P_T$

(9) All of the following are conclusions of the Kinetic Theory of Gases except

(a) derivation of the van der Waals equation
(b) derivation of Boyle's and Charles' Law
(c) relation of average kinetic energy of gases to temperature
(d) Graham's Law of Diffusion

(10) In the van der Waals equation for nonideal gases,
$\left(P + \dfrac{n^2 a}{V^2}\right)(V-nb) = nRT$, it is *not true* that

(a) $\dfrac{n^2 a}{V^2}$ corrects for intermolecular forces

(b) nb corrects for the volume occupied by gas molecules
(c) at high densities the equation reduces to the Ideal Gas Law
(d) all of the above are correct

(11) The pressure on a sample of gas is tripled, the volume is

(a) 9 times the original
(b) 3 times the original
(c) ⅓ of the original
(d) ⅑ of the original

(12)  If the temperature of a gas is increased by a factor of 4, the volume is

(a) increased by a factor of 16
(b) increased by a factor of 4
(c) increased by a factor of 2
(d) decreased by a factor of 4

(13)  One mole of an ideal gas occupies 3 liters at 37°C. Approximately what pressure, in atmospheres, does the gas exert?

(a) 1.1 atm
(b) 4.2 atm
(c) 8.5 atm
(d) 12.3 atm

(14)  What volume will 2 liters of a gas at 27°C and 2 atm occupy at S.T.P.?

(a) 3.6 liters
(b) 5.1 liters
(c) 1.1 liters
(d) cannot be determined

(15)  Two moles of an ideal gas occupy what volume at S.T.P.?

(a) 22.4 liters
(b) 44.8 liters
(c) 67.2 liters
(d) cannot be determined

(16)  It is found that 2 grams of a vaporized liquid occupy 0.82 liters at S.T.P. What is the molecular weight of the gas?

(a) 13.5 grams
(b) 27 grams
(c) 54 grams
(d) cannot be determined

(17)  A container of pure oxygen has a pool of water at its bottom. The atmospheric pressure is 760 torrs and equals the total pressure of the container. If the temperature is 37°C and the vapor pressure of water is 47 torrs at this temperature, what is the pressure of the dry oxygen?

(a) 700 mm Hg
(b) 684 mm Hg
(c) 807 mm Hg
(d) 713 mm Hg

(18)  A mixture of 2 moles of $O_2$, 3 moles of $N_2$, and 5 moles of $H_2$ exerts a pressure of 700 torrs. The partial pressure of $N_2$ is:

(a) 700 torrs
(b) 210 torrs
(c) 490 torrs
(d) 760 torrs

(19)  A mixture of 5 moles of $O_2$, 4 moles of $N_2$, and 1 mole of CO is collected above water at a temperature of 27°C. The total pressure is 760 torrs and the vapor pressure of water at 27°C is 27 torrs. What is the partial pressure exerted by $O_2$?

(a) 76 torrs
(b) 100 torrs
(c) 367 torrs
(d) 380 torrs

(20) Oxygen (molecular weight = 32) diffuses at a rate of 10 mls/min. Under the same conditions of temperature and pressure, how fast will hydrogen (molecular weight = 2) diffuse?

(a) 20 mls/min
(b) 40 mls/min
(c) 160 mls/min
(d) need more information

### 3.3.3    Answers to Questions in Section 3.3.2

( 1) d   ( 2) b   ( 3) c   ( 4) b   ( 5) d   ( 6) a   ( 7) c   ( 8) d   ( 9) a   (10) c   (11) c
(12) b   (13) c   (14) a   (15) b   (16) c   (17) d   (18) b   (19) c   (20) b

### 3.3.4    Discussion of Answers to Questions in Section 3.3.2

*Questions #1 to #10:* Adequately discussed in Section.

*Question #11* (Answer: c) This is a direct application of Boyle's Law. Volume varies inversely as pressure. So, if pressure is increased by a factor of 3, the volume is decreased by a factor of 3. That is, the volume is $\frac{1}{3}$ of the original.

*Question #12* (Answer: b) A direct application of Charles' Law. Volume varies directly as temperature. Since temperature is increased by a factor of 4, the volume is increased by a factor of 4.

*Question #13* (Answer: c) This problem deals with one gas under one set of n-P-V-T; this suggests that the equation to use is $PV = nRT$. Solving for pressure, one gets,

$$P = nRT/V$$

The value of R is required. By knowing the units used, this can be determined as follows:

$$R = \frac{PV}{nT} = \frac{(1 \text{ atm}) (22.4 \text{ liters})}{(1 \text{ mole}) (273°K)} = 0.082 \quad \frac{\text{atm-liters}}{\text{mole-}°K}$$

(Because 1 mole of an ideal gas at STP—273°K, 1 atm—occupies 22.4 liters.)

Also, remember, that the temperature is the absolute temperature: $T = 37° + 273° = 310°K$
Then,

$$P = \frac{(1)(0.082)(310)}{(3)} \approx 8.2 \text{ atms}$$

note $\frac{310}{3} \approx 100$ and then $(100)(0.082) \approx 8.2$.

Note the approximations made. The 8.2 is closest to 8.5 atms.

*Question #14* (Answer: a) Note that this problem requires the gas be compared at two different conditions of P-V-T; the best equation to use in this instance is,

$$\frac{P_2 V_2}{T_2} = \frac{P_1 V_1}{T_1}$$
$$(\text{STP}) \quad (\text{Original})$$

Solving for $V_2$,

$$V_2 = V_1 \left(\frac{T_2}{T_1}\right) \left(\frac{P_1}{P_2}\right) = (2) \left(\frac{273}{300}\right) \left(\frac{2}{1}\right) \approx 3.6$$

$$T_1 = 27 + 273 = 300$$

the approximation is made as follows

$$\frac{273}{300} \approx \frac{270}{300} \approx \frac{27}{30} \approx \frac{9}{10}$$

then, $(2)\left(\frac{9}{10}\right)(2) = \left(\frac{36}{8}\right) = 3.6$

*Question #15* (Answer: b) Since one mole of an ideal gas occupies 22.4 liters at STP, two moles would occupy twice as much or $2 \times 22.4 = 44.8$ liters.

*Question #16* (Answer: c) First the number of moles is determined. Since the substance is a gas and there is one set of PV-T conditions use:

$$PV = nRT.$$

Solving for n,

$$n = \frac{PV}{RT} = \frac{(1)(0.82)}{(0.082)(273)} \approx \frac{1}{27}$$

the approximation for n is as follows

$$\frac{0.82}{0.082} = 10, \text{ then } \frac{10}{273} \approx \frac{10}{270} \approx \frac{1}{27}.$$

The definition of moles (n) in (Section 3.6.1):

$$\text{moles} = \frac{\text{weight}}{\text{molecular weight}} \text{ or,}$$

$$\text{molecular weight} = \frac{\text{weight}}{\text{moles}} \approx \frac{2}{1/27} \approx (2)\left(\frac{27}{1}\right) \approx 54 \text{ gms.}$$

alternate: Since $n = \text{wt/mw}$, $PV = (\text{wt/mw})RT$; $mw = \text{wt}(RT/PV)$.

*Question #17* (Answer: d) The only point of this problem is to stress that when gases are collected over a liquid (e.g. water), the vapor pressure of that liquid must be subtracted from the total pressure to get the pressure of the gases without the added effect of the liquid's vapor pressure. The vapor pressure varies with temperature. Note that the total pressure of the gases is still the sum of the partial pressures (Dalton's Law),

$$P_{tot} = P_{O_2} + P_{H_2O} \text{ vapor}$$

$$P_{O_2} = P_{tot} - P_{H_2O} \text{ vapor} = 760 - 47 = 713.$$

*Question #18* (Answer: b) This is a direct application of Dalton's Law of partial pressures. The partial pressure of $N_2(P_{N_2})$ is,

$$P_{N_2} = X_{N_2}P_T$$
$$P_T = 700 \text{ torrs}$$
$$X_{N_2} = \frac{n_{N_2}}{n_{N_2} + n_{O_2} + n_{H_2}} = \frac{3}{3+5+2} = \frac{3}{10}$$
$$P_{N_2} = \frac{3}{10}(700) = 210 \text{ torrs.}$$

*Question #19* (Answer: c) This is just a combination of the principles of questions #17 and #18. First, the effect of the water vapor on the total pressure is taken into account:

$P_T(\text{Total pressure of gases}) = \text{total pressure} - \text{water vapor pressure}$

$$P_T = 760 - 27 = 733 \text{ torrs.}$$

Then Dalton's Law is applied using this 733 torrs:

$$P_{O_2} = X_2 P_T$$

$$X_2 = \frac{n_{O_2}}{n_{O_2} + n_{N_2} + n_{CO_2}} = \frac{5}{5+4+1} = \frac{5}{10} = \frac{1}{2}$$

$$P_{O_2} = (\tfrac{1}{2})(733) = 367 \text{ torrs.}$$

*Question #20* (Answer: b) In general, the lighter gas will diffuse faster. Using the formulation of Graham's Law of Diffusion,

$$\frac{V_{H_2}}{V_{O_2}} = \sqrt{\frac{MW_{O_2}}{MW_{H_2}}}$$

$$\frac{V_{H_2}}{10} = \sqrt{\frac{32}{2}} = \sqrt{16} = 4$$

$$V_{H_2} = (10)(4) - 40 \text{ mls/min.}$$

### 3.3.5    Vocabulary Checklist for the Gas Phase

_____ pressure
_____ ideal gas
_____ nonideal gas
_____ Boyle's Law
_____ Charles' Law
_____ Avogadro's Principle

_____ Dalton's Law
_____ partial pressure
_____ mole fraction
_____ Graham's Law of Diffusion
_____ van der Waals Equation

### 3.3.6    Concepts, Principles, etc. Checklist for the Gas Phase

_____ characteristics of ideal gases
_____ concept of partial pressures
_____ Ideal Gas Law
_____ Kinetic Theory of Gases
_____ volume-mole relationship of ideal gas at STP
_____ characteristics of nonideal gases

## 3.4    CONDENSED PHASES

### 3.4.1    Review of the Condensed Phases

The *condensed phases* are the liquids and the solids as opposed to the vaporized phase (i.e. gas). *The intermolecular forces* are forces that exist between the molecules of the liquid or solid. These forces depend upon the chemical characteristics of the molecules and play a large part in determining the physical behavior (e.g., phase changes, solubility) of the liquid or solid. The types of forces that exist between molecules are van der Waals, hydrogen bonds, and hydrophobic. *Van der Waals forces* are very weak attractive forces due to the net attraction between the nucleus of one atom and the electrons in another. These forces are effective only over short distances and increase as the molecular weights increase, i.e., as the number of atoms or electrons in a molecule increases. This type of van der Waals force merges with the slightly stronger forces (may also be considered van der Waals) that exist between polar molecules or between molecules that are inductible (i.e., a separation of charge in a molecule can be induced by the presence of a second). *Polar molecules* are those made up of elements differing in electronegativity, e.g.,

$$\overset{\delta+}{C}—\overset{\delta-}{O}, \overset{\delta+}{C}—\overset{\delta-}{Cl}, \text{ and are asymmetric in geometry.}$$

*Hydrogen bonds* are weak attractive bonds, but stronger than van der Waals, between the hydrogens on chlorine, fluorine, nitrogen or oxygen and the nonbonding electrons on these same elements. These are the only elements for which hydrogen bonding exists. Bonding becomes stronger when the electronegativity of the atoms increases and when the hydrogen bond can have a 180° orientation. (Fig. 3.6.)

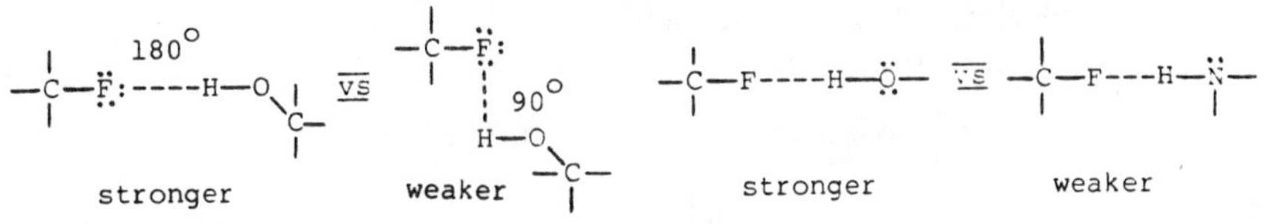

*Fig. 3.6—Hydrogen Bonding*

*Hydrophobic bonds* are weak attractive bonds between molecules that are nonpolar (no net separation of charges in molecules). These bonds exist because nonpolar molecules (e.g. hydrocarbons, fats, aromatics) decrease the entropy (see Section 3.8.1) of water when the molecules are apart. When these nonpolar molecules come together and form hydrophobic bonds, the entropy increases and the free energy is lowered and the bonds become stable. *Ionic forces* exist between ions, i.e., positive and negative ions. These can be very strong forces and are exemplified in ionic solids (e.g. NaCl, table salt). Ionic forces are due to Coulomb forces (see Section 5.7.1)

The weak forces (van der Waals, hydrogen bonds and hydrophobic), although very weak individually, are very strong when many exist between molecules as in proteins or nucleic acids. A large part of the stability of these and other polymers is due to the multitude of these weak forces. When solids melt or liquids evaporate, these are the forces that must be overcome. The greater the number of these intermolecular bonds, or the more diferent types these bonds present, the greater the stability of the substance and the more difficult it is to melt or evaporate. Temperature increases tend to disrupt these weak intermolecular forces easily, especially when they are few in number.

Also, molecules of similar types (e.g. hydrophobic or polar or with hydrogen bonding) tend to be soluble in each other because the forces are similar. Similarly, molecules of different types, especially polar versus nonpolar, tend to be insoluble.

The basic organization of *ionic crystals* is based on attempts to maximize the stability of the crystal by maximizing the attractive forces between cations (positive) and anions (negative) and minimizing the respulsive forces between ions of the same charge. Hence, anions and cations try to be as close together as possible while minimizing anion-anion repulsion.

### 3.4.2    Questions to Review Condensed Phases

(1)    Which of the following is not considered as an intermolecular force between molecules?

(a) covalent bonds
(b) hydrogen bonds
(c) hydrophobic bonds
(d) van der Waals forces

(2)  van der Waals forces depend upon

(a) repulsion of the molecules from water
(b) Coulomb attractions between ions
(c) attraction between the nucleus of one atom and the electrons of another
(d) none of the above

(3)  All of the following factors increase the strength of van der Waals forces between molecules except by an

(a) increase in the molecular weight of the molecules
(b) increase in the number of atoms in the molecule
(c) increase in the number of electrons in the molecule
(d) increase in the ionic strength of the molecule

(4)  The weakest (in strength) of the following intermolecular forces is:

(a) hydrogen bonding
(b) the typical van der Waals
(c) forces between polar molecules
(d) ionic

(5)  Hydrogen bonds are possible between all the following elements except:

(a) carbon
(b) nitrogen
(c) oxygen
(d) fluorine

(6)  Hydrophobic bonds

(a) are interactions between polar molecules
(b) do not occur for hydrocarbons
(c) are due to an increase in entropy of the system
(d) all of the above

(7)  The strongest of the forces between molecules is:

(a) van der Waals
(b) hydrogen bonding
(c) hydrophobic
(d) polar

(8)  For the three atoms involved in the hydrogen bond (e.g., $-\ddot{A}:$ and $H-\ddot{B}-$), the angle that allows the greatest strength (using H as the vertex) is:

(a) less than 90°
(b) 90°
(c) 90° to 180°
(d) 180°

(9)  The stability of some polymers may be due to

(a) many of the weak intermolecular forces (bond)
(b) a few of the weak intermolecular bonds
(c) cannot be due to the weak intermolecular bonds
(d) none of the above

### 3.4.3   Answers to Questions in Section 3.4.2

(1) a    (2) c    (3) d    (4) b    (5) a    (6) c    (7) d    (8) d    (9) a

### 3.4.4 Discussion of Answers to Questions in Section 3.4.2

All questions adequately discussed in Section.

### 3.4.5 Vocabulary Checklist for Condensed Phases

_____ intermolecular forces
_____ van der Waals forces
_____ polar molecules

_____ hydrogen bonds
_____ hydrophobic bonds
_____ ionic forces

### 3.4.6 Concepts, Principles, etc. Checklist for Condensed Phases

_____ weak intermolecular forces
_____ general idea or ionic forces in crystals
_____ role of weak forces in stability of molecules
_____ role of weak forces in phase changes and solubility

## 3.5 PHASE EQUILIBRIA

### 3.5.1 Review of Phase Equilibria

The *three phases* are gases, liquids and solids. Following are the conversions between the three states:

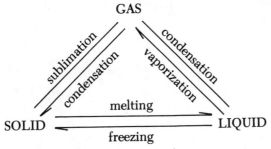

energies:          $\Delta H_f$          $\Delta H_v$
                 f = fusion      v = vaporization

*As a substance moves from solid to liquid to gas*, several changes occur: (1) the molecules become more disordered, (2) the kinetic energy of the molecules increase, (3) the intermolecular forces become weaker, and (4) the molecules become farther separated (density decreases).

The relative sizes of the heats of phase changes ($\Delta H_v > \Delta H_f$) imply that the liquid state is more like the solid state than the gaseous state. When going in the forward direction, heat must be put into the system and the surroundings become cooler (e.g. vaporization of sweat cools the body). When going in the reverse direction, heat is given off from the system and the surroundings become warmer (e.g., condensation of water vapor from the air warms the body). *Brownian motion* (e.g. the random motion of a pollen grain due to collision with the liquid molecules) is evidence for the motion and kinetic energies of liquid molecules. Molecules have a range of kinetic energies. The number in a given energy range ($\Delta E$) is proportional to $e^{-\Delta E/kT}$ (from the Boltzman distribution). Those molecules above a certain kinetic energy level can escape into the vapor phase (i.e., evaporate). To evaporate, the molecules must have enough energy to overcome the intermolecular forces (the stronger the attractive forces, the more energy required—see Section 3.4.1 for intermolecular forces). The molecules that evaporate become gases and exert a pressure called the *vapor pressure*. Solids also have a vapor pressure based on a similar argument. Generally, substances with stronger intermolecular attractive forces have lower vapor pressures. Substances with weak intermolecular forces tend to have high vapor pressures. Note: as the temperature increases, the average kinetic energy per molecule increases, and the liquid (or solid) evaporates faster (Fig. 3.7).

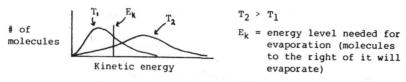

Note: as Temperature (T) increases ($T_1 \rightarrow T_2$) more molecules have $E_k$'s high enough to evaporate.

**Fig. 3.7—*Kinetic Energy of Molecules***

The *boiling point* (BP) of a liquid is the temperature at which the vapor pressure of the liquid equals the atmospheric (opposing) pressure. For the standard BP, this pressure is taken to be one atmosphere. Note, as the atmospheric pressure decreases, the liquid can boil at lower temperatures. Boiling points have great dependence upon intermolecular forces. Remember that nonpolar molecules have weaker forces. Note that symmetric molecules tend to have smaller intermolecular attractive forces also. The *freezing point* (FP) of the liquid (or melting point, MP, of the solid) is that temperature at which the vapor pressure of the solid equals the vapor pressure of the liquid.

Another way of describing the relationships above is the *phase diagram* (Fig. 3.8).

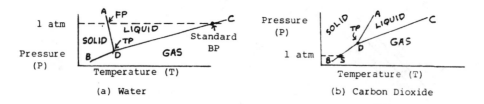

**Fig. 3.8—*Phase Diagrams: Water (a) and Carbon Dioxide (b)***

(1)　this is a plot of *pressure (P) versus temperature (T)*,
(2)　TP = *Triple point* which is the value of P and T where solid, liquid and gas all coexist in equilibrium,
(3)　*regions* marked solid, liquid and gas signify the existence of only that phase,
(4)　the *lines* represent the coexistence of two phases in equilibrium and the vapor pressures (below)
　　　AD = solid and liquid in equilibrum, transition is melting (freezing)
　　　BD = solid and gas in equilibrium, transition from solid to gas is called sublimation (reverse is condensation)
　　　CD = liquid and gas in equilibrium, transition is vaporization (condensation),
　　　CD = vapor pressure of the liquid at different temperatures
　　　BD = vapor pressure of the solid at different temperatures
(5)　Note that all the lines except AD for $H_2O$ have *positive slopes*. This means that as the pressure is increased on solid $H_2O$ (ice), its melting point decreases and ice can melt at a lower temperature. This is the basis for ice skating.
(6)　*The location of the 1 atmosphere of pressure relative to the TP* determines if a solid melts at atmospheric pressure or sublimes. If 1 atm is above the TP, get solid → liquid as for water. If the 1 atm is below the TP get solid → gas (sublimation) as for $CO_2$.

### 3.5.1.1 COLLIGATIVE PROPERTIES AND FREEZING POINT DEPRESSION

A solute added to a pure liquid changes some properties of that liquid. The effect of a solute on a pure liquid depends, primarily, on the relative number of particles present and not their identity. Properties that are affected by the number of particles present and not by the characteristics of the particles are called *colligative properties* (boiling point elevation, freezing point depression, vapor pressure and osmotic pressure). See Section 2.5.1.1 for osmosis. The effect of the number of solute particles (usually non-volatile, so there is no contribution to the overall vapor pressure) on the boiling point (BP) and freezing point (FP) can be understood by considering their effect on vapor pressure (VP) and using the phase diagram. When a solute is dissolved in a pure liquid, the solute molecules are bound by liquid molecules. This represents an increase in potential energy which must be overcome by kinetic energy if the molecules are to escape. This causes fewer to have enough kinetic energy to escape into the vapor phase, resulting in a lowering of the VP (Fig. 3.9).

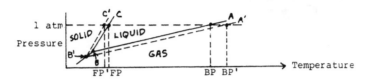

*Fig. 3.9—Effect of Solutes on BP and FP*

AB   = original VP line of the liquid
CB   = original FP line of the solid
A'B'  = lowering of the VP of the liquid by added solute
C'B'  = lowering the FP of the solid by the solute
ΔBP  = BP' – BP = boiling point elevation
FP   = original freezing
FP'  = new FP caused by solute
ΔFP  = FP' – FP = freezing point depression

Equations can be derived by thermodynamics to calculate the effect of a solute on the FP or BP of a liquid. These are (simplified):

$$\Delta T = + k_b m$$
$$\Delta T = - k_f m$$

$\Delta T$ = elevation (for BP) or depression (for FP) of BP or FP respectively

$$m = \text{molality} = \frac{\text{moles of solute particles}}{\text{kilogram of solvent}}$$

Note that the equation calls for moles of solute particles. This means that if a solute dissociates (e.g. NaCl), the moles of particles are greater than the moles of solute. If the solute dimerizes, the moles of particles are less. An alternative way to write the formula to take this into account is:

$$\Delta T = - i\, k_f\, m$$

i    = # of particles the solute dissociates into

$$m = \frac{\text{moles of solute}}{\text{kilogram of solvent}}$$

$k_b$   = boiling point elevation constant—depends on the pure liquid being used.
   $k_b = 0.51$ for $H_2O$
   $k_f$ = freezing point depression constant depends on the pure liquid being used
   $k_f = 1.86$ for $H_2O$

The above equations can be used for a variety of purposes:

(1)    k's can be calculated,     $k = \dfrac{\Delta T}{m}$

(2) The number of actual particles can be inferred—make a known $m$ for a liquid with a known k and calculate the expected $\Delta T$. If $\Delta T$ (by experiment) is greater than that calculated, then more particles than expected were present and the solute must have dissociated. If $\Delta T$ (by experiment) is less than that calculated, then fewer particles than expected were present, and the solute must have aggregated (e.g. dimerized). The actual molality of the particles can then be calculated because $\Delta T$ (from experiment) and k are known.

(3) Most often, the equations are used to estimate molecular weights = MW (given that corrections are made for dissociation or aggregation)

> take a liquid with a known k
> dissolve $x$ grams of solute (MW unkown)
>    in $y$ kg's of the liquid (solvent)
> then determine the $\Delta T$ experimentally
> the MW is found by going through these calculations

(a) $m = \dfrac{\Delta T}{k}$      $\Delta T$, k are known

(b) $m = \dfrac{\text{moles of solute}}{\text{kg of solvent}} = \Delta T/k$

(c) $m = (\text{g solute/MW solute})/\text{Kg of solvent} = \Delta T/k$

(d) MW solute $= (\text{g solute})(k)/(\text{Kg solvent})(\Delta T)$

## 3.5.2    Questions to Review Phase Equilibria

(1) The conversion of a gas to a liquid is called:

(a) melting
(b) vaporization
(c) freezing
(d) condensation

(2) As a solid changes to a liquid, all of the following occur except

(a) molecules become more disordered
(b) kinetic energy of the molecules decreases
(c) intermolecular forces become weaker
(d) molecules become farther separated

(3) The liquid state is more like the _____ state than the _____ state.

(a) gas; solid
(b) solid; gas
(c) equally similar to both

(4) Vaporization of a liquid from the skin will cause the skin to become:

(a) cooler
(b) warmer
(c) no change in temperature

(5) Which of the following liquids will have the highest vapor pressure?

(a) strong intermolecular forces
(b) weak intermolecular forces
(c) intermolecular forces have no effect on vapor pressure

(6) As the temperature of a substance increases, the average kinetic energy per molecule

(a) decreases
(b) increases
(c) is not affected
(d) cannot be determined

(7)    As the atmospheric pressure decreases, the boiling point of a liquid

(a) cannot be determined
(b) is not affected
(c) increases
(d) decreases

Use the following data for questions #8 to #12.

Phase Diagram for a Compound

(8)    Gas is represented by:

(a) 1
(b) 3
(c) 4
(d) 7

(9)    The vapor pressure of the liquid is represented by:

(a) 3
(b) 4
(c) 6
(d) 7

(10)   The triple point is:

(a) 1
(b) 4
(c) 5
(d) 7

(11)   Liquid can exist only in region _____.

(a) 1
(b) 2
(c) 3
(d) 5

(12)   At atmospheric pressure the solid phase of this substance will only:

(a) remain a solid
(b) melt
(c) freeze
(d) vaporize

(13)   Colligative properties depend upon

(a) the chemical properties of the solute
(b) the physical properties of the solute
(c) the chemical properties of the solvent
(d) the number of solute particles present in solution

(14)   Examples of colligative properties include all except:

(a) boiling point elevation
(b) solubility
(c) vapor pressure
(d) osmotic pressure

(15)    The effect of a solute on the vapor pressure of a liquid is to:

    (a) have no effect
    (b) increase it
    (c) decrease it
    (d) cannot be determined

(16)    The equation relating the freezing point depression ($\Delta T$) with the freezing point constant ($k_f$) and the molality (m) of the solution is (excluding the minus sign and i):

    (a) $\Delta T = k_f/m$
    (b) $\Delta T = m/k_f$
    (c) $\Delta T = 1/k_f m$
    (d) $\Delta T = k_f m$

Use the following for Questions #17 to #19:

Five grams of a compound with a molecular weight of 80 is placed in 500g of a liquid which has a normal freezing point of 58.5°C. The freezing point of the solution is now 57°C. Next, 2g of an unknown compound is placed in 250g of the same liquid, and the freezing point is now 58°C.

(17)    What is the freezing point depression constant ($k_f$) of the liquid?

    (a) 12
    (b) 6
    (c) 3
    (d) 1.5

(18)    What is the expected molecular weight of the unknown compound by freezing point analysis?

    (a) 192
    (b) 96
    (c) 48
    (d) cannot be determined

(19)    A mass spectograph analysis shows the true molecular weight of the compound to be 384. What inference can be made about the compound's behavior in the liquid?

    (a) it dissociates
    (b) it forms dimers
    (c) it forms tetramers
    (d) no inference can be made

## 3.5.3    Answers to Questions in Section 3.5.2

( 1) d  ( 2) b  ( 3) b  ( 4) a  ( 5) b  ( 6) b  ( 7) d  ( 8) b  ( 9) d  (10) c  (11) b
(12) d  (13) d  (14) b  (15) c  (16) d  (17) a  (18) a  (19) a

## 3.5.4    Discussion of Answers to Questions in Section 3.5.2

*Questions #1 to #16:* Adequately discussed in Section.

*Question #17* (Answer: a) Use the formula:

$$k = \Delta T/m$$

    Note: the complete formula is:

$$k = \Delta T/ - im$$

where i = the number of particles the substance dissociates into and the negative in the denominator offsets the negative temperature drop. If the absolute value of $\Delta T$ is taken the minus sign may be ignored, and if the molecule does not dissociate the i = 1 and may be ignored.

Then,

$$m = \text{moles/Kg of solvent} = (1/16)/(1/2) = (1/16)(2/1)$$
$$= 2/16 = 1/8$$

(moles = weight/molecular weight = 5/80 = 1/16, and Kgs = grams of substance/1000 grams = 500/1000 = 1/2).

And,

$$\Delta T = 58.5°C - 57°C = 1.5°C = 1\tfrac{1}{2} = 3/2$$

(Note, if the formula,

$$k = \Delta T/ - im$$

is used, the $\Delta T$ must be determined as follows,
$$\Delta T = T_f - T_i = 57 - 58.5 = -1.5°C$$
f = final, i = initial).

Finally,

$$k = (3/2)/(1/8) = (3/2)(8/1) = 24/2 = 12$$

*Question #18* (Answer: a) Use the results from #17 and the procedure outlined in the Section:

(a) $\quad m = \Delta T/k = \tfrac{1}{2}/12 = \tfrac{1}{2} \cdot 1/12 = 1/24$
$$\Delta T = 58.5 - 58 = 0.5 = \tfrac{1}{2}$$

(b) $\quad$ moles of solute = (m)(y) = (1/24)(1/4) = 1/96
$$y = \text{Kg's of solute} = 250/1000 = 1/4$$

(c) $\quad$ MW = x/moles of solute = 2/(1/96) = (2)(96/1) = 192
$$x = \text{weight of solute} = 2g$$

*Question #19* (Answer: a) The expected freezing point depression using the molecular weight given is

$$\Delta T = km = (12)(1/48) = 12/48 = 1/4 = 0.25°C$$
$$m = \text{moles/kg's solvents} = (2/384)/(1/4) = (2/384)(4/1)$$
$$= (2)(4)/384 = 1/48$$

So, the expected $\Delta T$ is 0.25°C. Since the actual is 0.5°C, this means there must have been more particles present than expected, and that the compound must have dissociated, or,

$$i = \Delta T/ - km = -(1/2)/ - (12)(1/48) = (1/2)(48/12) = 48/24 = 2.$$

This means 2 particles per original molecule.

## 3.5.5 Vocabulary Checklist for Phase Equilibria

_____ vaporization
_____ condensation
_____ heat of fusion
_____ heat of vaporization
_____ Brownian motion
_____ vapor pressure
_____ boiling point

_____ sublimation
_____ colligative properties
_____ molality
_____ boiling point elevation
_____ freezing point depression
_____ freezing point
_____ phase diagram

### 3.5.6    Concepts, Principles, etc. Checklist for Phase Equilibria

_____ changes that occur during phase changes
_____ interpretation of phase diagrams
_____ triple point
_____ colligative properties
_____ freezing point depression determinations


## 3.6    CHEMICAL COMPOUNDS

### 3.6.1    Review of Chemical Compounds

Compounds are made of discrete individual atoms (which, however, can be divided into neutrons, protons and electrons). These atoms then combine in specific ratios with each other, depending upon their chemical characteristics, to form compounds. The elements (a set of atoms with the same atomic number) have a constant weight, and these weights are maintained when combined into chemical compounds (a combination of two or more elements).

A *mole* of any substance contains $6.023 \times 10^{23}$ particles (*Avogadro's Number*). A mole of an element contains this many atoms. A mole of a compound contains this many molecules. For an element, the number of moles present is,

$$\text{moles} = \frac{\text{weight of sample in grams}}{\text{atomic weight of element in grams (GAW)}}$$

$$\text{GAW} = \text{gram-atomic weight.}$$

For a compound, the *gram-molecular weight* (GMW) is found by adding the (GAWs) of all the elements that make it up (need the molecular formula). Then, the moles of a compound is found as follows:

$$\text{moles} = \frac{\text{weight of sample in grams}}{\text{GMW}}$$

Moles can be calculated in many other ways (see below) and all of these are interconvertible via moles. *Mole is important* because it gives the number of molecules (or atoms) in a given weight of a substance, whereas the weight itself does not. Mole is the key to solving most quantitive mass problems in chemistry. In general, think about how to get the number of moles, and, usually the rest of the problem will be easier to complete.

Often, the number of molecules or atoms in a given weight of a sample is not sufficient. This is because different substances have differing combining powers with each other. That is, one molecule may be two or more times more potent than another for a specific purpose. A familiar example should be $H_2SO_4$ (a diprotic acid) and HCl (a monoprotic acid) in terms of donation of hydrogen ions ($H+$). A mole would contain the same number of molecules of $H_2SO_4$ and HCl, but this does not give us their relative potency in giving $H+$. What is needed is a measure, like mole, which would give us the relative or equivalent effectiveness of given weights of substances for specific charcteristics. For this reason, the measure called *equivalents* was established. When weights are converted to equivalents, one can be sure, for example, that one equivalent of an acid will react completely and equally with one equivalent of a base. It cannot be stated, without additional information, that one mole of an acid will react exactly with one mole of a base for the reasons above. Note that in one equivalent of a substance there are $6.023 \times 10^{23}$ particles of interest (e.g. $H+$ or $OH-$ for acids and bases). The formula for calculating equivalents is:

$$\text{equivalents} = \frac{\text{weight of sample in grams}}{\text{gram equivalent weight (GEW)}}$$

The GEW is calculated as follows:

$$GEW = \frac{\text{gram molecular weight}}{n}$$

*The value of n* depends on the situation. For acids, it is the number of hydrogens used in the reaction per molecule. For bases, it is the number of exchangeable $OH^-$s used in the reaction per molecule. For oxidation-reduction reactions, it depends on the number of electrons transferred by a given compound in a *given* reaction. For examples and further explanation of n, refer to 3.10.1, 3.11.1 and 3.12.1.

The percentage composition of compounds is the percent of the total weight of a given element in that compound:

$$\% \text{ composition of element A} = \frac{\text{total weight in grams of A}}{\text{GMW of the compound}} \times 100.$$

An example is: % of oxygen (O) in $KClO_3$ (K = 39, Cl = 36, O = 16)

$$\% \text{ of O} = \frac{(3)(16)}{39 + 36 + 3(16)} \times 100 = 39\%.$$

Of course, the percentages of all components should sum to 100%. An *empirical formula* is the formula with the smallest ratio of atoms to each other. The *molecular formula* is the actual formula of the molecule of the substance. For example, for benzene:

structural formula

molecular formula = $C_6H_6$
empirical formula = $C_1H_1$

Of course, it is possible for the empirical formula to be the same as the molecular formula. It is possible to determine empirical formulas if the percentage composition of the compound is known. This is done as follows:

(1)     Assume the percent of each element is the grams of each element (i.e., assume you are given 100 grams = 100% of the compound);
(2)     Divide the percentage composition of each element by its atomic weight to give the moles of each in the compound;
(3)     Divide each of these numbers by the smallest of the numbers gotten from step #2;
(4)     Determine what small number (to multiply the result of #3), usually 2–5, if any, is needed to convert the numbers from #3 into (approximately) whole numbers. These whole numbers are the ratio of the elements to each other.

What has been done is to convert weights (from percent) into moles by step #2. These moles are, themselves, the ratios of elements to each other. Steps #3 and #4 are just manipulations to get whole numbers because elements are made of atoms and not fractions of atoms. To *determine the molecular formula* from the empirical formula, the gram-molecular weight (GMW) must be known from some other source (can find GMW if weight of compound and number of moles is known—see below). Then determine the gram-empirical formula weight (i.e., add up the elements in the empirical formula) and then divide the GMW by the gram-empirical formula weight. The resulting number is how many times each element in the empirical formula is to be multiplied to get the molecular formula. An example is:

A compound of 2.04% H, 32.65% S, and 65.31% O has a GMW = 98 (from other experiments).
What is the empirical formula and molecular formula?

(H = 1, S = 32, O = 16)

By the steps above:

(1) H = 2.04g    S = 32.5g    O = 65.31g

(2) H: 2.04/1 = 2.04

    S: 32.65/32 = 1.02

    O: 65.31/16 = 4.08

(3) H: 2.04/1.02 = 2

    S: 1.02/1.02 = 1

    O: 4.08/1.02 = 4

(4) Not needed because already have whole numbers. Therefore, empirical formula is $H_2SO_4$.

Then, gram-empirical formula weight is:

$$2 (1) + (32) + 4(16) = 98.$$

Then, divide gram-molecular weight by the gram-empirical formula weight:

$$98/98 = 1$$

Then multiply each element in the empirical formula by the 1 to get the molecular formula which is the same as the empirical formula in this case.

Various means of determining the mole of substances are discussed in other Sections. The methods are:

(1) mole = weight in grams/GMW;

(2) MV = mole; M = molarity; V = liters (Section 3.10.1);

(3) NV = equivalents; N = normality, V = liters (Section 3.10.1);

(4) mV = mole; m = molality, V = kg's of solvent (Section 3.10.1);

(5) freezing point depression (or boiling point elevation) calculations (Section 3.5.1.1)
    T = km
first determine m, then use m to determine mole as in #4 above;

(6) one mole of any gas at STP occupies 22.4 liters (Section 3.3.1);

(7) at the same temperature and pressure, equal volumes of ideal gases contain equal numbers of moles (Avogadro's Principle) (Section 3.3.1);

(8) PV = nRT (Section 3.3.1)
Ideal Gas Equation;

(9) $P_1 = X_1 P_T$ (Section 3.3.1)
$P_1$ = partial pressure of gas #1
$P_T$ = total pressure
$X_1$ = mole fraction of gas #1;

(10) one mole of electrons is one faraday, a faraday is 96,500 coulombs; an ampere (measure of current) is 1 coulomb/sec (Section 3.12.1);

(11) Law of Dulong and Petit:
6.3 = (SH)(GAW)
SH = specific heat in cals/gram
GAW = gram-atomic weight of element.

Note that from the moles, the gram-molecular weight can be calculated, and that moles provide a means of conversion between the diverse situations above.

### 3.6.2    Questions to Review Chemical Compounds

(1)    A chemical compound

(a) is made of discrete individual atoms
(b) is made of atoms (of different elements) combined with each other in specific ratios
(c) has the weight equal to sum of the weights of the elements that make it up
(d) all of the above

(2)    Avogadro's number:

(a) the number of liters that make up one mole of gas
(b) there are $6.023 \times 10^{23}$ particles per mole
(c) the number of molecules in a chemical compound
(d) none of the above

(3)    Given that mole = m and the weight = w of a compound with a gram-molecular weight = GMW, which is the correct relationship between these?

(a) m = (w) (GMW)
(b) m = w/GMW
(c) m = GMW/w
(d) m = 1/(w)(GMW)

(4)    Equivalents

(a) are the same as the mole of a substance
(b) contain $\dfrac{6.023 \times 10^{23}}{n}$ particles, n = number of atoms under concern
(c) depend on the specific number of groups of interest, e.g., $H^+$ or electrons transferred, by a molecule
(d) none of the above

(5)    If equivalents = E, weight of sample = W and the gram equivalent weight = GEW, the correct relation between these is

(a) E = 1/(W)(GEW)
(b) E = GEW/W
(c) E = W/GEW
(d) E = (W)(GEW)

(6)    If gram-molecular weight = GMW, gram equivalent weight = GEW and the number of groups of interest per molecule = n, the correct relationship between these is:

(a) GEW = (n)(GMW)
(b) GEW = 1/(n)(GMW)
(c) GEW = n/GMW
(d) GEW = GMW/n

(7)    If the percent composition of element B in a compound = P, the number of atoms of element B in the compound = $n_1$, the gram atomic weight of element B = GAW, and the gram molecular weight of the compound = GMW, then the correct relationship between these is:

(a) P = (n)(GAW)/(GMW) × 100
(b) P = (n)(GAW)/(GMW)
(c) P = (n)(GAW)(GMW)
(d) P = GMW/(n)(GAW) × 100

(8)    All of the following formulas give moles except:

(a) (normality)(volume) = moles
(b) (molality) (kilograms of solvent) = moles
(c) liters of gas at STP/22.4 = moles
(d) (Pressure)(Volume)/(Ideal gas constant)(Temperature) = moles

(9) Moles may be calculated from all of the following types of data except:

(a) freezing point depressions
(b) partial pressures
(c) electrochemistry (Faradays of charge consumed)
(d) all of the above can give moles

The following information is provided for the remainder of the questions. Atomic weights: $H = 1$, $C = 12$, $N = 14$, $O = 16$, $F = 19$, $Na = 23$, $Al = 27$, $P = 31$, $S = 32$, $Cl = 35$, $K = 39$, $Ca = 40$, $Cr = 52$, $Fe = 56$, $Cu = 63$, $Br = 80$, $Ag = 108$, and $Pb = 207$.

(10) What is the gram-molecular weight of $NH_4Cl$?

(a) 53
(b) 50
(c) 49
(d) none of the above

(11) What is the gram-molecular weight of $C_6H_{12}O_6$?

(a) 180
(b) 130
(c) 29
(d) none of the above

(12) How may moles are 34g of $AgNO_3$?

(a) 0.20
(b) 0.30
(c) 0.40
(d) none of the above

(13) How many grams are there in 0.5 mole of $NaOH$?

(a) 5g
(b) 20 g
(c) 30 g
(d) none of the above

(14) It is known that 5g of a compound is 0.1 mole of that substance. What is its gram-molecular weight (GMW)?

(a) 25
(b) 100
(c) 150
(d) none of the above

(15) The gram-equivalent weight (GEW) of $HNO_3$ when it acts as an acid (donation of $H^+$) is approximately:

(a) 21
(b) 63
(c) 126
(d) none of the above

(16) The gram-equivalent weight of $H_3PO_4$ when it acts as an acid (donation of $H^+$) is approximately:

(a) 33
(b) 49
(c) 98
(d) all of the above

(17) In a reaction where $HNO_3$ is used, the nitrogen of the $HNO_3$ gains 5 electrons. The equivalent weight of $HNO_3$ in terms of its ability to exchange electrons is approximately:

(a) 3
(b) 13
(c) 63
(d) none of the above

(18) In a reaction where $KNO_3$ is used, the nitrogen gains 2 electrons. The equivalent weight of $KNO_3$ in terms of its ability to gain electrons is approximately:

(a) 21
(b) 32
(c) 63
(d) none of the above

(19) In a reaction, the Cr of $K_2Cr_2O_7$ gains 6 electrons. The equivalent weight of $K_2Cr_2O_7$ in this reaction in terms of its ability to exchange electrons is approximately:

(a) 147
(b) 49
(c) 25
(d) none of the above

(20) How many equivalents of base ($OH^-$) are there in 5g of $Al(OH)_3$ if all OHs react?

(a) 0.10
(b) 0.20
(c) 0.75
(d) none of the above

(21) Two equivalents of $H^+$ would require what weight of $H_2SO_4$?

(a) 196
(b) 98
(c) 49
(d) none of the above

(22) Approximately what percentage of $CuSO_4$ is sulfur?

(a) 20
(b) 30
(c) 40
(d) none of the above

(23) The approximate percentage of H in $(NH_4)_2 SO_4$ is:

(a) 6
(b) 7
(c) 4
(d) none of the above

(24) What is the empirical formula of the following compound?

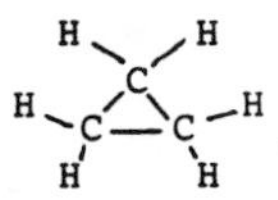

(a) $C_3H_6$
(b) $C_2H_2$
(c) $C_1H_2$
(d) none of these

(25)   A compound contains 39.8% Cu, 20.1% S and 40.1% O. Its empirical formula is:

(a) $CuSO_2$
(b) $Cu_2SO_3$
(c) $CuSO_4$
(d) none of these

(26)   A compound contains 39.9% C, 6.7% H and 53.4% O. The empirical formula is:

(a) $CH_2O$
(b) $C_2H_2O$
(c) CHO
(d) none of the above

(27)   A compound contains 2.6 gms of N, 0.8 gms of H, and 6.6 gms of Cl. The empirical formula is

(a) $N_2H_2Cl$
(b) $N(HCl)_2$
(c) $NH_4Cl$
(d) none of the above

(28)   A compound of carbon and hydrogen contains 92.3% C. The molecular weight (from other experiments) is known to be 52. What is the molecular formula?

(a) $C_2H_2$
(b) $C_4H_4$
(c) $C_3H_6$
(d) none of these

(29)   The specific heat of an element is 0.03, its gram atomic weight is:

(a) 18.9
(b) 210
(c) 189
(d) need more information

### 3.6.3     Answers to Questions in Section 3.6.2

( 1) d   ( 2) b   ( 3) b   ( 4) c   ( 5) c   ( 6) d   ( 7) a   ( 8) a   ( 9) d   (10) a   (11) a
(12) a   (13) b   (14) d   (15) b   (16) d   (17) b   (18) d   (19) c   (20) b   (21) b   (22) a
(23) a   (24) c   (25) c   (26) a   (27) c   (28) b   (29) b

### 3.6.4     Discussion of Answers to Questions in Section 3.6.2

*Questions #1 to #9:* Adequately discussed in this Section.

*Question #10* (Answer: a)   $GMW = N + 4\ (H) + Cl = 14 + 4(1) + 35 = 53$

*Question #11* (Answer: a)   $GMW = 6C + 12H + 60 = 6(12) + 12(1) + 6(16)$
$$= 72 + 12 + 96 = 180$$

*Question #12* (Answer: a)   $Moles = \dfrac{weight}{GMW} = 34/169 = 0.20$

$$GMW = Ag + N + 3(O) = 107 + 14 + 3(16)$$
$$= 121 + 48 = 169$$

*Question #13* (Answer: b)   $weight = (moles)(GMW) = (0.5)(40) = 20$ g
$$GMW = Na + O + H = 23 + 16 + 1 = 40$$

*Question #14* (Answer: d)   GMW = weight/moles = 5/0.1 = 50.

*Question #15* (Answer: b)   GEW = GMW/n = 63/1 = 63
$$GMW = H + N + 3(O) = 1 + 14 + 3(16)$$
$$= 15 + 48 = 63$$
n = # of exchangeable H's per molecule = 1

*Question #16* (Answer: d) $H_3PO_4$ can give 1, 2, or 3 protons in a reaction; therefore the reaction must be specified. $3(1) + 31 + 4(16) = 98 = GMW$. Then 98/1 = 98, 98/2 = 49, $98/3 \approx 33$.

*Question #17* (Answer: b)   $GEW = \dfrac{GMW}{n} = 63/5 \approx 13$
$$GMW = H + N + 3(O) = 1 + 14 + 3(16)$$
$$= 15 + 48 = 63$$
n = # of exchangeable electrons per molecule = 5

*Question #18* (Answer: d)   $GEW = \dfrac{GMW}{n} = 101/2 \approx 50$
$$GMW = K + N + 3(O) = 39 + 14 + 3(16)$$
$$= 53 + 48 = 101$$
n = # of exchangeable electrons per molecule = 2

*Question #19* (Answer: c)   $GEW = \dfrac{GMW}{n} = 294/12 \approx 25$
$$GMW = 2(K) + 2(Cr) + 7(O) = 2(39) + 2(52) + 7(16)$$
$$= 78 + 104 + 112 = 294$$
n = # of exchangeable electrons per molecule
$$= (2)(6) = 12 \text{ because there are two Cr's per molecule}$$

*Question #20* (Answer: b)  Equivalents $= \dfrac{weight}{GEW} \approx 5/26 \approx 0.20$
$$GEW = \dfrac{GMW}{n} = 78/3 \approx 26$$
$$GMW = Al + 3(O) + 3(H) = 27 + 3(16) + 3(1)$$
$$= 27 + 48 + 3 = 78$$
n = # of exchangeable OH's per molecule = 3

*Question #21* (Answer: b) Weight = (GEW)(Equivalents) = (49)(2) = 98
$$GEW = GMW/n = 98/2 = 49$$
$$GMW = 2(H) + S + 4(O) = 2(1) + 32 + 4(16)$$
$$= 2 + 32 + 64 = 98$$
n = # of exchangeable H's per molecule = 2

*Question #22* (Answer: a)   % S = (weight of S/GMW)(100) = (32/159)(100) $\approx$ 20
weight of S = (1)(S) = (1) (32) = 32
$$GMW = Cu + S + 4(O) = 63 + 32 + 4(16) = 95 + 64 = 159$$

*Question #23* (Answer: a)   % H = (weight of H/GMW)(100) = (8/132)(100) $\approx$ 6
weight of H = 8(H) = 8(1) = 8
$$GMW = 2(N) + 8(H) + S + 4(O) = 2(14) + 8(1) + 32 + 4(16)$$
$$= 28 + 8 + 32 + 64 = 132$$

*Question #24* (Answer: c) The molecular formula is $C_3H_6$ (by counting all the atoms). The smallest ratio of this is $C_1H_2$.

*Question #25* (answer: c)   By these steps enumerated in the section,
(1) Cu 39.8 g   S = 20.1g   O = 40.1g
(2) moles Cu = 39.8/63 = 0.63
    moles   S = 20.1/32 = 0.63
    moles   O = 40.1/16 = 2.51
    this gives $Cu_{0.63}$   $S_{0.63}$   $O_{2.51}$
(3) dividing each number by 0.63:
    $Cu_{\frac{0.63}{0.63}}$        $S_{\frac{0.63}{0.63}}$        $O_{\frac{2.51}{0.63}} = Cu_1S_1O_{3.98}$
(4) not needed since $3.98 \approx 4$, and this yields $CuSO_4$

*Question #26* (Answer: a)  Follow the same steps as in #25,

(1) $C = 39.9g$   $H = 6.7g$   $O = 53.4g$
(2) moles $C = 39.9/12 = 3.33$
    moles $H = 6.7/1 = 6.7$
    moles $O = 53.4/16 = 3.34$
    this gives $C_{3.33}$  $H_{6.7}$  $O_{3.34}$
(3) dividing each number by 3.33:

$$C_{\frac{3.33}{3.33}} \qquad H_{\frac{6.7}{3.33}} \qquad O_{\frac{3.34}{3.33}} = C_1H_2O_1 = CH_2O$$

(4) not needed

*Question #27* (Answer: c)  (1) just use the grams as given

$N = 2.6g$   $H = 0.8g$   $Cl = 6.6g$
(2) moles $N = 2.6/14 = 0.19$ $(\approx 0.20!)$
    moles $H = 0.8/1 = 0.80$
    moles $Cl = 6.6/35 = 0.19$ $(\approx 0.20!)$
$N_{0.2}$  $H_{0.8}$  $Cl_{0.2}$
(3) Divide all by 0.2

$$N_{\frac{0.2}{0.2}} \quad H_{\frac{0.8}{0.2}} \quad Cl_{\frac{0.2}{0.2}} = N_1H_4Cl_1 = NH_4Cl$$

(4) not needed

*Question #28* (Answer: b) The correct answer can be obtained just by determining the molecular weights of the options. The procedure outlined in the Section is first to determine the empirical formula and then the molecular formula from it:

(1) $C = 92.3g$   $H = 100 - 92.3 = 7.7g$
(2) moles $C = 92.3/12 = 7.7$
    moles $H = 7.7/1 = 7.7$
        $C_{7.7}$  $H_{7.7}$
(3) Divide both by 7.7

$$C_{\frac{7.7}{7.7}} \quad H_{\frac{7.7}{7.7}} = C_1H_1 = CH$$

(4) not needed

The gram-empirical formula weight is $C + H = 12 + 1 = 13$. This goes into the gram-molecular weight $52/13 = 4$ times. This means the ratios of elements in the empirical formula must be multiplied by 4 and this gives

$$C_4H_4.$$

*Question #29* (Answer: b) This is a direct application of the Law of Dulong and Petit (see Section)

$$6.3 = (SH)(GAW)$$
$$GAW = 6.3/SH = \frac{6.3}{0.03} = 210$$

## 3.6.5     Vocabulary Checklist for Chemical Compounds

_____ mole
_____ Avogadro's Number
_____ equivalent
_____ gram-molecular weight

_____ gram atomic weight
_____ gram-equivalent weight
_____ percent composition

## 3.6.6     Concepts, Principles, etc. Checklist for Chemical Compounds

_____ mole concept and calculations using moles
_____ concept of equivalents and calculations using equivalents
_____ empirical versus molecular formulas
_____ alternative methods of determining mole

## 3.7  MASS CHANGES IN CHEMICAL REACTIONS—STOICHIOMETRY

### 3.7.1  Review of Stoichiometry

Stoichiometry refers to the use of atomic theory to make quantitative assessments of atoms, compounds and chemical reactions.

*Chemical equations* should be balanced prior to doing stoichiometric calculations. Balancing is by trial and error (for non-redox), and the check is to see if there are equal numbers of each element on each side of the equation. A hint to aid in balancing equations is:

> balance the element(s) which appear in only one compound on each side of the equation, save elements which appear in more than one compound until last.

Practice is the key to balancing equations. An example of a balanced equation is:

$$N_2(g) + 3H_2(g) \rightarrow 2NH_3(g).$$

The numbers in front of the molecules give the smallest ratios of these molecules that will react with each other. That is, they are the number of moles of each that must be present to get a complete reaction. If there is too much (or too little) of a reactant present, then that reactant is in excess (or is deficient), and the reaction when finished will have some reactants left over. The amount and which reactant left over is calculated from the balanced equation using the *ratio of moles*. Note again that moles are the intermediary between weights, volumes, etc. and that the numbers in the equations reflect ratios of moles and nothing else. Other points will be stressed in the questions. See also Section 3.12.1 for oxidation-reduction reactions.

### 3.7.2  Questions to Review Stoichiometry

(1)  Given the following equation, the coefficient in front of $KClO_3$ is (balance the equation):

$$KClO_3 \rightarrow KCl + KClO_4$$

(a) 1
(b) 2
(c) 3
(d) 4

(2)  The coefficient in front of Zn in the following equation, when balanced, is:

$$Zn + HCl \rightarrow ZnCl_2 + H_2$$

(a) 1
(b) 2
(c) 3
(d) 4

(3)  Which of the following species has the largest coefficient in the balanced equation?

$$C_{12}H_{22}O_{11} + O_2 \rightarrow CO_2 + H_2O$$

(a) $O_2$
(b) $CO_2$
(c) $H_2O$
(d) $O_2$ and $CO_2$

(4)  What is the coefficient in front of $Ca(OH)_2$ in the following equation when balanced?

$$(NH_4)_2SO_4 + Ca(OH)_2 \rightarrow NH_3 + H_2O + CaSO_4$$

(a) 1
(b) 2
(c) 3
(d) 4

(5)    What is the sum of coefficients in the following equation when balanced?

$$CuO + H_3PO_4 \rightarrow Cu_3(PO_4)_2 + H_2O$$

(a) 6
(b) 7
(c) 8
(d) 9

(6)    What is the sum of coefficients in the following equation when balanced?

$$Na_2O_2 + H_2O \rightarrow NaOH + O_2$$

(a) 5
(b) 7
(c) 9
(d) 11

Use the following unbalanced equation for questions #7 through #10.

$$N_2H_4(l) + N_2O_4(l) \rightarrow N_2(g) + H_2O(l)$$

$$(H = 1, N = 14, O = 16)$$

(7)    The sum of coefficients in the balanced equation is:

(a) 4
(b) 6
(c) 8
(d) 10

(8)    How many moles of $N_2$ will be produced if 3 moles of $N_2H_4$ is used up in the reaction?

(a) 2
(b) 3
(c) 4½
(d) 9

(9)    There are 8 gms of $N_2H_4$ and 92 gms of $N_2O_4$ available. What weight of water in grams can be made from this?

(a) 4½
(b) 9
(c) 18
(d) 36

(10)   If 36g of $H_2O$ is produced in the above reaction, what volume of nitrogen is also produced assuming the reaction is at STP?

(a) 1.5 liters
(b) 10 liters
(c) 33.6 liters
(d) 44.8 liters

Use the following information for questions #11 through #14.

$$FeS(s) + O_2(g) + H_2O(l) \rightarrow Fe_2O_3(s) + H_2SO_4(l)$$

$$(H = 1, O = 16, S = 32, Fe = 56)$$

(11)   The sum of the coefficients in the balanced equation is:

(a) 8
(b) 13
(c) 18
(d) 23

(12) If 22.4 liters of $O_2$ are allowed to react with 44g of FeS, approximately what weight of $H_2SO_4$ is produced (assume reaction run at STP)?

(a) 98g
(b) 49g
(c) 44g
(d) 2g

(13) If 5 moles of FeS are used in the reaction, what is the maximum number of moles of $Fe_2O_3$ that can be produced?

(a) 1.0
(b) 2.5
(c) 5.0
(d) 7.5

(14) If 98g of $H_2SO_4$ are desired, what volume of $O_2$ must be used in the reaction (assume STP)?

(a) 50.4 liters
(b) 22.4 liters
(c) 11.2 liters
(d) 1 liter

### 3.7.3   Answers to Questions in Section 3.7.2

(1) d  ( 2) a  ( 3) d  ( 4) a  ( 5) d  ( 6) c  ( 7) d  ( 8) c  ( 9) b  (10) c  (11) d
(12) c  (13) b  (14) a

### 3.7.4   Discussion of Answers to Questions in Section 3.7.2

*Question #1* (Answer: d) The O's appear in only one compound on each side of the equation, so balance it first. In this type of situation, simply multiply each compound by the number of atoms of the element (i.e., O in this case) in the other compound:

$$\text{unbalanced: } KClO_3 \rightarrow KCl + KClO_4$$
$$\text{balanced O: } 4KClO_3 \rightarrow KCl + 3KClO_4$$

There is no apparent clear choice between K or Cl so just pick one to balance. Luckily both K and Cl are already balanced. Check by counting total number of each element on each side of the equation:

| check: | $4KClO_3$ | $+$ | $KCl + 3KClO_4$ |
|---|---|---|---|
| K: | 4 | | 4 |
| Cl: | 4 | | 4 |
| O: | 12 | | 12 |

*Question #2* (Answer: a) Can select Zn, H or Cl because all appear in only one compound on each side. In this case, select the one that appears most complicated which is H or Cl in this case:

| unbalanced: | $Zn + HCl \rightarrow ZnCl_2 + H_2$ |
|---|---|
| balanced H: | $Zn + 2HCl \rightarrow ZnCl_2 + H_2$ |
| Zn and Cl: | both are balanced also |

| check: | $Zn + 2HCl$ | $+$ | $ZnCl_2 + H_2$ |
|---|---|---|---|
| Zn: | 1 | | 1 |
| Cl: | 2 | | 2 |
| H: | 2 | | 2 |

*Question #3* (Answer: d)

$$\text{unbalanced:} \quad C_{12}H_{22}O_{11} + O_2 \rightarrow CO_2 + H_2O$$
$$\text{balance C:} \quad C_{12}H_{22}O_{11} + O_2 \rightarrow 12CO_2 + H_2O$$
$$\text{balance H:} \quad C_{12}H_{22}O_{11} + O_2 \rightarrow 12CO_2 + 11H_2O$$
$$\text{balance O:} \quad C_{12}H_{22}O_{11} + 12O_2 \rightarrow 12CO_2 + 11H_2O$$

check: $C_{12}H_{22}O_{11} + 12O_2$ | $12CO_2 + 11H_2O$

| | | |
|---|---|---|
| C: | 12 | 12 |
| H: | 22 | 22 |
| O: | $11 + 24 = 35$ | $24 + 11 = 35.$ |

*Question #4* (Answer: a)

unbalanced: $(NH_4)_2SO_4 + Ca(OH)_2 \rightarrow NH_3 + H_2O + CaSO_4$
Note: Treat $SO_4^{-2}$ as a group in this case.

$SO_4^{-2}$ and Ca are already balanced

balance N: $(NH_4)_2SO_4 + Ca(OH)_2 \rightarrow 2NH_3 + H_2O + CaSO_4$

balance O: $(NH_4)_2SO_4 + Ca(OH)_2 \rightarrow 2NH_3 + 2H_2O + CaSO_4$
(note that the O's in the $SO_4^{-2}$'s balance themselves and do not have to be accounted for in this balancing of the O's)

balance H: already balanced.

check: $(NH_4)_2SO_4 + Ca(OH)_2$ | $2NH_3 + 2H_2O + CaSO_4$

| | | |
|---|---|---|
| N: | 2 | 2 |
| H: | $8 + 2 = 10$ | $6 + 4 = 10$ |
| S: | 1 | 1 |
| O: | $4 + 2 = 6$ | $2 + 4 = 6.$ |

*Question #5* (Answer: d)

unbalanced: $CuO + H_3PO_4 \rightarrow Cu_3(PO_4)_2 + 2H_2O$
Note: the $PO_4^{-3}$ can be treated as a group since it is not changed in the reaction.
Can select Cu, $PO_4^{-3}$ or H to balance first, the H's appear the most complicated so do them first.

balance H: $CuO + 2H_3PO_4 \rightarrow Cu_3(PO_4)_2 + 3H_2O$
balance $PO_4$: already balanced
balance Cu's: $3CuO + 2H_3PO_4 \rightarrow Cu_3(PO_4)_2 + 3H_2O$
balance O: already balanced (note again that the O's on the $PO_4^{-3}$'s were balanced by balancing the $PO_4^{-3}$'s)

check: $3CuO + 2H_3PO_4$ | $Cu_3(PO_4)_2 + 3H_2O$

| | | |
|---|---|---|
| Cu: | 3 | 3 |
| O: | $3 + 8 = 11$ | $8 + 3 = 11$ |
| H: | 6 | 6 |
| P: | 2 | 2 |

*Question #6* (Answer: c)

unbalanced: $Na_2O_2 + H_2O \rightarrow NaOH + O_2$
balance Na: $Na_2O_2 + H_2O \rightarrow 2NaOH + O_2$
balance H: already balanced
balance O: $Na_2O_2 + H_2O \rightarrow 2NaOH + \frac{1}{2}O_2$
remove fractions by multiplying through by 2:

check: $2Na_2O_2 + 2H_2O$ | $4NaOH + O_2$

| | | |
|---|---|---|
| Na: | 4 | 4 |
| O: | $4 + 2 = 6$ | $4 + 2 = 6$ |
| H: | 4 | 4 |

*Question #7* (Answer: d)

$$\text{unbalanced:} \quad N_2H_4 + N_2O_4 \;\rightarrow\; N_2 + H_2O$$
$$\text{balance O:} \quad N_2H_4 + N_2O_4 \;\rightarrow\; N_2 + 4H_2O$$
$$\text{balance H:} \quad 2N_2H_4 + N_2O_4 \;\rightarrow\; N_2 + 4H_2O$$
$$\text{balance N:} \quad 2N_2H_4 + N_2O_4 \;\rightarrow\; 3N_2 + 4H_2O$$

| check: | $2N_2H_4 + N_2O_4$ | $\rightarrow 3N_2 + 4H_2O$ |
|---|---|---|
| N: | $4 + 2 = 6$ | 6 |
| H: | 8 | 8 |
| O: | 4 | 4 |

*Question #8* (Answer: c) These types of problems are solved by using the known ratios of the moles of the compounds from the balanced equation.

Known ratios from equation

$$\frac{x \text{ moles } N_2}{3 \text{ moles } N_2H_4} = \frac{3 \text{ moles } N_2}{2 \text{ moles } N_2H_4}$$

$$x = (3/2)(3) = 9/2 = 4\tfrac{1}{2}.$$

*Question #9* (Answer: b) First convert weights to moles:

GMWs (gram-molecular weight):
$$N_2H_4 = 2(14) + 4(1) = 28 + 4 = 32$$
$$N_2O_4 = 2(14) + 4(16) = 28 + 64 = 92$$
$$H_2O = 2(1) + 16 = 2 + 16 = 18$$

$$\text{moles} = \frac{\text{weight}}{\text{GMW}}$$

$$\text{moles of } N_2H_4 = \frac{8}{32} = \frac{1}{4}$$

$$\text{moles of } N_2O_4 = \frac{92}{92} = 1$$

Then determine if one of these is in limiting amount by using the ratios of the compounds in the balanced equation:

if all of the $N_2H_4$ were used up, then:

$$\frac{x \text{ moles } N_2O_4}{\tfrac{1}{4} \text{ mole } N_2H_4} = \frac{1 \text{ mole } N_2O_4}{2 \text{ moles } N_2H_4}$$

$$\frac{x}{\tfrac{1}{4}} = \frac{1}{2}$$

$$x = (\tfrac{1}{2})(\tfrac{1}{4}) = \frac{1}{8} \text{ moles of } N_2O_4 \text{ would be required.}$$

if all of the $N_2O_4$ were used up, then:
$$\frac{x \text{ moles } N_2H_4}{1 \text{ mole of } N_2O_4} = \frac{2 \text{ moles } N_2H_4}{1 \text{ mole } N_2O_4}$$

$$\frac{x}{1} = \frac{2}{1}$$

$$x = \left(\frac{2}{1}\right)(1) = 2 \text{ moles of } N_2H_4 \text{ would be required.}$$

Since only ¼ mole of $N_2H_4$ is available, and not 2 moles as would be required to use up all of the $N_2O_4$, the $N_2H_4$ is the limiting reagent. Then, using the moles of the limiting reagent, calculate the expected moles of the desired product.

$$\frac{x \text{ moles of } H_2O}{\frac{1}{4} \text{ mole of } N_2H_4} = \frac{4 \text{ moles } H_2O}{2 \text{ moles } N_2H_4}$$

$$\frac{x}{\frac{1}{4}} = \frac{4}{2}$$

$$x = \left(\frac{4}{2}\right)(\tfrac{1}{4}) = \tfrac{1}{2} \text{ mole } O_2.$$

Now calculate the grams of $O_2$:

$$\text{moles} = \frac{\text{weight}}{\text{GMW}}$$

$$\text{weight} = (\text{moles})(\text{GMW}) = (\tfrac{1}{2})(18) = 9 \text{ gms.}$$

*Question #10* (Answer: c) Again use moles as the intermediary. First need GMWs where they can be determined:

GMWs:

$$H_2O = 2(1) + 16 = 18$$
$$N_2 \quad = 2(14) = 28$$
$$\text{moles} = \frac{\text{weight}}{\text{GMW}}$$

$$\text{moles of } H_2O = \frac{36}{18} = 2$$

Then use equation to find moles of $N_2$:

$$\frac{x \text{ moles } N_2}{2 \text{ moles of } H_2O} = \frac{3 \text{ moles } N_2}{4 \text{ moles } H_2O}$$

$$\frac{x}{2} = \frac{3}{4}$$

$$x = (\tfrac{3}{4})(2) = 1\tfrac{1}{2} \text{ moles of } N_2$$

Then since at STP and 22.4 liters = 1 mole of gas:

$$\frac{x \text{ liters of } N_2}{3/2 \text{ moles of } N_2} = \frac{22.4 \text{ liters of } N_2}{1 \text{ mole of } N_2}$$

$$\frac{x}{3/2} = \frac{22.4}{1}$$

$$x = (22.4)(3/2) = 33.6 \text{ liters.}$$

*Question #11* (Answer: d)

| | |
|---|---|
| unbalanced: | $FeS + O_2 + H_2O \rightarrow Fe_2O_3 + H_2SO_4$ |
| balance H, S: | already balanced |
| balance Fe: | $2FeS + O_2 + H_2O \rightarrow Fe_2O_3 + H_2SO_4$ |
| rebalance S: | $2FeS + O_2 + H_2O \rightarrow Fe_2O_3 + 2H_2SO_4$ |
| rebalance H: | $2FeS + O_2 + 2H_2O \rightarrow Fe_2O_3 + 2H_2SO_4$ |
| balance O: | $2FeS + 9/2\ O_2 + 2H_2O \rightarrow Fe_2O_3 + 2H_2SO_4$ |
| multiply by 2: | $4FeS + 9O_2 + 4H_2O \rightarrow 2Fe_2O_3 + 4H_2SO_4$ |

check: $4FeS + 9O_2 + 4H_2O \rightarrow 2Fe_2O_3 + 4H_2SO_4$

| | | |
|---|---|---|
| Fe: | 4 | 4 |
| S: | 4 | 4 |
| O: | 18 + 4 = 22 | 6 + 16 = 22 |
| H: | 8 | 8 |

*Question #12* (Answer: c) Again convert to moles:

moles of $O_2$: $\dfrac{x \text{ moles } O_2}{22.4 \text{ liters } O_2} = \dfrac{1 \text{ mole } O_2}{22.4 \text{ liters } O_2}$

$$\frac{x}{22.4} = \frac{1}{22.4}$$

$$x = \left(\frac{1}{22.4}\right)(22.4) = 1 \text{ mole}$$

moles of FeS: GMW of FeS = 56 + 32 = 88

moles of Fe = $\dfrac{\text{weight}}{\text{GMW}} = \dfrac{44}{88} = \dfrac{1}{2}$

Then determine if either reagent is in limiting amounts;

if all the $O_2$ is used up

$$\frac{x \text{ moles FeS}}{1 \text{ mole } O_2} = \frac{4 \text{ moles FeS}}{9 \text{ moles } O_2}$$

$$\frac{x}{1} = \frac{4}{9}$$

x = 4/9 mole of FeS would be required

if all the FeS is used up

$$\frac{x \text{ moles } O_2}{\frac{1}{2} \text{ mole FeS}} = \frac{9 \text{ moles } O_2}{4 \text{ moles FeS}}$$

$$\frac{x}{\frac{1}{2}} = \frac{9}{4}$$

$$x = \left(\frac{9}{4}\right)\left(\frac{1}{2}\right) = \frac{9}{8} \text{ moles of } O_2 \text{ would be required}$$

So, the $O_2$ is in limiting amounts because less than 9/8 mole is available. Note that more than 4/9 mole of FeS is available to react with the $O_2$. Then use moles of $O_2$ to determine how much of $H_2SO_4$ will be produced:

$$\frac{x \text{ moles } H_2SO_4}{1 \text{ mole } O_2} = \frac{4 \text{ moles } H_2SO_4}{9 \text{ moles } O_2}$$

$$\frac{x}{1} = \frac{4}{9}$$

x = 4/9 makes $H_2SO_4$

since moles = $\dfrac{\text{weight}}{\text{GMW}}$ and

GMW of $H_2SO_4$ = 2(1) + 32 + 4(16) = 2 + 32 + 64 = 98

then,

weight of $H_2SO_4$ = (moles)(GMW) = $\left(\dfrac{4}{9}\right)(98) \approx (4)(11) = 44$ gms.

*Question #13* (Answer: b)

$$\frac{x \text{ moles } Fe_2O_3}{5 \text{ moles FeS}} = \frac{2 \text{ moles } Fe_2O_3}{4 \text{ moles FeS}}$$

$$\frac{x}{5} = \frac{2}{4}$$

$$x = \left(\frac{2}{4}\right)(5) = \frac{5}{2} = 2\frac{1}{2} \text{ moles of } Fe_2O_3$$

*Question #14* (Answer: a)

$$\text{GMWs: } H_2SO_4 = 2(1) + 32 + 4(16) = 2 + 32 + 64 = 98$$
$$O_2 = 2(16) = 32$$

moles: moles $H_2SO_4 = \dfrac{98}{98} = 1$ mole

moles of $O_2$ required:

$$\frac{\text{x moles } O_2}{1 \text{ mole } H_2SO_4} = \frac{9 \text{ moles } O_2}{4 \text{ moles } H_2SO_4}$$

$$\frac{x}{1} = \frac{9}{4}$$

$$x = \left(\frac{9}{4}\right)(1) = \frac{9}{4} = 2\tfrac{1}{4} \text{ moles of } O_2$$

Volume of $O_2$:

$$\frac{\text{x liters of } O_2}{9/4 \text{ moles of } O_2} = \frac{22.4 \text{ liters of } O_2}{1 \text{ mole of } O_2}$$

$$\frac{x}{9/4} = \frac{22.4}{1}$$

$$x = \left(\frac{22.4}{1}\right)\left(\frac{9}{4}\right) = 50.4 \text{ liters}$$

## 3.7.5    Vocabulary Checklist for Stoichiometry

None

## 3.7.6    Concepts, Principles, etc. Checklist for Stoichiometry

_____ symbolism of chemical equations
_____ balancing of chemical equations
_____ use of chemical equations in solving problems

## 3.8    ENERGY CHANGES IN REACTIONS

### 3.8.1    Review of the Energy Changes in Reactions

Enthalpy ($\Delta H$) is the energy change (in terms of heat content) in a chemical reaction that occurs at constant pressure. The natural tendency of systems is toward minimum energy—the lower the energy of the system, the more stable the system. This means that a reaction that occurs with loss of energy (or negative energy) is a favorable reaction. The *standard enthalpy of formation* ($\Delta H_f^{\circ}$) is the enthalpy change when one mole of a compound is formed from its elements at $298°k$. An example is:

$$C + \tfrac{1}{2}O_2 \text{ (g)} \rightarrow CO(g) \quad \Delta H_f^{\circ} \text{ (CO)} = -26.4 \text{ kcal.}$$

The *standard enthalpy change of a reaction* ($\Delta H°$) is:

$$\Delta H° = \Sigma \Delta H_f^{\circ} \text{ (products)} - \Sigma \Delta H_f^{\circ} \text{ (reactants)}$$

That is, the $\Delta H_f^{\circ}$ of all the products are added together and the $\Delta H_f^{\circ}$ of all the reactants are subtracted from them. Note: the enthalpy of elements as they exist at $298°k$ is zero. *Hess's Law of Constant Heat Summation* states that $\Delta H°$'s of the reactions can be added algebraically to get the overall $\Delta H°$ for the overall reaction. Note that when the direction of a reaction is reversed, the sign of the $\Delta H°$ is changed (from $+ \rightarrow -$, or from $- \rightarrow +$). Also, if the reaction, as written is multiplied (or divided) by a number, the $\Delta H°$ must also be multiplied (or divided) by the same number. An example:

Q:    Find the enthalphy of formation ($\Delta H_f^o$) of $Ca(OH)_2(s)$ given the following:

$$2H_2(g) + O_2(g) \rightarrow 2H_2O(l) \qquad \qquad \Delta H = -136.6 \text{ kcal}$$
$$CaO(s) + H_2O(l) \rightarrow Ca(OH)_2(s) \qquad \Delta H = -15.3 \text{ kcal}$$
$$2CaO(s) \rightarrow 2Ca(s) + O_2(g) \qquad \qquad \Delta H = +303.6 \text{ kcal}$$

A:    $\Delta H_f^o$ of $Ca(OH)_2$ means its formation from $Ca(s)$, $H_2(g)$ and $O_2(g)$. The answer by using the principles above is:

$$\frac{1}{2} [2H_2(g) + O_2(g) \rightarrow 2H_2O(l)] \qquad \Delta H = \frac{1}{2}(-136.6 \text{ kcal})$$
$$CaO(s) + H_2O(l) \rightarrow Ca(OH)_2(s) \qquad \Delta H = -15.3 \text{ kcal}$$
$$\frac{1}{2}[2Ca(s) + O_2(g) \rightarrow 2CaO(s)] \qquad \Delta H = \frac{1}{2}(-303.6 \text{ kcal})$$

rewriting the above,

$$H_2(g) + \frac{1}{2}O_2(g) \rightarrow H_2O(l) \qquad \Delta H = -68.3 \text{ kcal}$$
$$CaO(s) + H_2O(l) \rightarrow Ca(OH)_2(s) \qquad \Delta H = -15.3 \text{ kcal}$$
$$Ca(s) + \frac{1}{2}O_2(g) \rightarrow CaO(s) \qquad \Delta H = -151.8 \text{ kcal}$$

---

net:

$$Ca(s) + H_2(g) + O_2(g) \rightarrow Ca(OH)_2(s) \qquad \Delta H = -235.4 \text{ kcal}$$

(Note: the $CaO(s)$ and $H_2O(l)$ cancel because they are on opposite sides of the equation.)

*Entropy* ($\Delta S$) is another measure of the stability of a system. It represents that part of the total energy not available for useful work. Entropy can be viewed as a measure of the number of microscopic states associated with a given macroscopic state. The more microscopic states a given macroscopic state has, the higher its entropy. This is also the same as saying the more probable (in the sense of probability) a state is, the higher its entropy. This is also the same as saying the more random a state, the higher its entropy. Systems tend toward maximum entropy for the greatest stability.

$\Delta H$ and $\Delta S$ represent two tendencies of systems. These may oppose each other or be in the same direction. *Free energy* ($\Delta G$) is a measure of the tendency of a system which takes into account $\Delta H$ and $\Delta S$. It gives the net tendency of the system. The formulation of $\Delta G$ is

$$\Delta G = \Delta H - T\Delta S$$
T = absolute temperature.

For chemical reactions, the following conditions hold:

if $\Delta G = 0$,    then the reaction is at equilibrium
$\Delta G < 0$,    then a spontaneous reaction (no energy input) is possible
$\Delta G > 0$,    then no reaction spontaneously

The system tends toward a minimal value of $\Delta G$ which is the maximal stability.

The more negative $\Delta G$, the more probable the reaction will go as written. In summary, the $\Delta G$ represents the useful energy the system has to do work. As before, with $\Delta H$

$$\Delta G° = \Sigma \Delta G_f^o \text{ (products)} - \Sigma \Delta G_f^o \text{ (reactants)}.$$

Bonded molecules have lower energy than separate atoms; therefore, when atoms combine to form molecules, they lose energy (when spontaneous). The *bond dissociation energy* (D) is the enthalpy change of the reaction in which a specific bond in a gaseous molecule is broken. The D is positive (i.e., it requires input of energy to break a bond). The *average bond energy* (E) is the approximate energy required to break a bond of a particular type (e.g., C-H) in any compound it may occur in. Note that each C-H in $CH_4$ has a different D, but the E would be the average of all four of these. The larger the numerical value (all are positive by definition) of the bond energy, the stronger the bond.

*Exothermic* reactions proceed with a negative $\Delta H$, and *endothermic* reactions proceed with a positive $\Delta H$.

That is:  exothermic:  reactants → products + heat
endothermic:  heat + reactants → products.

### 3.8.2    Questions to Review Energy Changes in Reactions

(1)    A measure of the heat of a reaction:

(a) entropy
(b) enthalpy
(c) free energy
(d) none of these

(2)    The more stable systems with regard to $\Delta H$ are systems that have

(a) zero $\Delta H$
(b) maximum $\Delta H$
(c) minimum $\Delta H$

(3)    A measure of the total energy not available for useful work is the:

(a) entropy
(b) enthalpy
(c) free energy
(d) none of the above

(4)    The more stable systems with regard to entropy are systems that have

(a) minimum $\Delta S$
(b) maximum $\Delta S$
(c) zero $\Delta S$
(d) none of these

(5)    High values of entropy are associated with all of the following except:

(a) a large number of microscopic states for a given macroscopic state
(b) high probability of a state
(c) high randomness of a state
(d) all of the above are correct

(6)    The net energy available to a system is given by the:

(a) entropy
(b) enthalpy
(c) free energy
(d) none of the above

(7)    The relationship between free energy ($\Delta G$), enthalpy ($\Delta H$), entropy ($\Delta S$) and absolute temperature (T) is

(a) $\Delta G = \Delta H + \Delta S$
(b) $\Delta G = \Delta H + T\Delta S$
(c) $\Delta G = \Delta H - T\Delta S$
(d) $\Delta G = T\Delta H - \Delta S$

(8)    If $\Delta G < 0$, then

(a) the reaction is at equilibrium
(b) a spontaneous reaction is possible
(c) no reaction is possible
(d) none of the above

(9) With regard to ΔG a system is most stable when

(a) ΔG is a maximum
(b) ΔG is a minimum
(c) ΔG is zero
(d) none of the above

(10) The larger the numerical value of a bond energy, the

(a) stronger the bond
(b) weaker the bond
(c) no relation to strength of bond

(11) The following reaction is:   reactants → products    $\Delta H = $ negative

(a) exothermic
(b) endothermic
(c) neither

Use the following information for the remainder of the Questions.

Enthalpies of Formation, $\Delta H_f^\circ$ (kcals/mole) at 298°K

| | | | | | | | |
|---|---|---|---|---|---|---|---|
| $H_2O(g)$ | $-58$ | $NO_2(g)$ | $8$ | $Ca(OH)_2$ | $-236$ | $CH_3CH_2OH(l)$ | $-66$ |
| $H_2O(l)$ | $-68$ | $NH_3(g)$ | $-11$ | $CaCO_3(s)$ | $-288$ | $C_2H_4(g)$ | $13$ |
| $SO_3(g)$ | $-94$ | $CO_2(g)$ | $-94$ | $C_2H_6(g)$ | $-20$ | $C_4H_{10}(g)$ | $-30$ |
| $NO(g)$ | $19$ | $CaO(s)$ | $-152$ | $CH_3OH(l)$ | $-57$ | | |

Bond Energies (ΔH in kcals/mole)

| | | | | | | | | | |
|---|---|---|---|---|---|---|---|---|---|
| H-H | 104 | O-H | 111 | N=N | 226 | C-Cl | 79 | C=C | 194 |
| H-Cl | 103 | O=O | 118 | C-C | 83 | C-N | 70 | C=O | 170 |
| C-H | 99 | Cl-Cl | 58 | C-O | 84 | C≡C | 147 | | |

(12) Calculate the $\Delta H_f^\circ$ of $H_2SO_4(l)$ given the following equation:

$H_2O(l) + SO_3(g) \rightarrow H_2SO_4(l)$    $\Delta H^\circ = -32$ kcals

(a) $-6$
(b) $-58$
(c) $-162$
(d) $-194$

(13) Calculate the heat (ΔH°) of reaction for the following reaction:

$CaO(s) + CO_2(g) \rightarrow CaCO_3(s)$

(a) $-534$
(b) $+534$
(c) $+42$
(d) $-42$

(14) Calculate the heat (ΔH°) of reaction for the following reaction:

$C_2H_4(g) + H_2O(l) \rightarrow CH_3CH_2OH(l)$

(a) $-121$
(b) $+15$
(c) $-15$
(d) $-11$

(15) Calculate the heat (ΔH°) of a reaction for the combustion of n-butane ($C_4H_{10}$)

$$C_4H_{10}(g) + O_2(g) \rightarrow CO_2(g) + H_2O(l)$$
(unbalanced)

(a) $-132$
(b) $-192$
(c) $-310$
(d) $-686$

(16)   Which of the following steps requires the most energy?

$$\text{(I)} \quad C = 0 \rightarrow C - O$$
$$\text{(II)} \quad C = C \rightarrow C - C$$

(neglect other bonds that might be formed)

(a) I
(b) II
(c) both equal

(17)   Which of the following steps releases the most energy?

(a) I
(b) II
(c) neither releases energy


## 3.8.3   Answers to Questions in Section 3.8.2

( 1) b   ( 2) c   ( 3) a   ( 4) b   ( 5) d   ( 6) c   ( 7) c   ( 8) b   ( 9) b   (10) a   (11) a
(12) d   (13) d   (14) d   (15) d   (16) a   (17) a


## 3.8.4   Discussion of Answers to Questions in Section 3.8.2

*Questions #1 to #11:* Adequately discussed in Section.

*Question #12* (Answer: d) The $\Delta H_f^{\circ}$ is the formation of one mole of the $H_2SO_4(l)$ from its elements:

$$H_2(g) - S(s) + 2O_2(g) \rightarrow H_2SO_4(l) \qquad \Delta H_f^{\circ} = ?$$

Now using the information given, a set of equations must be put together that adds up to this net equation. This is done as follows:

(1) $H_2(g) + \frac{1}{2}O_2(g) \rightarrow H_2O(l)$ $\qquad \Delta H_f^{\circ} = -68$

(2) $S(s) + \frac{3}{2}O_2(g) \rightarrow SO_3(g)$ $\qquad \Delta H_f^{\circ} = -94$

Rearrange these to show how they add up to the equation wanted:

$H_2(g) + \frac{1}{2}O_2(g) \rightarrow H_2O(l)$ $\qquad \Delta H_f^{\circ} = -68$ kcals

$S(s) + \frac{3}{2}O_2(g) \rightarrow SO_3(g)$ $\qquad \Delta H_f^{\circ} = -94$ kcals

$H_2O(l) + SO_3(g) \rightarrow H_2SO_4(l)$ $\qquad \Delta H_f^{\circ} = -32$ kcals

---

sum: $H_2(g) + 2O_2(g) + S(s) \rightarrow H_2SO_4(l)$ $\qquad \Delta H_f^{\circ} = -194$ kcals

Or, an alternative method:

$$\Delta H^{\circ} \text{ (product)} - \Delta H^{\circ} \text{ (reactant)} = \Delta H^{\circ} \text{ reaction}$$

$$\Delta H_f^{\circ} H_2SO_4 - \{\Delta H_f^{\circ} H_2O(l) + \Delta H_f^{\circ} SO_3(g)\} = -32 \text{ kcal}$$

$$\Delta H_f^{\circ} H_2SO_4 - (-68 \text{ kcal} - 94 \text{ kcal}) = -32 \text{ kcal}$$

$$\Delta H_f^{\circ} H_2SO_4 = -194 \text{ kcal}$$

*Question #13:* (Answer: d) This is a direct application of Hess' Law.

$$\Sigma\Delta H_f^\circ \text{ (products)} = -288$$

$$\Sigma\Delta H_f^\circ \text{ (reactants)} = -94 - 152 = -246$$

then,

$$\Delta H^\circ = \Sigma\Delta H_f^\circ \text{ (products)} - \Sigma\Delta H_f^\circ \text{ (reactants)}$$

$$\Delta H^\circ = -288 - (-246) = -288 + 246 = -42.$$

*Question #14:* (Answer: d) This is also a direct application of Hess' Law.

$$\Sigma\Delta H_f^\circ \text{ (products)} = -66$$

$$\Sigma\Delta H_f^\circ \text{ (reactants)} = -68 + 13 = -55$$

and,

$$\Delta H = \Sigma\Delta H_f^\circ \text{ (products)} - \Sigma\Delta H_f^\circ \text{ (reactants)}$$

$$= -66 - (-55) = -66 + 55 = -11.$$

*Question #15* (Answer: d) First balance the equation (Section 3.7):

$$\begin{array}{lll} \text{unbalanced:} & C_4H_{10} + O_2 & \rightarrow \quad CO_2 + H_2O \\ \text{balance H:} & C_4H_{10} + O_2 & \rightarrow \quad CO_2 + 5H_2O \\ \text{balance C:} & C_4H_{10} + O_2 & \rightarrow \quad 4CO_2 + 5H_2O \\ \text{balance O:} & C_4H_{10} + \dfrac{13}{2}O_2 + & 4CO_2 + 5H_2O \end{array}$$

(leave as 1 mole $C_4H_{10}$ because $\Delta H^\circ$ based on one mole of the substance)

$$\begin{array}{lll} \text{check:} & \text{C:} & 4 & | & 4 \\ & \text{H:} & 10 & | & 10 \\ & \text{O:} & 13/2(2) = 13 & | & 13 \end{array}$$

Now apply Hess' Law:

$$\Sigma\Delta H_f^\circ \text{(products)} = 4\,\Delta H_f^\circ \text{ of } CO_2(g) + 5\Delta H_f^\circ \text{ of } H_2O(l)$$

$$= 4(-94) + 5(-68) = -376 - 340 = -716$$

$$\Sigma\Delta H_f^\circ \text{(reactants)} = \Delta H_f^\circ \text{ of } C_4H_{10} + 13/2\Delta H_f^\circ \text{ of } O_2(g)$$

$$= -30 + 13/2(O) = -30$$

and,

$$\Sigma\Delta H^\circ = \Delta H_f^\circ \text{ (products)} - \Delta H_f^\circ \text{ (reactants)}$$

$$= -716 - (-30) = -716 + 30 = -686 \text{ kcals.}$$

*Question #16* (Answer: a) This is an application of Hess' Law using bond energies:

| | | $\Delta H$ |
|---|---|---|
| C=O | $\rightarrow$ C+O | 170 |
| C+O | $\rightarrow$ C−O | −84 |
| C=O | $\rightarrow$ C−O | 86 |
| | | |
| C=C | $\rightarrow$ 2C | 147 |
| 2C | $\rightarrow$ C−C | −83 |
| C=C | $\rightarrow$ C−C | 64 |

*Question #17* (Answer: a) Again apply Hess' Law to each by adding all bond energies in products and reactants:

$$
\begin{array}{lll}
\text{I} & H_2 + C_2H_4 \rightarrow 6H + 2C & \Delta H \\
& 104 + 4(99) + 147 & \\
& \text{H-H} \quad \text{4C-H} \quad\quad C = C & 647 \text{ kcal} \\
& 6H + 2C \rightarrow C_2H_6 & \\
& \quad\quad\quad 83 + 6(99) & -677 \text{ kcal} \\
& \quad\quad\quad \text{C-C} + 6CH & \\
\text{net} & H_2 + C_2H_4 \rightarrow C_2H_6 & -\ 30 \text{ kcal} \\
\\
\text{II} & H_2 + CH_2O \rightarrow 4H + C + O & \\
& 104 + 2(99) + 170 & 472 \text{ kcal} \\
& \text{H-H} + CH \quad\quad C = O & \\
& 4H + C + O \rightarrow CH_3OH & \\
& \quad\quad\quad 3(99) + 84 + 111 & -492 \text{ kcal} \\
& \quad\quad\quad 3\text{C-H} + \text{C-O} + OH & \\
\text{net} & H_2 + CH_2O \rightarrow CH_3OH & -\ 20 \text{ kcal}
\end{array}
$$

### 3.8.5 Vocabulary Checklist for Energy Changes in Reactions

_____ enthalpy
_____ standard enthalpy of formation
_____ standard enthalpy of a reaction
_____ Hess' Law
_____ entropy

_____ free energy
_____ bond energy
_____ exothermic
_____ endothermic

### 3.8.6 Concepts, Principles, etc. Checklist for Energy Changes in Reactions

_____ relation between $\Delta H$, $\Delta S$ and $\Delta G$ and meaning of each
_____ use of Hess' Law
_____ use and meaning of bond energies

## 3.9 RATE PROCESSES IN CHEMICAL REACTIONS—KINETICS & EQUILIBRIUM

### 3.9.1 Review of Rate Processes in Chemical Reactions

#### 3.9.1.1 KINETICS

*Kinetics* is concerned with the rates (how fast) of chemical reactions. This means it is concerned with the activation energy (see below) rather than the $\Delta H$ (enthalpy change) of a reaction as in thermodynamics (Section 3.8.1).

*For a chemical reaction to occur*, several conditions must be met. They are:

(1)  the molecules must *collide* (make contact). The more they collide, the greater the chance of a reaction.

(2)  The molecules must have enough energy to react once they have collided. Remember that molecules have a distribution of kinetic energies (Boltzman distribution), and only some of the molecules will have enough energy to react. Note: Kinetic energy is proportional to the average temperature of the molecules.

(3)  Given a collision and sufficient energy, a molecule may not react unless the *orientation* is correct. The energy requirements and orientation are related in that some orientations require less energy for reaction to occur.

The three factors above help determine the *activation energy* ($E_A$). The $E_A$ is the energy barrier which must be overcome for a reaction to occur. The higher the $E_A$, the slower the reaction. A *catalyst* (a substance not used up or changed in a reaction) speeds up reactions by lowering the $E_A$. This is how *enzymes* work (Section 2.1.1).

Most reactions proceed as a series of steps which are exemplified by chain reactions. *Chain reactions* are exemplified by radical reactions such as halogenation. The steps are as follows:

(1)    *Initiation* — the production of radicals
$$Cl_2 \rightarrow 2Cl'$$

(2)    *Propagation* — the production of radicals by reaction with radicals, this keeps the reaction going:

$$Cl^- + R_3CH \rightarrow R_3C + HCl$$
$$R_3C + Cl_2 \rightarrow R_3CCl + Cl$$

(3)    *Termination* — the destruction of radicals by the reactions of two radicals with each other or by the reactions of radicals with the walls of the container:

$$Cl^- R_3C \rightarrow R_3CCl$$
$$R_3C + R_3C \rightarrow R_3C - CR_3$$

There are many possible overall paths (reaction coordinates) which may be taken by reactants being converted to products. The path taken will be the one with the lowest $E_A$. Each step, i.e., each $E_A$ in an overall path, is called an *elementary process*. The elementary process with the highest $E_A$ is the *slowest step (rate determining* step) and determines the overall rate of the reaction. If one molecule is involved in an elementary process, it is said to be *unimolecular*. If two molecules, it is said to be bimolecular; if three, then *trimolecular*, etc. Given an overall path (with its composite elementary processes), the *principle of microscopic reversibility* states that the elementary processes of the reverse reaction are the same as the forward reaction (Fig. 3.10).

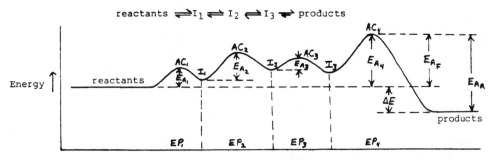

Fig. 3.10 - A Reaction Coordinate

EP  = elementary process
AC  = activated complex, a transient species that may be converted to products or reactants, cannot be isolated; also called the *transition state complex*
I   = intermediates, transient species that may be isolated in some instances; note they are like "rest points" between the EP's
$E_A$  = activation energies
$E_{A_F}$ = overall $E_A$ for forward reaction
$E_{A_R}$ = overall $E_A$ for reverse reaction
$\Delta E$ = energy of the reaction = $E_{A_R} - E_{A_F}$

The *rates of reactions* are quantified in terms of *rate expressions* which relate the change in concentration of one reactant (or product) with time to the concentration of other reactants (or products):

for,

$$aA + bB \rightarrow cC + dD \qquad \text{(overall reaction)}$$

the rate expression might be,

$$\text{rate} = \frac{\Delta[A]}{\Delta t} = -k\,[A]^m\,[B]^n$$

the minus sign $(-)$ is because [ A ] is decreasing with time,

$k$ = rate constant for the reaction
[ ] = concentration in moles/liter (molarity).

Note that the exponents of $A(m)$ and $B(n)$ do not, in general, equal the coefficients of $A(a)$ and $B(b)$. This points out that rate expressions cannot be determined from the stoichiometric equations; they must be determined by experiment. The rate of reaction, and hence, the rate expression, varies during the course of the reaction. This is because the net reaction rate is,

net rate = forward rate − reverse rate,

forward rate = $k_f\,[A]^m[B]^n$
reverse rate  = $k_r\,[C]^x[D]^y$.

The *forward rate* depends on the concentration of the reactants, and the *reverse rate* depends on the concentration of the products. Early (initially) in the reaction, there are more reactants and the forward rate dominates. As reactants are converted to products, there accumulates more products and the reverse rate increases until it equals the forward rate. This point is equilibrium (Fig. 3.11).

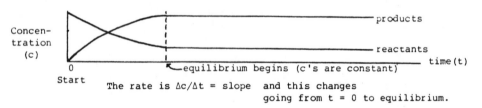

Fig. 3.11 - Course of a Reaction

For the reason above, most rate expressions are for *initial rates* (reactants present but no products) and, hence, are forward rates and take the form:

$$\text{rate} = k[A]^m[B]^n$$

The problem then is to determine the values of m and n. This is done by varying the concentration of one reactant while holding other reactants constant and determining how the rate is affected by this. The *order* of the reaction (contrasted with molecularity) is the sum of the exponents in the experimentally derived rate expression. For example:

given: rate = $k[A]^2[B]^{1/2}$

then: order of reaction = $2 + \frac{1}{2} = 2\frac{1}{2}$
order of reactant in $\underline{A}$ = 2
order of reactant in $\underline{B}$ = $\frac{1}{2}$

First order kinetics means the order is one, second order is two, etc. The rate constant can be calculated once the orders in each reactant is known:

$$k = \frac{\text{rate}}{[A]^2[B]^{1/2}}$$

From the collision theory of gaseous reactions, the following equation is derived:

$$k = Ae^{-Ea/RT}$$

k   = rate constant
A   = a constant which includes collision, orientation, and molecular factors
e   = base of natural logs
Ea  = activation energy
R   = 1.99 cal/mole − °K
T   = absolute temperature

The $E_a$ can be calculated by determining the rate constant at a number of different temperatures and making this plot:

$$lnk = lna - \frac{E_A}{R} \cdot \frac{1}{T}$$

$(y = b + m \cdot x)$     $lnk$     slope $= -E_A/R$     $1/T$

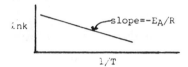

(Review also Vol. II: *Skills Development for the Medical College Admission Test*, the section on semi-log graphs.)

## 3.9.1.2   EQUILIBRIUM

All chemical reactions proceed toward an equilibrium state. The *equilibrium state* exists when the forward rate equals the reverse rate: hence, there is no change in the components of the reaction (see 3.9.1.1). This points out that the equilibrium state is a dynamic state; i.e., the reactions have not ceased, and reactants are being converted to products and products are being converted to reactants. At equilibrium, $\Delta G$ (free energy) is zero, $\Delta H$ (enthalpy) is a minimum, and $\Delta S$ (entropy) is maximum (see Section 3.8.1). This means that there is a *minimum energy* and *maximum randomness* in a system at equilibrium.

The *equilibrium constant (K)* is a quantitative way of describing the interrelationships of the concentrations of components at equilibrium. It is:

given the reaction: $aA + bB \underset{k_2}{\overset{k_1}{\rule{0.6cm}{0.4pt}}} cC + dD$

forward rate    $= k_1 [A]^a[B]^b$

backward rate  $= k_2 [C]^c[D]^d$

then the equilibrium constant is:

forward rate = backward rate

$$K_1 = [A]^a[B]^b = K_2[C]^c[D]^d$$

$$K = \frac{k_1}{K_2} = \frac{[C]^c[D]^d}{[A]^a[B]^b}$$ depends only on temperature

[   ] = concentration in moles/liter (molarity)
[gases] = atmospheres
[pure solids] = constant and are essentially = 1.

The K is a measure of the capacity of reactants to be converted to products. The larger the K, the more reactants will be converted to products. The expression:

$$\frac{[C]^c[D]^d}{[A]^a[B]^b}$$

can be determined *at points other than equilibrium. The direction the reaction must proceed to get to equilibrium* can be determined by comparing the values of the expression with the K:

if $\frac{[C]^c[D]^d}{[A]^a[B]^b} < K$

then the reaction proceeds to equilibrium from left to right as written (the numerator, products, must increase and/or the denominator, reactants, must decrease for the expression to equal K);

if $\frac{[C]^c[D]^d}{[A]^a[B]^b} > K$

then the reaction proceeds to equilibrium from right to left as written (the reverse of the above).

Note that the equilibrium constant for the reverse ($K_R$) of a given reaction (K) is:

$$K_R = 1/K.$$

The overall equilibrium constant (K) for a series of reactions that sum to this overall reaction is:

$$K = K_1 K_2 K_3 \ldots$$

When a reaction is *exothermic* ($\Delta H$ is negative), the K actually decreases as the temperature increases. The reverse is true for an endothermic reaction (see 3.8.1).

*Le Chatelier's Principle* is a good way to determine what the effect of a change in condition (e.g., concentration) will do the relative concentrations of reactants/products and other factors (e.g., heat, volume) in a reaction. The Principle is:

> Any perturbation (change) to a system initially at equilibrium will cause that system (if left alone) to adjust in such a way as to offset that perturbation.

This means the system will go toward a new equilibrium but with concentrations and other factors appropriately adjusted. A practical way of using Le Chatelier's Principle is:

(1)    Write all the components and conditions of the reaction on the appropriate side of the equation. This includes all the reactants, products, heat and volume. The heat is the heat of the reaction. If positive, it is a reactant; if negative, it is a product (see 3.8.1). Remember that an increase in temperature is like increasing the energy (heat) and vice versa. The volume can be related to the moles (in the balanced equation) of gases in the reaction. Put the volume on the side with the fewer moles of gas ("balances" out the volume). Remember that as pressure increases, the volume decreases and vice versa.

(2)    Apply these rules (from Le Chatelier's) to determine how the equilibrium will shift:

(a) if a component or condition increases, the reaction is shifted to the opposite side; i.e., components/conditions on the other side will increase and those on the same side will decrease;

(b) if a component/condition decreases, the reaction is shifted to its side, the other components/conditions on that side increase and the components/conditions on the opposite decrease.

An example is:

given the reaction,

$$M_2(g) + 3 E_2 (g) — 2 ME_3(g) \qquad \Delta H = + 10 \text{ kcals}$$

Rewrite using the rules above.

$$\text{heat} + M_2(g) + 3E_2(g) — 2ME_3(g) + \text{volume}$$

Examples of effects of perturbations are:

if ↑M$_2$,
   reaction shifts to right

if ↓E$_2$,
   reaction shifts to left

if ↑pressure,
   this causes volume to decrease
   reaction shifts to right

if ↓temperature,
   same as decreasing heat and decreasing volume
   reaction shift is indeterminate

if add a catalyst
   no shift in equilibrium by a catalyst,
   catalyst *only affects rate of reaction.*


## 3.9.2    Questions to Review Kinetics and Equilibrium

(1)    All of the following conditions must be met in order for a chemical reaction to occur except:

(a) collisions between molecules
(b) sufficient energy per molecule to react
(c) appropriate orientation of colliding molecules
(d) all of the above are necessary

(2)    The energy that must be overcome for a chemical reaction to occur is called the

(a) enthalpy
(b) activation energy
(c) entropy
(d) free energy

(3)    The steps in a chain reaction include all except

(a) initiation
(b) propagation
(c) acceleration
(d) termination

(4)    The step in which radicals already present are used to generate new radicals is called

(a) initiation
(b) propagation
(c) acceleration
(d) none of the above

Use the following diagram to answer Questions #5 through #7.

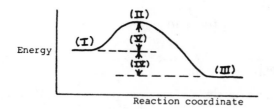

Energy | Reaction coordinate

(5) The activation energy of the forward reaction is given by:

(a) II
(b) III
(c) IV
(d) V

(6) The heat of the reaction is given by:

(a) II
(b) III
(c) IV
(d) V

(7) The activated complex would be located at:

(a) I
(b) II
(c) III
(d) none of the above

(8) The rate determining step of a reaction with a series of steps is characterized by:

(a) the lowest energy of activation
(b) the highest energy of activation
(c) the highest enthalpy
(d) none of the above

(9) The role of a catalyst is to:

(a) shift the equilibrium of the reaction in favor of products
(b) speed up the reaction by raising the activation energy
(c) speed up the reaction by lowering the activation energy
(d) none of the above

(10) At equilibrium:

(a) the forward reaction continues
(b) the reverse reaction continues
(c) there is minimum energy and maximum randomness
(d) all of the above

(11) As the value of K (the equilibrium constant) becomes larger:

(a) more products will be present at equilibrium
(b) less products will be present at equilibrium
(c) the faster the reaction will proceed
(d) the slower the reaction will proceed

(12) Given the reaction symbolized as:   $A \xrightleftharpoons{K} B$

if   $\dfrac{[B]}{[A]} = 2 \times 10^{-5}$ and it is known that $K = 5 \times 10^{-4}$ from other experiments, in what direction must the reaction proceed to reach equilibrium?

(a) [B] must increase and/or [A] decrease
(b) [B] must decrease and/or [A] decrease
(c) cannot be determined from the information given

(13) For the reaction: $A + 2B \overset{K}{\rightleftharpoons} 2C$, the concentrations, in moles/liters, of the components at equilibrium are:

$$[A] = 1 \times 10^{-2}M, [B] = 2 \times 10^{-3}M, [C] = 5 \times 10^{-6}M.$$

What is the equilibrium constant (K) of the reaction?

(a) $6.25 \times 10^{-4}$
(b) 0.225
(c) 25
(d) none of the above

Use the following information for Questions #14 through #17.

$$C_2H_5OH(l) + 3O_2(g) \rightleftharpoons 2CO_2(g) + 3H_2O(l) \quad \Delta H^\circ = -327 \text{ kcals}$$

(14) If the temperature is increased, the equilibrium:

(a) shifts to the left
(b) shifts to the right
(c) is unchanged

(15) If the pressure is increased, the equilibrium:

(a) shifts to the left
(b) shifts to the right
(c) is unchanged

(16) If $O_2(g)$ is added, the equilibrium:

(a) shifts to the left
(b) shifts to the right
(c) is unchanged

(17) A chemical is added which absorbs $CO_2(g)$. This will cause the equilibrium to be:

(a) shifted to the left
(b) shifted to the right
(c) unchanged

Use the following information for Questions #18 through #21.

$$CH_4(g) + H_2O(l) \rightleftharpoons CH_3OH(l) + H_2(g) \quad \Delta H = +29 \text{ kcal}$$

(18) If the $H_2(g)$ formed is allowed to escape from the reaction, the equilibrium will be:

(a) shifted to the left
(b) shifted to the right
(c) unchanged

(19) If the pressure is doubled, the equilibrium:

(a) shifts to the left
(b) shifts to the right
(c) is unchanged

(20) Suppose $CO^{+2}$ catalyzes this reaction. If it is added, the equilibrium:

(a) shifts to the left
(b) shifts to the right
(c) is unchanged

(21) The temperature is decreased, this causes the equilibrium to:

    (a) shift to the left
    (b) shift to the right
    (c) be unchanged

### 3.9.3    Answers to Questions in Section 3.9.2

( 1) d  ( 2) b  ( 3) c  ( 4) b  ( 5) d  ( 6) c  ( 7) b  ( 8) b  ( 9) c  (10) d  (11) a
(12) a  (13) a  (14) a  (15) b  (16) b  (17) b  (18) b  (19) c  (20) c  (21) a

### 3.9.4    Discussion of Answers to Questions in Section 3.9.2

*Questions #1 to #11:* Adequately discussed in the text.

*Question #12* (Answer: a) In this case $[B]/[A]<K$ because $2\times10^{-5}<5\times10^{-4}$. Then for $[B]/[A]$ to become equal to K, the $[B]$ must increase and the $[A]$ must decrease.

*Question #13* (Answer: a) The equilibrium constant (K) is,

$$K = \frac{[C]}{[A][B]^2} = \frac{[5\times10^{-6}]^2}{[1\times10^{-2}][2\times10^{-3}]^2} = \frac{25\times10^{-12}}{(10^{-2})(4\times10^{-6})}$$

$$K = \frac{25\times10^{-12}}{4\times10^{-8}} = \frac{25}{4}\times10^{-12+8} = 6.25\times10^{-4}$$

*Question #14* (Answer: a) The complete equation is

$$C_2H_5OH(l) + 3O_2(g) \rightleftharpoons 2CO_2(g) + 3H_2O(l) + vol. + heat.$$

Volume goes on the right side because there are fewer moles of gas on that side. Heat goes on the right because the reaction is exothermic, i.e., heat is a product. Then an increase in temperature causes an increase in heat which shifts the reaction to the opposite side (the left). Increased temperature also increases the volume (Charles' Law). This also shifts the reaction to the left.

*Question #15* (Answer: b) See #14. An increase in pressure causes a decrease in volume. A decrease in volume pulls a reaction to its side (the right).

*Question #16* (Answer: b) The added $O_2$ shifts the reaction to the opposite side (the right). Increased temperature also increases the volume (Charles' Law). This also shifts the reaction to the left.

*Question #17* (Answer: b) The $CO_2(g)$ decreases and this pulls the reaction to its side (the right).

*Question #18* (Answer: b) the overall equation is:

$$heat + CH_4(g) + H_2O(l) \rightleftharpoons CH_3OH(l) + H_2(g).$$

The heat is on the left because the reaction is endothermic which means heat is used as a reactant. There is no volume factor because there is an equal number of moles of gases on both sides. Since the $H_2$ is being removed, the reaction is pulled to its side (the right).

*Question #19* (Answer: c) See #18. There is no volume factor so the pressure has no effect.

*Question #20* (Answer: c) Catalysts do not affect the equilibrium of a reaction.

*Question #21* (Answer: a) A decrease in temperature is like decreasing the heat which shifts the reaction to that side (the left).

## 3.9.5 Vocabulary Checklist for Kinetics & Equilibrium

_____ kinetics
_____ Le Chatelier's Principle
_____ activation energy
_____ equilibrium constant
_____ propagation
_____ intermediates

_____ transition states
_____ catalyst
_____ chain reactions
_____ initiation
_____ termination


## 3.9.6 Concepts, Principles, etc. Checklist for Kinetics and Equilibrium

_____ requirements for a chemical reaction to occur
_____ steps in chain reactions
_____ meaning of equilibrium and the equilibrium constant
_____ use of Le Chatelier's Principle


## 3.10 SOLUBILITY

### 3.10.1 Review of Solubility

#### 3.10.1.1 CONCENTRATION UNITS

A *liquid solution* is a homogenous, continuous liquid of variable composition over a limited range consisting of two or more components. Note that a solution may also be gaseous or solid. Given a two component solution, the *solvent* is the component in greater amount (herein, usually a pure liquid), and the *solute* is the component in lesser amount (herein, usually a solid or second liquid). Note that solids, gases or other liquids can be dissolved in a given pure liquid to make a solution.

There are many possible ways of *measuring the composition of solutions*. The common ones are:

(1) *Percent composition* can be weight/volume, weight/weight, volume/volume, etc. It must be designated as to the type and the units of mass and volume used.

$$\% = \frac{\text{amt. of solute}}{\text{total amt. of solution}} \times 100 \text{ (usual form)}.$$

(2) *Density* ($\varrho$)

$$\varrho = \frac{\text{mass of solution}}{\text{total volume of solution}}$$

(3) *Mole Fraction* (X)

$$x_1 = \frac{\text{moles of one component}}{\text{moles of all components}} = \frac{n}{\sum_{i=1}^{i=m} n_i}$$

$n_1$ = moles of component #1. $i = 1$

$\sum_{i=1}^{i=m} n_i$ = sum over moles of all m components.
$i = 1$    $(i = 1, 2, \ldots, m)$.

This is useful when emphasizing the relation between concentration-dependent properties of solutions and the relative amounts of the components (see below).

(4) *Molarity* (M)

$$M = \frac{\text{moles of solute}}{\text{liter of solution}}$$

Varies with the temperature.

(5) *Molality (m)*

$$m = \frac{\text{moles of solute}}{\text{kilogram of solvent}}$$

Does not vary with temperature.

(6) *Formality (F)*

$$F = \frac{\text{moles of solute}}{\text{liter of solution}}$$

Essentially the same as M. Technically more correct for substances that do not exist as molecules, and the formula is used to calculate the gram-formula weight (e.g., NaCl is the formula for "salt" which has no discrete molecules).

The following concept is important for solving problems dealing with solutions and concentrations. Most problems can be solved by realizing there is usually a *conservation of mass*. This means:

given: $C = \text{concentration unit} = \frac{\text{amt. of solute}}{\text{volume of solution}}$

(all of the above are like this except for molality; just substitute kilograms for volume and solvent for solution)

$V$ = volume of solution

then: $(C)(V)$ = amount of solute
amount = gms, moles, equivalents, etc., depending on the concentration unit $(C)$ used

then: this amount of solute is conserved

(1) as solutions are diluted,
$C_1V_1 = C_2V_2 = \text{amount}$
e.g., $M_1V_1 = M_2V_2 = \text{moles}$
$(\%_1)(V_1) = (\%_2)(V_2) = \text{grams if } \% \text{ is (W/V)}$.
(2) as solutions are made from solid and liquids,
$CV$ = amount of solute used to make the solution, e.g.,

$$(M)(V) = \text{moles} = \frac{\text{weight}}{\text{gram-molecular weight}}$$

$(\%)(V) = \text{grams} (\% \text{ is w/v here})$.

Then the correct combination of formulas is chosen depending upon the problem.

## 3.10.1.2   IONS IN SOLUTION, SOLUBILITY, CHEMICAL SEPARATIONS

*Electrolytes* are substances that dissociate into positive and negative ions when dissolved in solvent. The ions are positive (cations) and negative (anions) and are surrounded by solvent molecules in solution (a process called solvation; when the solvent is $H_2O$, this is hydration). Our discussion will refer to water as a solvent.

Some substances are only partially soluble in water. The *ion product* is a means of quantifying the solubility:

$$M_mA_a + H_2O \rightarrow mM^{+a}(aq) + aA^{-m}(aq)$$

$$(aq) = \text{dissolved in water}$$

$$\text{ion product} = [\,M^{+a}\,]^m[\,A^{-m}\,]^a$$

$$[\ \ ] = \text{concentration in moles/liter, i.e. molarity.}$$

The ion product can be calculated for any solution. The *solubility product* ($K_{sp}$) is the ion product for a *saturated solution* (as much as possible of the solute has been dissolved at a given temperature):

$$K_{sp} = [\ M^{+a}\ ]^m [\ A^{-m}\ ]^a$$

for a saturated solution. The smaller the $K_{sp}$, the less soluble is a solid. The $K_{sp}$ is larger than the ion product except at saturation where they are equal. As long as the ion product is less than the $K_{sp}$, more solute can be dissolved.

The *common ion effect* on solubility can be understood in terms of Le Chatelier's Principle (Section 3.9.1.2). Explanation of the effect is based on analysis of the following equation:

$$M_mA_a + H_2O \rightleftharpoons mM^{+a}(aq) + aA^{-m}(aq).$$

The common ions would be $M^{+a}$ or $A^{-m}$. These are increased by adding compounds that dissociate into them and add them to solution, and they are decreased by adding species that react with them and remove them from solution. If $M^{+a}$ or $A^{-m}$ are increased, the reaction shifts to the left and less of $M_mA_a$ dissolves. If $M^{+a}$ or $A^{-m}$ are decreased, the reaction shifts to the right and more of the $M_mA_a$ dissolves. Note that $K_{sp}$ is not affected—the ion not changed compensates (by increasing or decreasing) for the ion changed (the common ion). For example:

for $CaSO_4$ $\quad K_{sp} = 2.4 \times 10^{-5}$

$$CaSO_4(s) + H_2O \rightarrow Ca^{+2}(aq) + SO_4^{-2}(aq)$$

if, given $NaSO_4$ which gives $SO_4^{-2}$, the reaction shifts to the left and more solid $CaSO_4$ forms, this leaves less $Ca^{+2}(aq)$ in solution.

if, given $Na_3PO_4$, the $PO_4^{-3}$ reacts with $Ca^{+2}(aq)$ to form $Ca_3(PO_4)_2$ which has a $K_{sp} = 1.3 \times 10^{-32}$ and is very insoluble, this removes $CA^{+2}(aq)$ from the solution which causes the reaction to shift to the right, this causes more of the $CaSO_4(s)$ to dissolve and this results in more $SO_4^{-2}(aq)$ in solution.

### 3.10.2 Questions to Review Solubility

(1)  Fifty grams of sugar are dissolved in enough water (approximately 168 ml) to make 200 ml of solution. The percent composition of sugar in solution in terms of gms/ml is:

(a) 40%
(b) 0.25%
(c) 2.5%
(d) 25%

(2)  The density of the sugar solution in question #1 in gms/ml (assume water weighs 1 gm/ml) is:

(a) 0.8
(b) 1.00
(c) 1.05
(d) 1.09

(3)  What weight of salt is in 50 mls of solution with a density of 1.05 gms/ml? Assume the volume is due mostly to water and water weighs 1 gm/ml.

(a) 1.05
(b) 2.5
(c) 3.25
(d) 5.0

(4)     A gas mixture contains 84g of $N_2$ (N = 14), 64g of $O_2$ (O = 16), and 10g of $H_2$ (H = 1). What is the mole fraction of $O_2$ in this mixture?

(a) 0.4
(b) 0.3
(c) 0.2
(d) need more information

(5)     A solution is made by dissolving 23g of ethyl alcohol ($C_2H_5OH$; C = 12, O = 16, H = 1) in 500 mls of water. Water has a density of 1 gm/ml. What is the molality of ethyl alcohol?

(a) 0.25
(b) 0.5
(c) 1.0
(d) none of the above

(6)     Seventy-five grams of $Na_2CO_3$ (Na = 23, C = 12, O = 16) are dissolved in enough water to make 1 liter of solution. What is the molarity of the solution?

(a) 1.1
(b) 1.0
(c) 0.71
(d) none of the above

(7)     One-hundred milliliters of a 2M solution of $H_2SO_4$ contains how many moles of $H_2SO_4$?

(a) 0.2
(b) 2
(c) 200
(d) none of the above

(8)     A 3M solution of $H_3PO_4$ (all H's react) contain how may equivalents of $H_3PO_4$ in 500 mls?

(a) 1
(b) 2
(c) 6
(d) none of the above

(9)     What weight of NaCl (Na = 23, Cl = 35) would be required to make 2 liters of a 1.5F solution?

(a) 174
(b) 116
(c) 58
(d) none of the above

(10)    How many mls will need to be added to 500 mls of a 1.5M solution in order to make a 1.0M solution:

(a) 100 mls
(b) 250 mls
(c) 5000 mls
(d) none of the above

(11)    Given the following data:

| Ion | Radius (A) | Charge |
| --- | --- | --- |
| Li | 0.68 | +1 |
| K | 1.33 | +1 |
| Cs | 1.67 | +1 |

Which ion would *most likely* have the largest hydration shell in solution?

(a) Li+
(b) K+
(c) Cs+
(d) cannot be predicted

Use the following information for Questions #16 through #19. (The numbers are $K_{sp}$'s)

| | |
|---|---|
| $BaSO_4$..........$1 \times 10^{-10}$ | $BaF_2$...........$2 \times 10^{-6}$ |
| $PbS$...........$7 \times 10^{-29}$ | $PbSO_4$..........$1 \times 10^{-8}$ |
| $PbCO_3$.........$2 \times 10^{-13}$ | $AgCl$..........$3 \times 10^{-10}$ |
| $Ag_2S$...........$1 \times 10^{-51}$ | $FeS$...........$1 \times 10^{-19}$ |
| $HgS$...........$3 \times 10^{-53}$ | |

(12) If a saturated solution of $Cu(OH)_2$ contains $[Cu^{+2}] = 3.4 \times 10^{-7}$ and $[OH^-] = 6.8 \times 10^{-7}$ the $K_{sp}$ is:

(a) $8.2 \times 10^{-21}$
(b) $1.6 \times 10^{-19}$
(c) $4.6 \times 10^{-13}$
(d) none of the above

(13) A saturated solution of $Cu(IO_3)_2$ is $3.0 \times 10^{-3}$ moles/liters (m). The $K_{sp}$ is:

(a) $6 \times 10^{-6}$
(b) $2.7 \times 10^{-8}$
(c) $9 \times 10^{-9}$
(d) none of the above

(14) A saturated solution of $BaSO_4$ contains what concentration of $Ba^{+2}$?

(a) $2 \times 10^{-10}$
(b) $1 \times 10^{-5}$
(c) $0.5 \times 10^{-10}$
(d) none of the above

(15) If enough $Na_2SO_4$ is added to a saturated solution of $PbSO_4$ to make the total $[SO_4^{-2}] = 2 \times 10^{-2}M$, how much $[Pb^{+2}]$ is in solution?

(a) $2 \times 10^{-16}$
(b) $1 \times 10^{-4}$
(c) $5 \times 10^{-7}$
(d) none of the above

## 3.10.3    Answers to Questions in Section 3.10.2

( 1) d  ( 2) d  ( 3) b  ( 4) c  ( 5) c  ( 6) c  ( 7) a  ( 8) d  ( 9) a  (10) b  (11) a
(12) b  (13) d  (14) b  (15) c

## 3.10.4    Discussion of Answers to Questions in Section 3.10.2

*Question #1* (Answer: d)
$$\% = \frac{\text{weight of solute}}{\text{volume of solution}} \times 100 = \frac{50}{200} \times 100 = \frac{50}{2} = 25\%$$

*Question #2* (Answer: d)
$$\text{density} = \frac{\text{total mass of solution}}{\text{total volume of solution}} = \frac{\text{weight of sugar} + \text{weight of water}}{\text{total volume of solution}}$$
$$= \frac{50 + 168}{200} = \frac{218}{200} = \frac{25}{20} = \frac{5}{4} = 1.09 \text{ gms./ml.}$$

*Question #3* (Answer: b)

$$\text{density (d)} = \frac{\text{total weight (w)}}{\text{total volume (v)}}$$

$$d = \frac{w}{v}$$

$$w = (v)(d) = (50 \text{ mls})(1.05 \text{ gm/ml}) = 52.5 \text{ gms total}$$

w = total weight = weight of salt + weight of water
weight of water = (1gm/ml)(50 mls) = 50 gms
52.5 = weight of salt + 50
weight of salt = 2.5 gms.

*Question #4* (Answer: c)

$$X_{O_2} = \frac{n_{O_2}}{n_{O_2} + n_{N_2} + n_{H_2}} = \frac{2}{2+3+5} = \frac{2}{10} = 0.2$$

$$n_{O_2} = \frac{\text{weight}}{\text{GMW}} = \frac{64}{32} = 2; \quad n_H = \frac{10}{2} = 5; \quad n_H = \frac{84}{28} = 3$$

*Question #5* (Answer: c)

$$m = \frac{\text{moles of solute}}{\text{kg's of solvent}} = \frac{\frac{1}{2}}{\frac{1}{2}} = 1.0$$

$$\text{moles of } C_2H_5OH = \frac{\text{weight}}{\text{GMW}} = \frac{23}{46} = \frac{1}{2}$$

$$\text{GMW} = C_2H_5OH = 2(12) + 5(1) + 16 + 1 = 24 + 5 + 17 = 46$$

$$\text{kg's of water} = (500 \text{ mls}) \left(\frac{1 \text{ gm}}{1 \text{ ml}}\right) \left(\frac{1 \text{ kg}}{1000 \text{ gm}}\right) = \frac{500}{1000} \text{ kg} = \frac{1}{2} \text{ kg}$$

*Question #6* (Answer: c)

$$m = \frac{\text{moles of solvent}}{\text{liters of solution}} = \frac{.71}{1} = 0.71$$

$$\text{moles of } Na_2CO_3 = \frac{\text{weight}}{\text{GMW}} = \frac{75}{106} = .71$$

$$\text{GMW of } CaCO_3 = 2(23) + 12 + 3(16) = 52 + 48 = 106$$

*Question #7* (Answer: a)

$$\text{moles} = (M)(V) = (2)(0.1) = 0.2$$

$$V = (100 \text{mls}) \left(\frac{1l}{1000 \text{ mls}}\right) = \frac{100}{1000} = \frac{1}{10} = 0.1$$

*Question #8* (Answer: d)

$$\text{equivalents} = (N)(V) = (9)(\tfrac{1}{2}) = 9/2 = 4.5$$

$$N = nM = (3)(3) = 9$$

$$V = (500 \text{ mls}) \left(\frac{1l}{1000 \text{ mls}}\right) = \frac{500}{1000} = 1/2$$

*Question #9* (Answer: a) First find the number of moles that are required, then find the weight from this:

$$\text{moles} = (F)(V) = (1.5)(2) = 3$$

$$\text{since moles} = \frac{\text{weight}}{\text{GMW}}$$

$$\text{weight} = (\text{GMW})(\text{moles}) = (58)(3) = 174$$
$$\text{GMW of } NaCl = 23 + 35 = 58$$

*Question #10* (Answer: b)

$$M_2 V_2 = M_1 V_1$$

$$V_2 = \frac{M_1 V_1}{M_2} = \frac{(1.5)(500)}{1.0} = 750 \text{ mls is the total volume.}$$

Then $750 - 500 = 250$ mls for the added volume (pure water, e.g.).

*Question #11* (Answer: a) In general, the ion with the highest charge to volume (or radius) will be the most hydrated. Since all the charges are the same, the ion with the smallest radius will be the most densely charged and have the greatest hydration—this is Lithium.

*Question #12* (Answer: b)

$$Cu(OH)_2 \rightleftharpoons Cu^{+2} + 2OH^-$$

$$Ksp = [Cu^{+2}][OH^-]^2 (3.4 \times 10^{-7})(6.8 \times 10^{-7})^2$$

$$\approx (3 \times 10^{-7})(7 \times 10^{-7})^2 \approx (3 \times 10^{-7})(49 \times 10^{-14})$$
$$\approx (3 \times 10^{-7})(50 \times 10^{-14}) \approx 150 \times 10^{-21} \approx 1.5 \times 10^{-19}$$

Note that estimation works well here.

*Question #13* (Answer: d)

$$Cu(IO_3)_2 \rightleftharpoons Cu^{+2} + 2IO_3^-$$

$$Ksp = [Cu^{+2}][IO_3^-]^2$$

$$[Cu^{+2}] = \text{amt dissolved} = 3 \times 10^{-3}$$

$$[IO_3^-] = \text{twice the amount dissolved} = 2(3 \times 10^{-3}) = 6 \times 10^{-3}$$

$$Ksp = (3 \times 10^{-3})(6 \times 10^{-3})^2 = (3 \times 10^{-3})(36 \times 10^{-6}) = 108 \times 10^{-9}$$
$$= 108 \times 10^{-7}$$

Notice that the options are very nearly equal and estimation might prove hazardous.

*Question #14* (Answer: b)

$$BaSO_4 \rightleftharpoons Ba^{+2} + SO_4^{-2}$$

$$Ksp = [Ba^{+2}][SO_4^{-2}]$$

$$[Ba^{+2}] = [SO_4^{-2}]$$

$$Ksp = 1 \times 10^{-10} = [Ba^{+2}][Ba^{+2}] = [Ba^{+2}]^2$$

$$[Ba^{+2}] = (1 \times 10^{-10})^{1/2} = 1 \times 10^{-5}$$

*Question #15* (Answer: c)

$$PbSO_4 \rightleftharpoons Pb^{+2} + SO_4^{-2}$$

$$Ksp = [Pb^{+2}][SO_4^{-2}] = 1 \times 10^{-8}$$
$$[Pb^{+2}][2 \times 10^{-2}] = 1 \times 10^{-8}$$
$$[Pb^{+2}] = \frac{1 \times 10^{-8}}{2 \times 10^{-2}} = 0.5 \times 10^{-6} = 5 \times 10^{-7}$$

Note that since each $PbSO_4$ gives only one $Pb^{+2}$ per molecule, the $[Pb^{+2}]$ in solution is the same as the amount of $PbSO_4$ that dissolves in the solution. The above is an example of the common ion in effect.


## 3.10.5 Vocabulary Checklist for Solubility

_____ solvent          _____ mole fraction          _____ ion product
_____ solute           _____ molality               _____ percent composition
_____ solubility product  _____ molarity            _____ common ion effect
_____ density          _____ formality

### 3.10.6     Concepts, Principles, etc. Checklist for Solubility

_____ concentration units and their use in solving problems
_____ ions in solution
_____ common ion effect


## 3.11     ACIDS, BASES, AND BUFFERS

### 3.11.1     Review of Acids, Bases, and Buffers

#### 3.11.1.1   ACIDS AND BASES

There are three common definitions of acids and bases:

(1)   **Arrhenius**

Substances that can dissociate into $H^+$ are acids. Substances that can dissociate into $OH^-$ are bases.

(2)   **Bronsted-Lowry**

An acid is a substance that can donate $H^+$. A base is a substance that can accept $H^+$.

(3)   **Lewis**

An acid is an electron pair acceptor, so it needs a vacant orbital. A base is an electron pair donator, so it needs a free pair of electrons.

Certain acids or bases fall under one classification; others may fall under more than one. The Bronsted-Lowry concept is stressed herein.

The *strength* of an acid (protic, esp.) is determined by its ability to donate protons ($H^+$). The strength of a base is determined by its ability to accept protons. This strength is measured by the acid (or base) dissociation constant:

*Acid*

$$HA \rightleftharpoons H^+ + A^- \qquad \text{(neglecting solvent, } H^+(H_2O) \text{ or } H_3O \text{ is more realistic)}$$

$$K_A = \frac{[H^+][A^-]}{[HA]} \qquad \text{at equilibrium}$$

*Base*

$$MOH \rightleftharpoons M^+ + OH^- \qquad \text{(for hydroxy bases)}$$

$$K_B = \frac{[M^+][OH^-]}{[MOH]} \qquad \text{at equilibrium}$$

The larger the $K_A(K_B)$, the stronger the acid (base). The smaller the $pK_A$ ($pK_B$), the stronger the acid (base)—see below for pH. If an acid is strong its *conjugate base* is weak and vice versa. The same is true for bases and their *conjugate acids*. This terminology is:

$$\underset{\text{acid}_1}{HA} \quad + \quad \underset{\text{base}_2}{B} \quad \rightleftharpoons \quad \underset{\text{conjugate base}_1}{A^-} \quad \underset{\text{conjugate acid}_2}{HB^+}$$

A strong acid is one that dissociates completely. A weak acid is one that dissociates incompletely. The conjugate base (acid) of a weak acid (base) is also weak.

*Salts* of strong acids (bases) are neutral. Salts of weak acids or bases are basic and acidic, respectively. This is because they hydrolyze in water; the process is hydrolysis:

*a salt of a weak acid is basic*

$CH_3CO_2H$ (acetic acid) is a weak acid
$CH_3CO_2{}^-Na^+$ (sodium acetate) is the salt
$CH_3CO_2{}^-Na^+ + HOH \rightleftharpoons CH_3CO_2H + Na^+ + OH^-$ solution is basic

*a salt of a weak base is acidic*

$NH_4OH$ is a weak base
$NH_4Cl$ is the salt
$NH_4Cl + HOH \rightleftharpoons NH_4OH + H^+ + Cl^-$ solution is acidic

Examples of strong acids are $H_2SO_4$, HCl, $HNO_3$, HI, HBr, $HClO_4$. Examples of weak acids are $H_2CO_3$, $H_3PO_4$ and $CH_3CO_2H$. Examples of strong bases are NaOH, KOH, LiOH and $Ca(OH)_2$. The important weak base is $NH_3$ (ammonia) or $NH_4OH$. Organic acids (Section 4.10.1) and some phenols (Section 4.9.1) may be strong or weak acids. The organic bases are amines (Section 4.11.1) and are weak.

The *pH* is defined as follows:

$$pH = -\log[H^+] = \log(1/[H^+])$$

$[H^+]$ = hydrogen ion concentration in moles/liter as molarity or normality (both are the same in this case).

The $pK_A$ and pOH are similarly defined. The pH of water solutions at 25°C range from pH = 1 to pH = 14. A pH = 7 is neutral, a pH < 7 is acid and a pH > 7 is basic. The dissociation of water is:

$$H_2O \rightleftharpoons H^+ + OH^-$$

$$Kw = [H^+][OH^-] = 10^{-14}$$

Note that Kw is *not the equilibrium constant*. This results in this relationship:

$$pH + pOH = 14.$$

The $H^+$ *of a strong acid* or the $OH^-$ of a strong base can be calculated from the normality (discussed in Section 3.10.1) of the acid or base. The $H^+(OH^-)$ *from a weak acid (base)* cannot be calculated from the normality of the acid (base) because they are only partially dissociated. These problems are rigorously solved by using the equations below:

(1) $K_A = \dfrac{[H^+][A^-]}{[HA]}$

(2) $K_W = [H^+][OH^-]$

Equation (1) can be simplified if $K_A \ll [HA_O]$ (original concentration of acid), then:

$$[H^+] \approx \sqrt{K_A[HA_O]}$$

The $[H^+]$ can also be arrived at as follows:

$$HA \rightleftharpoons H^+ + A^-$$

original: $[HA_O]$   0   0
at equilibrium: $[HA_O] - x$   x   x   (assume negligible $H^+$ from $H_2O$)

then: $K_A = \dfrac{[H^+][A^-]}{[HA]} = \dfrac{(x)(x)}{[HA_O] - x}$

x = amount of HA that dissociates in moles/liter = $[H^+]$

The equation can be solved using the quadratic formula, or if the x is small relative to $[HA_O]$, then neglect x in the expression $[HA_O] - x$, and solve to get

$$[H^+] \approx \sqrt{K_A[HA_O]}$$

as before.

*Neutralization* reactions are solved using the following equation:

$$N_A V_A = N_B V_B$$

N     = normality (see Section 3.10.1.1)
V     = volume in liters
A     = acid
B     = base.

A neutralization reaction is one in which the number of equivalents of acid is exactly neutralized by an equal number of equivalents of base.

A *titration* reaction is one in which a given amount of acid (base) is neutralized by a base (acid) which is added step-wise. A titration reaction may be done as follows:

f     = fraction of acid neutralized = equivalents of base added/$n_0$
$n_0$ = original equivalents of acid
V     = original volume of acid
v     = volume of base added
$[H^+]$ (from acid and water) = $[OH^-]$ at the equivalence point

then,

$$[H^+] = (n_0)(1-f)/(V+v) + \text{contribution from the H}_2\text{0 (usually neglect)}$$
$$= \text{acid concentration at any given point during the titration up to neutralization by base (f = 1.0)}$$

note that $(n_0) (1-f)/(V+v)$ = amount of acid not neutralized by added base.

Titration reactions can be used to calculate the normality of unknown acid (base) solutions, the equivalent weights of an unknown base or acid or the $pK_A$'s ($pk_B$'s). Examples of titration curves are in Fig. 3.12.

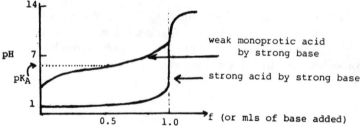

*Fig. 3.12 — Titration Curves*

Note that the curve differs for strong and weak acids, and that the $pK_A = pH$ where the acid is half neutralized.


## 3.11.1.2   BUFFERS

A *buffer solution* resists changes in pH. This means a buffer solution is able to hold the pH of a solution relatively constant when an acid or base is added to that solution. *Buffers* are mixtures of weak acids or bases and their salts. For example:

(1)   acetic acid                     sodium acetate
      $CH_3CO_2H$                      $CH_3CO_2^- Na^+$

(2)   carbonic acid                   sodium bicarbonate
      $H_2CO_3$                        $NaHCO_3$

(3)   ammonium hydroxide              ammonium chloride
      $NH_4OH$                         $NH_4Cl$

Most strong acids or bases and their salts do not make good buffers because they cannot hold the pH constant (see below).

A buffer works by having an acid component to neutralize added bases and a basic component to neutralize added acids. This can be accomplished by using weak acids or bases and their salts. For example:

for acetic acid-acetate buffer

$CH_3CO_2H$ combines with added base
$CH_3CO_2H + OH^- \rightleftharpoons CH_3CO_2^- + H_2O$
$CH_3CO_2^-$ combines with added acid
$CH_3CO_2^- + H^+ \rightleftharpoons CH_3CO_2H$

Hence the pH (depends on free $H^+$ or $OH^-$) is held nearly constant.

It may be obvious that it is the ratio of salt and weak acid or base that is important.

The *Henderson-Hasselbalch* relation points out the importance of the ratio:

$$HA + H_2O \xrightarrow{K_A} H_3O^+ + A^-$$
$$K_A = \frac{[H_3O^+][A^-]}{[HA]}$$

(HA = acid and $A^-$ = salt of the acid)

solving for $[H_3O^+]$

(1) $[H_3O^+] = \left(\frac{[HA]}{[A^-]}\right)(K_A)$ or,

(2) $pH = pK_A + \log\frac{[A^-]}{[HA]}$

(1) and (2) are equivalent expressions of the Henderson-Hasselbalch relation.

The *effectiveness of a buffer* can be understood in terms of this relation. The key points are:

(1) buffers are most effective when the desired pH (of the solution) is near the $pK_A$,

(2) ratios ($[A^-]$ / $[HA]$) in the range of 0.1 to 10 are where buffers are effective. Note that this is because the ratio changes slowly and, thus, the pH changes slowly when the ratio = 1 (i.e., $[A^-] = [HA]$).

Important buffers in the body are:

(1) phosphates—inorganic and organic (least important)
(2) carbonic acid—bicarbonate (most important)
(3) proteins—moderate importance.


### 3.11.2    Questions to Review Acids, Bases and Buffers

(1)    An acid is a substance that can donate hydrogen ion ($H^+$); this is a definition of acids given by:

(a) Lewis
(b) Arrhenius
(c) Bronsted-Lowry
(d) none of the above

(2)    A base is an electron pair donor; this is a definition of bases given by:

(a) Arrhenius
(b) Bronsted-Lowry
(c) Lewis
(d) none of the above

(3) The conjugate base of a weak acid (one that dissociates incompletely) is:

(a) strong
(b) weak

(4) Given the reaction of acid (HA) and base (B) below: $HA + B \rightleftharpoons A^- + HB^+$

(a) $A^-$ is the conjugate of acid of HA
(b) $A^-$ is the conjugate base of B
(c) $HB^+$ is the conjugate acid of B
(d) $HB^+$ is the conjugate base of HA

(5) The salt of a strong acid is:

(a) basic
(b) neutral
(c) acidic

(6) The salt of a weak acid is:

(a) basic
(b) neutral
(c) acidic

(7) The salt of a weak base is:

(a) basic
(b) neutral
(c) acidic

(8) Select the weak acid:

(a) HCl
(b) $HNO_3$
(c) $H_2SO_4$
(d) $CH_3CO_2H$

(9) Select the strongest acid:

(a) $CH_3CO_2H$
(b) $H_3PO_4$
(c) $H_2CO_3$
(d) $H_2SO_4$

(10) Select the weak base:

(a) NaOH
(b) KOH
(c) $NH_3$
(d) $Ca(OH)_2$

(11) All of the following are important buffer systems of the body except:

(a) carbonic acid-bicarbonate
(b) phosphates
(c) proteins
(d) nucleic acids

(12) A buffer solution is most effective when

(a) a strong acid or base and its salt are used
(b) the desired pH is near the pK of the acid or base
(c) the ratio of salt to acid (base) is less than 1/10 or greater than 10
(d) all of the above

(13) A buffer solution

(a) is made of strong acids and their salts
(b) is made of strong bases and their salts
(c) resists changes in pH when acids or bases are added
(d) all of the above

(14) Borane, 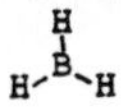 with boron having an atomic number of five and B-H bonds being relatively strong covalent bonds, is a(n):

(a) acid by Bronsted-Lowry
(b) acid by Lewis
(c) acid by Arrhenius
(d) base by Lewis

(15) Ammonia, $H-\overset{..}{\underset{H}{N}}-H$ is a(n):

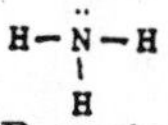

(a) acid by Bronsted-Lowry
(b) base by Bronsted-Lowry
(c) base by Lewis
(d) both (b) and (c)

(16) Pyruvic acid is a weak acid. Sodium hydroxide is a strong base. These are combined to form water and sodium pyruvate (a salt). If this salt is placed in water, the solution will be:

(a) basic
(b) neutral
(c) acidic

(17) Given the acid HA that dissociates into $H^+$ and $A^-$, the acid dissociation constant ($K_A$) is:

(a) $K_A = \dfrac{[H^+][A^-]}{[HA]}$

(b) $K_A = \dfrac{[HA]}{[H^+][A^-]}$

(c) $K_A = [HA][H^+][A^-]$

(d) $K_A = \dfrac{[HA][H^+]}{[A^-]}$

(18) Acid #1 has an acid dissociation constant ($K_{A_1}$) of $5 \times 10^{-5}$. Acid #2 has a $K_{A_2} = 9 \times 10^{-7}$:

(a) acid #1 is a weaker acid than acid #2
(b) the conjugate base of acid #1 is a weaker base than the conjugate base of acid #2
(c) both (a) and (b)
(d) neither (a) or (b)

(19) Fifty mls of a 2M solution of HCl contains how many milliequivalents of acid?

(a) 100
(b) 10
(c) 1
(d) 0.1

(20) What volume of an 0.1M acid would be required to neutralize 50 mls of an 0.3M base?

(a) about 17 mls
(b) 150 mls
(c) 300 mls
(d) 450 mls

(21) If 100 mls of a 2M solution of acid neutralizes 25 mls of a solution of base, the normality of the base is:

(a) 0.5M
(b) 2M
(c) 4M
(d) 8M

(22) Select the incorrect expression of pH ($[H^+]$ = hydrogen ion concentration):

(a) $pH = -\log [H^+]$
(b) $pH = \log [H^+]^{-1}$
(c) $pH = 1/\log [H^+]$
(d) $pH = \log(1/[H^+])$

(23) A solution has a hydroxide ion concentration of $10^{-8}$, the pH is

(a) 0
(b) 1
(c) 6
(d) 8

(24) A solution has a hydrogen ion concentration ($[H^+]$) of $2 \times 10^{-6}$; the pH is ($\log 2 = 0.30$):

(a) 4.3
(b) 5.7
(c) 6.3
(d) 12.3

(25) A solution has a pH = 9.3. The hydrogen ion concentration is: (antilog $0.30 = 2$, antilog $0.70 = 5$):

(a) $5 \times 10^{-9}$
(b) $2 \times 10^{-9}$
(c) $5 \times 10^{-10}$
(d) $2 \times 10^{-10}$

(26) A solution has a pOH = 9, the hydrogen ion concentration is:

(a) $10^{-9}$
(b) $10^9$
(c) $10^5$
(d) $10^{-5}$

(27) The pH of a 0.01M solution of HCl (strong acid) is:

(a) 1
(b) 2
(c) $-1$
(d) need more information

(28) Calculate the pH of a 0.001M solution of NaOH (strong base):

(a) 11
(b) 4
(c) 1
(d) 3

(29) A 0.10M solution of monoprotic weak acid is 10% ionized, the pH is:

(a) 0.01
(b) 0.1
(c) 1
(d) 2

(30) If the $K_A$ is much less than the original concentration $HA_O$ of a *weak* acid in solution, and $H^+$ = hydrogen ion concentration, then:

(a) $K_A \approx [H^+] + [HA_O]$
(b) $[H^+] \approx \sqrt{K_A[HA_O]}$
(c) $K_A \approx [H^+]/[HA_O]$
(d) $[H^+] \approx \sqrt{K_A/[HA_O]}$

(31) The acid dissociation constant ($K_A$) of a weak monoprotic acid is $4 \times 10^{-5}$. The $[H^+]$ of a 0.1M solution is:

(a) $4 \times 10^{-6}$
(b) $4 \times 10^{-5}$
(c) $2 \times 10^{-4}$
(d) $2 \times 10^{-3}$

(32) Which point (or line) on the graph below showing the titration of a weak monoprotic acid by a base represents the $pK_A$ of the acid?

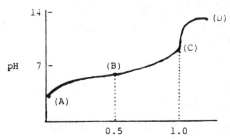

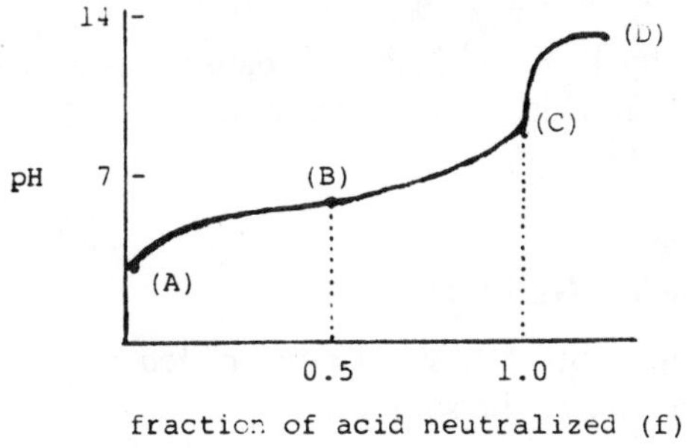

(a) A
(b) B
(c) C
(d) D

(33) All of the following could be used to make a buffer solution except:

(a) $H_2CO_3$
(b) $H_2SO_4$
(c) $NH_4OH$
(d) $CH_3CO_2H$

(34) A buffer solution that is 0.1M in an acid (with a $pK_A = 5$) and its salt which is 1.0M would have a pH of:

(a) 5.1
(b) 6
(c) 6.1
(d) 7

(35) A buffer solution with a pH = 3.3 is desired. An acid (with a $pK_A = 4.3$) and its salt are available. What ratio of salt to acid is required?

(a) 10
(b) 1
(c) 1/10
(d) 1/100

## 3.11.3     Answers to Questions in Section 3.11.2

( 1) c   ( 2) c   ( 3) b   ( 4) c   ( 5) b   ( 6) a   ( 7) c   ( 8) d   ( 9) d   (10) c   (11) d
(12) b   (13) c   (14) b   (15) d   (16) a   (17) a   (18) b   (19) a   (20) b   (21) d   (22) c
(23) c   (24) b   (25) c   (26) d   (27) b   (28) a   (29) d   (30) b   (31) d   (32) b   (33) b
(34) b   (35) c


## 3.11.4     Discussion of Answers to Questions in Section 3.11.2

*Questions #1 to #13:* Adequately discussed in Section.

*Question #14* (Answer: b) Since the atomic number is five, the electron configuration is $1s^2$ $2s^2$ $2p^1$. Then there are only 3 bonding electrons ($2s^2$ $2p^1$) to fill the four possible bonding orbitals ($2s$, $2p_x$, $2p_y$, $2p_z$). This means there is one vacant orbital that can accept an electron pair. Lewis' definition of an acid is an electron pair acceptor. The information about the covalent bond is to suggest that the H's do not dissociate, and, therefore, the Arrhenius and Bronsted-Lowry definitions do not hold.

*Question #15* (Answer: d) Ammonia is a base by Bronsted-Lowry because it is a proton acceptor. It is also a base by Lewis because it is an electron pair donator.

*Question #16* (Answer: a) The reaction is,

$$\text{pyruvic acid} + NaOH \rightarrow H_2O + Na \text{ pyruvate}$$
$$Na \text{ pyruvate} + HOH \rightleftharpoons \text{pyruvic acid} + Na^+ + OH^-$$

It is the free $OH^-$ in solution that makes the solution basic. Undissociated acid (e.g., pyruvic acid) has no effect on the acidity or basicity of the solution.

*Question #17* (Answer: a) The $K_A$ is defined as the equilibrium constant of this reaction:

$$HA \rightleftharpoons H^+ + A^- \text{ at equilibrium}$$

This is given as:
$$K_A = \frac{[H^+][A^-]}{[HA]}$$

*Question #18* (Answer: b) The larger the $K_A$, the stronger the acid. Also, stronger acids have weaker conjugate bases (see Section for terminology). Note that $10^{-5} > 10^{-7}$, this means acid #1 is stronger than acid #2 and its conjugate base is weaker.

*Question #19* (Answer: a)

| | |
|---|---|
| MV = moles | if V = liters, M = moles/liter |
| MV = millimoles (mm) | if V = mls, M = mm/ml |
| (2mm/ml)(50 mls) = 100 mm. | |

*Question #20* (Answer: b)

$$M_A V_A = M_B V_B$$
$$V_A = \frac{M_B V_B}{M_A} = \frac{(0.3)(50)}{(0.1)} = (3)(50) = 150 \text{ mls.}$$

*Question #21* (Answer: d)

$$M_A V_A = M_B V_B$$
$$M_B = \frac{M_A V_A}{V_B} = \frac{(2)(100)}{(25)} = (2)(4) = 8 \text{ M}$$

*Question #22* (Answer: c) Recall that,

$$-\log x = \log x^{-1} = \log \left(\frac{1}{x}\right).$$

*Question #23* (Answer: c) Since,

$$K_W = [H^+][OH^-] = 10^{-14}$$

$$[H^+] = \frac{10^{-14}}{[OH^-]} = \frac{10^{-14}}{10^{-8}} = 10^{-6}$$

then:

$$pH = -\log[H^+] = -\log 10^{-6} = -(-6) = +6$$
$$(\log 10^{-6} = -6 \text{ the log of any power of 10 is the exponent}).$$

Or:

$$pOH = -\log[OH^-] = -\log 10^{-8} = -(-8) = 8$$
$$pH + pOH = 14$$
$$pH = 14 - pOH = 14 - 8 = 6$$

*Question #24* (Answer: b)

$$pH = -\log[H^+] = -\log 2 \times 10^{-6} = -(\log 2 + \log 10^{-6})$$
$$= -(0.30 - 6) = -(-5.7) = 5.7$$

Note carefully the signs above.

*Question #25* (Answer: c)

$$pH = -\log[H^+]$$
$$9.3 = -\log[H^+] = \log[H^+]^{-1}$$
$$10^{9.3} = 10^{\log[H^+]-1} = [H^+]^{-1} = 1/[H^+]$$
$$[H^+] = 1/10^{9.3} = 10^{-9.3} = 10^{-10+0.7} = 10^{0.7} \times 10^{-10} = 5 \times 10^{-10}$$

(antilog of $0.7 = 5$ or $10^{0.7} = 5$).

Study the steps carefully. Several important log relationships are shown.

*Question #26* (Answer: d) First method:

Step (a):   $pH + pOH = 14$
$$pH = 14 - pOH = 14 - 9 = 5$$

Step (b):
$$pH = -\log[H^+]$$
$$5 = -\log[H^+]$$
$$-5 = \log[H^+]$$
$$10^{-5} = [H^+]$$

Second method,

Step (a):
$$pOH = -\log[OH^-]$$
$$9 = -\log[OH^-]$$
$$-9 = \log[OH^-]$$
$$10^{-9} = [OH^-]$$

Step (b): $[H^+][OH^-] = 10^{-14}$
$$[H^+] + 10^{-14}/[OH^-] = 10^{-14}/10^{-9} = 10^{-5}$$

*Question #27* (Answer: b) The $[H^+]$ of a strong acid is the normality of the acid. For HCl, the molarity and normality are equal. Then:

(a) $[H^+] = 0.01 = 1 \times 10^{-2}$

(b) $pH = -\log[H^+] = -\log(10^{-2}) = -(-2) = 2$

*Question #28* (Answer: a) The hydroxide concentration of a strong base is its normality. The molarity (M) is the same as normality (N) for NaOH. Then:

(a) $[OH^-] = 0.001 = 1 \times 10^{-3} = 10^{-3}$

(b) $[H^+][OH^-] = 10^{-14}$

$\quad [H^+] = 10^{-14}/[OH^-] = 10^{-14}/10^{-3} = 10^{-11}$

(c) $pH = -\log[H^+] = -\log 10^{-11} = -(-11) = 11$.

Or, the problem may be solved by:

(a) $pOH = -\log[OH^-] = -\log(10^{-3}) = -(-3) = 3$

(b) $pH + pOH = 14$
$\quad pH = 14 - pOH = 14 - 3 = 11$.

*Question #29* (Answer: d) For the reaction given:

|  | **HA** | **H**$^+$ | **A**$^-$ |
|---|---|---|---|
| original: | $HA_O$ | O | O |
| equilibrium: | $0.9HA_O$ | $0.1HA_O$ | $0.1HA_O$ |

Then:

$\quad [H^+] = (0.1)(0.1) = 0.01 = 10^{-2}$

Then:

$\quad pH = -\log[H^+]$
$\quad\quad = -\log(10^{-2}) = -(-2) = 2$.

*Question #30* (Answer: b) This serves to point out a formula that can be used in the often met situation described in this question. It is discussed in the Section.

*Question #31* (Answer: d) The $[H^+]$ of a weak acid must be calculated from $K_A$. Since $0.1 \gg 4 \times 10^{-5}$, use the formula:

$\quad [H^+] = \sqrt{K_A[HA_O]} = \sqrt{(4 \times 10^{-5})(10^{-1})} = \sqrt{4 \times 10^{-6}}$
$\quad\quad = \sqrt{4} \times \sqrt{10^{-6}} = 2 \times 10^{-3}$

and:

$2 \times 10^{-3} \ll 10^{-1} (0.002 \ll 0.1)$ so the assumption is correct. An alternative method to solve the problem is:

$$HA \rightleftharpoons H^+ + A^-$$

| start: | 0.1 | 0 | 0 |
|---|---|---|---|
| equilibrium: | $0.1 - x$ | x | x |

$K_A = \dfrac{[H^+][A^-]}{[HA]} = \dfrac{[x][x]}{[0.1-x]} = \dfrac{x^2}{0.1-x} = \dfrac{x^2}{0.1}$ (assume $x \ll 0.1$)

$\quad 4 \times 10^{-5} = x^2/10^{-1}$
$\quad\quad x^2 = (10^{-1})(4 \times 10^{-5}) = 4 \times 10^{-6}$
$\quad x = \sqrt{4 \times 10^{-6}} = \sqrt{4} \times \sqrt{10^{-6}} = 2 \times 10^{-3}$

*Question #32* (Answer: b) This is shown in the Section. The $pK_A$ of an acid is the pH at which it can be half neutralized or $f = 0.5$.

*Question #33* (Answer: b) $H_2SO_4$ is a strong acid. Strong acids or bases do not make good buffers.

*Question #34* (Answer: b) Use Henderson-Hasselbalch relation:

$\quad pH = pK_A + \log\dfrac{[A^-]}{[HA]} = 5 + \log\dfrac{1.0}{0.1} = 5 + \log 10 = 5 + 1 = 6$

*Question #35* (Answer: c) Use the Henderson-Hasselbalch relation,

$$pH = pK_A + \log \frac{[A^-]}{[HA]}$$

$$3.3 = 4.3 + \log \frac{[A^-]}{[HA]}$$

$$-1 = \log \frac{[A^-]}{[HA]}$$

$$10^{-1} = [A^-]/[HA]$$

$$\frac{1}{10} = \frac{[A^-]}{[HA]}.$$

## 3.11.5    Vocabulary Checklist for Acids, Bases, and Buffers

_____ Arrhenius  
_____ Bronsted-Lowry  
_____ Lewis  
_____ conjugate base  
_____ conjugate acid

_____ neutralization  
_____ buffers  
_____ Henderson-Hasselbalch  
_____ titration  
_____ pH

## 3.11.6    Concepts, Principles, etc. Checklist for Acids, Bases, and Buffers

_____ definitions of acids and bases  
_____ strengths of acids/bases and their salts  
_____ definition and calculations using pH  
_____ titrations  
_____ neutralizations  
_____ buffer solutions and calculations

## 3.12    ELECTROCHEMISTRY

### 3.12.1    Review of Electrochemistry

Electrochemistry is the study of chemical reactions in which the reactants undergo a change in oxidation state (i.e., there is a transfer of electrons between atoms). The *oxidation state* (OS) of an atom is a convenient bookkeeping device for keeping track of the electrons in a reaction. The atoms do not actually possess the charge (when in a molecule) designated by the OS. The following rules (general with exceptions) are useful for determining the OS:

(1)    all elements have an OS = 0 in the elemental form, e.g., $O_2$, Fe, Na (these can exist as ions but then they are not in the elemental form);

(2)    hydrogen is $+1$ except when combined with metals as hydrides ($-1$);

(3)    oxygen is $-2$ except when combined with fluorine, then it is $+2$, or in peroxides ($-1$), or in superoxides ($-\frac{1}{2}$);

(4)    Fluorine is always $= -1$;

(5)    Group I metals (Li, Na, K, etc.) are $+1$;

(6)    Group II metals (Mg, Ca, Sr, Ba) are $+2$;

(7)    Halogens (Cl, Br, I) are $-1$ unless combined with F or O;

(8)     $Al = +3$;

(9)     charges (not OS) of some common complex ions:

| $SO_4^{-2}$ | sulfate | $CO_3^{-2}$ | carbonate |
| $NO_3^{-1}$ | nitrate | $CH_3CO_2^-$ | acetate |
| $PO_4^{-3}$ | phosphate | $ClO_4^-$ | perchlorate |
| $OH^-$ | hydroxide | | |

In an oxidation-reduction reaction, one (or more) atom(s) is always oxidized, and one (or more) atoms is always reduced. *Oxidation* is the loss of electrons (or equivalently the loss of hydrogen in organic chemistry), and *reduction* is the gain of electrons (or equivalently the gain of hydrogen in organic chemistry). An *oxidizing agent* is a substance that can take electrons from other atoms and is reduced. A *reducing agent* is a substance that can give electrons to other atoms and is oxidized. The overall reaction can be divided into the *oxidation half-reaction* and the *reduction half-reaction*, for example:

overall reaction:           $Zn + CU^{+2} \rightleftharpoons Zn^{+2} + Cu$

oxidation half-reaction:    $Zn \rightleftharpoons Zn^{+2} + 2e^-$

reduction half-reaction:    $CU^{+2} + 2e^- \rightleftharpoons Cu$

Note:

(1) the $e^-$ (electrons) in the oxidation (loss) half-reaction are on the right side (of the arrow), and for the reduction (gain) half-reaction they are on the left;

(2) the sum of the electrons in the balanced half-reactions must cancel out when added (algebraically) to get the overall reaction.

These half-reactions may occur at *electrodes* (a substance, a metal or carbon, at which electrons may be exchanged). An *anode* is an electrode that attracts the "negative" (relatively) substance, is positive itself and is where reduction of electrode occurs and oxidation of the solution occurs. A *cathode* is an electrode that attracts the "positive" (relative to *less* positive) substance, is negative itself, and is where oxidation of electrode and reduction of the solution occurs. That is, electrons enter the anode by the oxidation of some substance and move to the cathode where they exit by reducing some substance. To get from the anode to the cathode there must be a conducting connector, e.g., a wire or a salt bridge.

The capacity of one substance to give or take electrons from another substance is complex. Suffice it to say that electron affinities, ionization potentials, concentrations, pressures and temperature are all important. Fortunately, the relative ability of a substance to give or take electrons can be quantified in one number symbolized by E. E is the potential difference (or voltage, Section 5.7) that is generated when two substances are connected. This potential, when standardized, is called the *standard half-cell potential* (E°) as follows:

(1)     a *reference half-reaction* is established and its $E° = 0$,
        $2H^+ (1M) + 2e^- \rightarrow H_2(1 \text{ atm})$
        atm = atmosphere and M = molar

(2)     all other half-reactions are compared to this and the E° for each of them is determined,

(3)     to be E°, these standard conditions must hold:
        concentration of all solutes is 1M (one molar),
        pressure of all gases is 1 atm,
        temperature is 25°C (298°K).

*The standard half-cell potential* (E°) can be written as an oxidation half-reaction,

        $A \rightarrow A^{+n} + ne^-$,
or, as a reduction half-reaction
        $A^{+n} + ne^- \rightarrow A$.

The first is called an *oxidation cell potential*; the second is called a *reduction cell potential*. Usually the reduction cell potentials are used. Regardless of which one is used, the *interpretation* of E° is the same. The more positive the E°, the more likely the reaction to proceed to the right as written. Please note:

(1)     if the direction of the equation is reversed, the sign of E° changes to the opposite $(+ \to -)$ or $(- \to +)$,

(2)     the value of E° *is not* affected by the stoichiometry of the reaction.

To determine the *potential for a reaction*, call it $\Delta E°$, the appropriate E° for the half-cell reactions must be looked up, given the correct sign, and then added up. For example, given the reaction,

$$2A + B^{+2} \to 2A^{+1} + B$$

the oxidation half-reaction (O) is,

$$(O): 2A \to 2A^{+1} + 2e^-$$

the reduction half-reaction (R) is,

$$(R): B^{+2} + 2e^- \to B.$$

Then if a table of reduction potentials is available, one will find these (in the table)

$$A^{+1} + e^- \to A \qquad E° = -1.10V$$
$$B^{+2} + 2e \to B \qquad E° = +0.50V$$

These half-reactions from the reduction potential table are rewritten as they occur (the direction) in the given reaction:

$$(O): 2A \to 2A^{+1} + 2e^- \qquad E° = +1.10V$$
$$\underline{(R): 2e^- + B^{+2} \to B \qquad E° = +0.50V}$$

overall:    $2A + B^{+2} \to 2A^{+1} + B \quad \Delta E° = +1.60V$

Note: (1) when balancing the half-reaction, the E°, is not affected as for the (O) above,

(2) when reversing the equation as found in the table, the sign of E° (from the table) is reversed as for the (R),

(3) if the overall $\Delta E°$ is positive, then the reaction proceeds from left to right as written,

(4) if the overall $\Delta E°$ is negative, then the reaction proceeds in the reverse direction and it should be rewritten as such.

The value of $\Delta E°$ determines the maximal amount of work the reaction can perform. The relation is:

work (joules) $= (\Delta E)(q) = (\Delta E)(I)(\Delta t)$
$\Delta E =$ volts        q = charge in coulombs
    I = current in amperes (coulombs/sec)
    t = time in seconds

The equation is valid for electrolysis (below).

*Galvanic cells* produce a current and voltage internally by a chemical reaction. For example, a lead storage battery. The size of the potential, $\Delta E°$, is as calculated by the methods above.

*Concentration cells* can produce a current and voltage by differences in concentrations of the same substance. The larger the concentration difference, the larger the potential produced by the cell.

*Electrolysis* is the process whereby electrons are pushed into a system by an external voltage, and a reaction can be forced to go in a direction it could not go spontaneously. This is one way metals may be recovered from their salts. Also, gold or silver electroplating is done this way. The key relations are:

1F (faraday) = 96,500 coulombs = 1 mole of electrons (Faraday's Relation)

1 ampere of current = 1 coulomb/sec.

These relations are used to determine how much of a metal can be plated out by a given current acting over a certain time, or they can be used to calculate the reverse.

The suggested sequence of steps to *balance oxidation-reduction equations is:*

(1)     identify which substance(s) is(are) oxidized and reduced in the net ionic equation,

(2)     write half-reactions for each substance oxidized and reduced,

(3)     balance each half-reaction,

(4)     add half-reactions and the electrons should cancel out (multiply each half-reaction by a small whole number as necessary),

(5)     check by counting elements on each side,

(6)     Note: for each half-reaction and the overall reaction, the charges should be equal on each side of the equation as should the mass (number of each element on each side); often $H^+$, $OH^-$, or $H_2O$ can be added as needed depending on the pH of the solution.

### 3.12.2     Questions to Review Electrochemistry

(1)     The oxidation state of an element in its elemental form is:

(a) +1
(b) 0
(c) −1
(d) need electron configuration

(2)     All of the following generally have an oxidation state of +1 except:

(a) F
(b) Na
(c) H
(d) K

(3)     All of the following generally have an oxidation state of +2 except:

(a) Al
(b) Ca
(c) Ba
(d) Mg

(4)     Which complex ion below has a charge of −2?

(a) $NO_3^-$?
(b) $PO_4^-$?
(c) $ClO_4^-$?
(d) $SO_4^-$?

(5)     Oxidation of a molecule

(a) results in a gain of electrons;
(b) results in a more negative oxidation state;
(c) may be viewed as the loss of hydrogen in some cases;
(d) all of the above

(6)    A oxidizing agent is a species that

(a) goes to a more negative oxidation state
(b) gains electrons
(c) is reduced
(d) all of the above

(7)    In the reduction half-reaction, the electrons appear on the _____ of the equation.

(a) right side
(b) left side
(c) either side

(8)    When the oxidation and reduction half-reactions are added, the sum of the electrons is:

(a) positive
(b) negative
(c) zero
(d) any of the above

(9)    Oxidation of the solution (or solute) occurs at the:

(a) anode
(b) cathode
(c) neither
(d) both

(10)   "Positive" substances are attracted to the:

(a) anode
(b) cathode
(c) neither
(d) both

(11)   The direction of electron flow is:

(a) from anode to cathode
(b) from cathode to anode
(c) either way

(12)   All of the half-cell potentials ($\Delta E$) use the _____ as the reference.

(a) hydrogen ($H_2$) half-cell
(b) oxygen ($O_2$) half-cell
(c) carbon (C) half-cell
(d) arbitrarily set zero point

(13)   The $\Delta E°$ depends on all the following variables except:

(a) temperature
(b) concentrations
(c) pressures of gases
(d) all of the above

(14)   Half-cell potentials are usually written as:

(a) oxidation half-reactions
(b) reduction half-reactions

(15)   The more negative the value of $\Delta E°$,

(a) the more likely the reaction is to proceed left to right (as written)
(b) the more likely the reaction is to proceed right to left (the reverse of the way it is written)
(c) either of the above

(16) If the coefficients in a half-reaction are doubled, the $\Delta E°$ is:

(a) doubled
(b) halved
(c) not affected

(17) If $\Delta E$ = electrical potential, I = current and $\Delta t$ = time the current is flowing, then the work (or energy) = W generated is:

(a) $W = \dfrac{(\Delta E)(I)}{\Delta t}$

(b) $W = \dfrac{\Delta E}{(I)(\Delta t)}$

(c) $W = (\Delta E)(I)(\Delta t)$
(d) none of the above

(18) If the potential created by a chemical reaction is used to move a current, the cell created is called a:

(a) concentration cell
(b) galvanic cell
(c) electrolytic cell
(d) none of the above

(19) One faraday corresponds to

(a) one volt of cell potential
(b) 96,487 amperes
(c) one mole of electrons
(d) all of the above

(20) What is the oxidation state of Pt in $PtCl_4^{-2}$?

(a) $+2$
(b) $-2$
(c) $+4$
(d) $-4$

(21) The oxidation state of Co in $Co_3(PO_4)_2$ is:

(a) $+2$
(b) $+3$
(c) $-2$
(d) $-3$

(22) The oxidation state of Cr in $K_2Cr_2O_7$ is:

(a) $+3$
(b) $+6$
(c) $+12$
(d) $-12$

(23) The oxidation state of Fe in $FeCl_2$ is:

(a) $-4$
(b) $-2$
(c) $+4$
(d) $+2$

(24) Which of the following would be considered a reduction half-reaction?

(a) $A^{+2} + 2e^- \rightarrow A$
(b) $A \rightarrow A^{+2} + 2e^-$
(c) both
(d) neither

(25) The reduction half-reaction of the following reaction is: $A^{+2} + 2B \rightarrow A + 2B^{+1}$

(a) $2B \rightarrow 2B^{+1} + 2e^-$
(b) $A \rightarrow A^{+2} + 2e^-$
(c) $A^{+2} + 2e^- \rightarrow A$
(d) $2B^{+1} + 2e^- \rightarrow 2B$

(26) Suppose A and $B^{+2}$ are placed in the same solution. Will there be a spontaneous reaction? If so, what is the balanced equation? Below are the pertinent reduction potentials:

$$A^{+1} + e^- \rightarrow A \qquad E° = -1.50 \text{ volts}$$
$$B^{+2} + 2e^- \rightarrow B \qquad E° = -1.00 \text{ volts}$$

(a) no, because the $\Delta E°$ of the reaction is negative
(b) yes, $A + B^{+2} \rightarrow A^{+1} + B$
(c) yes, $2A + B^{+2} \rightarrow 2A^{+1} + B$
(d) yes, $2A + B \rightarrow 2A^{+1} + B^{+2}$

Use the following data for the remainder of the problems.

## Standard Reduction Potentials at 25° C

| Acid Solutions: | Half-Reaction | E°(volts) |
|---|---|---|
| | $Ca^{+2} + 2e^- \rightarrow Ca$ | $-2.9$ |
| | $Na^+ + e^- \rightarrow Na$ | $-2.7$ |
| | $Al^{+3} + 3e^- \rightarrow Al$ | $-1.7$ |
| | $Mn^{+2} + 2e^- \rightarrow Mn$ | $-1.2$ |
| | $Zn^{+2} + 2e^- \rightarrow Zn$ | $-0.8$ |
| | $Cu^{+2} + 2e^- \rightarrow Cu$ | $+0.3$ |
| | $I_2(s) + 2e^- \rightarrow 2I^-$ | $+0.5$ |
| | $PtCl_4^{-2} + 2e^- \rightarrow Pt + 4Cl^-$ | $+0.7$ |
| | $Ag^+ + e^- \rightarrow Ag$ | $+0.8$ |
| | $O_2 + 4H^+ + 4e^- \rightarrow 2H_2O(l)$ | $+1.23$ |
| | $Cr_2O_7^{-2} + 6e^- \rightarrow Cr^{+3}$ | $+1.33$ |
| | $Cl_2 + 2e^- \rightarrow 2Cl^-$ | $+1.36$ |
| | $MnO_4^- + 5e^- \rightarrow Mn^{+2}$ | $+1.51$ |

**Equations:**

$$\Delta E = \Delta E° - \frac{0.059}{n} \log \frac{[C]^c[D]^d}{[A]^a[B]^b} = \Delta E° - \frac{0.059}{n} \log K \text{ at } 25°C$$

(the Nernst Equation)
for $aA + bB \rightarrow cC + dD$

Note [ solids ] = 1, [ gases ] = atmospheres

$\Delta E°$ = standard cell potential
$\Delta E$ = cell potential at new set of concentrations
$n$ = number of electrons exchanged in the reaction as written
$K$ = equilibrium constant

$$\Delta G° = -nF\Delta E° \qquad \text{or} \qquad \Delta G = -nF\Delta E$$

$F$ = faraday = 23,000 cals/volts ( = 96,5000 coulombs)
$n$ = number of electrons exchanged in reaction as written
$\Delta E$ = cell potential
$\Delta G$ = free energy of reaction = cals

(27) The sum of all the coefficients in the following equation when balanced (the solution is *acidic* and *aqueous*) is: $\quad Ag + NO^{-3} \rightarrow Ag^+ + NO$

(a) 9
(b) 14
(c) 15
(d) 18

(28) The sum of *all* the coefficients in the following equation when balanced (solution is *basic* and *aqueous*) is:

$$N_2H_4 + Cu(OH)_2 \rightarrow N_2 + Cu$$

(a) 8
(b) 10
(c) 12
(d) 14

(29) The sum of *all* the coefficients in the following equation when balanced (solution is *basic* and *aqueous*) is:

$$ClO_2 + OH^- \rightarrow ClO_2^- + ClO_3^-$$

(a) 5
(b) 7
(c) 9
(d) 10

Use the following information for Questions #30 to #39.

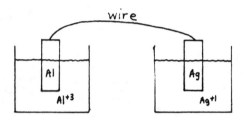

both solutions are acidic

(30) Which substances are the reactants in the above cell assuming concentrations are all standard (1M)?

(a) $Al + Ag$
(b) $Al^{+3} + Ag^+$
(c) $Al + Ag^+$
(d) $Ag + Al^{+3}$

(31) Write the balanced oxidation half-reaction of the above cell:

(a) $Ag^+ + e^- \rightarrow Ag$
(b) $Al^{+3} + 3e^- \rightarrow Al$
(c) $Ag \rightarrow Ag^+ + e^-$
(d) $Al \rightarrow Al^{+3} + 3e^-$

(32) Reduction of the solution is occurring at the _____ electrode.

(a) Al
(b) Ag
(c) neither
(d) both

(33) The Al electrode is _____ and is called the _____.

(a) positive, anode
(b) positive, cathode
(c) negative, anode
(d) negative, cathode

(34) The flow of electrons is from the _____ electrode to the _____ electrode.

(a) Al, Ag
(b) Ag, Al

(35)    The sum of coefficients in the balanced equation for the reaction is:

(a) 4
(b) 6
(c) 8
(d) 10

(36)    The *standard* cell potential ($\Delta E°$) for the reaction is _____ volts.

(a) $-0.9$
(b) 0.9
(c) 2.5
(d) 4.1

(37)    Using the Nernst equation, the cell potential ($\Delta E$), in volts, at 25°C as written in question #35 for $[Al^{+3}] = 0.1m$ and $[Ag^+] = 0.1m$

(a) $-1.14$
(b) 1.14
(c) 2.46
(d) 2.10

(38)    The free energy ($\Delta G$) of the reaction for the conditions, given in calories, is:

(a) $+169,740$
(b) $-169,740$
(c) $+56,580$
(d) $-56,580$

(39)    This type of cell may be *best* considered a(n):

(a) concentration cell
(b) galvanic cell
(c) electrolytic cell
(d) none of these

(40)    Which of the following substances will oxidize Mn?

(a) $Al^{+3}$
(b) Na
(c) $Zn^{+2}$
(d) $Ca^{+2}$

(41)    Which of the following substances will reduce $I_2(s)$?

(a) Pt
(b) $Ag^+$
(c) $Cl^-$
(d) Zn

(42)    Which of the following is a stronger oxidizing agent than $Cr_2O_7^{-2}$?

(a) $Cl^-$
(b) $MnO_4^-$
(c) $O_2$
(d) $Ag^+$

(43)    Which of the following is a stronger reducing agent than Zn?

(a) $Cu^{+2}$
(b) $Na^+$
(c) Al
(d) Pt

(44)    A current of 10 amps is passed through a solution of $Ag^+$ for one hour. What weight of Ag (GAW = 108) will be plated out?

   (a) 40.3g
   (b) 22.4g
   (c) 5.6g
   (d) 1.2g

## 3.12.3    Answers to Questions in Section 3.12.2

( 1) b   ( 2) a   ( 3) a   ( 4) d   ( 5) c   ( 6) d   ( 7) b   ( 8) c   ( 9) a   (10) b   (11) a
(12) a   (13) d   (14) b   (15) b   (16) c   (17) c   (18) b   (19) c   (20) a   (21) a   (22)b
(23) d   (24) a   (25) c   (26) c   (27) b   (28) b   (29) b   (30) c   (31) d   (32) b   (33) a
(34) a   (35) c   (36) c   (37) c   (38) b   (39) b   (40) c   (41) d   (42) b   (43) c   (44) a

## 3.12.4    Discussion of Answers to Questions in Section 3.12.2

*Questions #1 to #19:* Adequately explained in Section.

*Question #20* (Answer: a) An equation is:

   $Pt + 4Cl = -2$        ($Cl = -1$ from rules in Section)
   $Pt + 4(-1) = -2$
   $Pt - 4 = -2$
   $Pt = +2.$

*Question #21* (Answer: a) An equation is:

   $3Co + 2\,PO_4 = 0$        ($PO_4 = -3$ from Section)
   $3\,Co + 2(-3) = 0$
   $3\,Co - 6 = 0$
   $3\,Co = +6$
   $Co = +2$

*Question #22* (Answer: b) An equation is:

   $2K + 2Cr + 70 = 0$
   $2(+1) + 2Cr + 7(-2) = 0$
   $2Cr - 12 = 0$
   $2Cr = +12$
   $C = +6$

*Question #23* (Answer: d) The equation is:

   $Fe + 2Cl = 0$
   $Fe + 2(-1) = 0$
   $Fe - 2 = 0$
   $Fe = +2.$

*Question #24* (Answer: a) A reduction half-reaction has the electrons on the left side (so that there is a gain) as in (a).

*Question #25* (Answer: c) In the reaction as written, the $A^{+2}$ is being reduced to A: i.e., $A^{+2} \rightarrow A$ is a change to a more negative (less positive) oxidation state which is reduction.

*Question #26* (Answer: c) The half-reactions would be:

   $A \rightarrow A^{+1} + e^-$        $E° = +1.50$ V (because reversed)
   $B^{+2} + 2e^- \rightarrow B$        $E° = -1.00V,$

This is because A and $B^{+2}$ are the reactants given. Then balance electrons (by multiplying half-reactions as necessary) so they sum to zero:

$$2A \rightarrow 2A^{+1} + 2e^- \qquad E° = +1.50V \text{ (note } E° \text{ does not change)}$$
$$B^{+2} + 2e^- \rightarrow B \qquad E° = -1.0V$$

Sum: $2A + B^{+2} \rightarrow 2A^{+1} + B \qquad \Delta E° = +0.50V$

Since, the $\Delta E°$ is positive, the reaction will occur spontaneously as written.

*Question #27* (Answer: b) Follow the scheme given in the Section:

(1)   Ag is oxidized; the N in $NO_3^-$ is reduced

$$Ag + NO_3^- \rightarrow Ag^+ + NO$$
oxidation states: $0 \; +5, -2 \qquad +1 \quad +2, -2$

(2)   (a) oxidation half-reaction

$$Ag \rightarrow Ag^+ + e^-$$

(b) reduction half-reaction

$$3e^- + NO_3^- \rightarrow NO$$

(3)   (a) $Ag \rightarrow Ag^+ + e^-$        already balanced

(b) $NO_3^- + 3e^- \rightarrow NO$        N's are balanced

$4H^+ + NO_3^- + 3e^- \rightarrow NO$        Add $H^+$ to left to balance charge on *both* sides

$4H^+ + NO_3^- + 3e^- \rightarrow NO + 2H_2O$        Add $H_2O$ to right to balance H's and O's

(4)   $3\,Ag \rightarrow 3\,Ag^+ + 3e^-$

$$\underline{4H^+ + NO_3^- + 3e^- \rightarrow NO + 2H_2O}$$
$$4H^+ + 3Ag + NO_3^- \rightarrow 3Ag^+ + NO + 2H_2O$$
sum of coefficients $= 4 + 3 + 1 + 3 + 1 + 2 = 14$

(5)   everything checks

Note that for acidic or basic solutions the $H^+$ or $OH^-$, respectively, are usually on the left side of the equation. Also, the balancing of charge does not have to make the overall charge neutral but must make the net charge on one side equal the net charge on the other.

*Question #28* (Answer: b) As in #27 above,

(1)   N is oxidized, Cu is reduced

$$N_2H_4 + Cu(OH)_2 \rightarrow N_2 + Cu$$
oxidation states: $-2, +1 \quad -2, -2, +1 \qquad 0 \qquad 0$

(2)   (a) oxidation half-reaction
$$N_2H_4 \rightarrow N_2 + 4e^- \qquad \text{(each N loses two electrons)}$$

(b) reduction half-reaction
$$2e^- + Cu(OH)_2 \rightarrow Cu$$

(3)   balance each half-reaction

(a) $N_2H_4 \rightarrow N_2 + 4e^-$        N's are already balanced

$4\,OH^- + N_2H_4 \rightarrow N_2 + 4e^-$        Add $OH^-$ to left to balance charge

$4\,OH^- + N_2H_4 \rightarrow N_2 + 4e^- + 4\,H_2O$        Add $H_2O$ to right to balance the O's (and H's)

(b) $2e^- + Cu(OH)_2 \rightarrow Cu$        Cu's are balanced

$2e^- + Cu(OH)_2 \rightarrow Cu + 2OH^-$        balance charge by adding $OH^-$ to the right side, H's and O's are then balanced

(4)  $\quad$ $4OH^- + N_2H_4 \rightarrow N_2 + 4H_2O + 4e^-$
$\dfrac{4e^- + 2Cu(OH)_2 \rightarrow 2Cu + 4OH^-}{N_2H_4 + 2Cu(OH)_2 \rightarrow N_2 + 2Cu + 4H_2O}$ $\quad$ (multiply by 2)

sum of coefficients $= 1 + 2 + 1 + 2 + 4 = 10$.

(5)  $\quad$ everything checks out

*Question #29* (Answer: b) Follow steps as in #27:

(1)  $\quad$ Cl is oxidized, Cl is reduced

$\qquad$ $ClO_2 + OH^- \rightarrow ClO_2^- + ClO_3^-$

oxidation states: $\quad +4, -2 \quad -2, +1 \quad +3, -2 \quad +5, -2$

(2)  $\quad$ (a) oxidation half-reaction

$\qquad$ $ClO_2 \rightarrow ClO_3^- + e^-$

$\quad$ (b) reduction half-reaction

$\qquad$ $e^- + ClO_2 \rightarrow ClO_2^-$

(3)  $\quad$ balance each half-reaction

$\quad$ (a) $ClO_2 \rightarrow ClO_3^- + e^-$ $\qquad\qquad$ Cls already balanced, add $OH^-$ to
$\qquad\qquad\qquad\qquad\qquad\qquad\qquad\qquad$ left to balance charge

$\qquad$ $2\,OH^- + ClO_2 \rightarrow ClO_3^- + e^-$
$\qquad$ $2\,OH^- + ClO_2 \rightarrow ClO_3^- + H_2O + e^-$ $\quad$ Add $H_2O$ to right to balance O and H

$\quad$ (b) $e^- + ClO_2 \rightarrow ClO_2^-$ $\qquad\qquad$ Cl's, O and charge are already balanced

(4)  $\quad$ $2\,OH^- + ClO_2 \rightarrow ClO_3^- + H_2O + e^-$
$\dfrac{e^- + ClO_2 \rightarrow ClO_2^-}{2OH^- + 2ClO_2 \rightarrow ClO_2^- + ClO_3^- + H_2O}$

sum of coefficients $= 2 + 2 + 1 + 1 + 1 = 7$

*Question #30* (Answer: c) There are four possible substances for reactants Al, $Al^{+3}$, Ag and $Ag^+$; only two can be reactants. One will be oxidized and one will be reduced. The candidates for oxidation are Al and Ag; the candidates for reduction are $Al^{+3}$ and $Ag^{+1}$. Since the $\Delta E°$ for $Al \rightarrow Al^{+3} + 3e^-$ ($+1.7$) is larger than the $\Delta E°$ for $Ag \rightarrow Ag^+ + e^-$ ($+0.8$) which is larger than the $\Delta E°$ for $Al^{+3} + 3e \rightarrow Al$ ($-1.7$), the Al must be oxidized and the $Ag^+$ reduced.

*Question #31* (Answer: d) From #30, the Al is oxidized to get: $Al \rightarrow Al^{+3} + 3e^-$.

*Question #32* (Answer: b) From #30, the $Ag^+$ is being reduced so reduction must be occurring at the Ag electrode.

*Question #33* (Answer: a) Oxidation is occurring at the Al electrode from #32. Oxidation occurs at the anode which is positive.

*Question #34* (Answer: a) The Al electrode is losing electrons ($Al \rightarrow Al^{+3} + 3e^-$) which travel through the wire to the Ag electrode where they are used ($Ag^+ + e^- \rightarrow Ag$).

*Question #35* (Answer: c) Following the steps in the Section for balancing equations:

(1)  $\quad$ Al is oxidized, $Ag^+$ is reduced

$\qquad\qquad$ $Al + Ag^+ \rightarrow Al^{+3} + Ag$

oxidation states: $\qquad 0 \quad +1 \quad +3 \quad 0$

(2)  $\quad$ (a) oxidation half-reaction

$\qquad$ $Al \rightarrow Al^{+3} + 3e^-$

$\quad$ (b) reduction half-reaction

$\qquad$ $e^- + Ag^+ \rightarrow Ag$

(3)    both are already balanced

(4)    $Al \rightarrow Al^{+3} + 3e^-$

$\underline{3e^- + 3Ag^+ \rightarrow 3Ag}$    (multiplied by 3)

$Al + 3Ag^+ \rightarrow Al^{+3} + 3Ag$

sum of coefficients $= 1 + 3 + 1 + 3 = 8$

(5)    everything checks

*Question #36* (Answer: c) Using the balanced half-reactions from #35 and the E° from the table:

$Al \rightarrow Al^{+3} + 3e^-$    $E° = +1.7$ (sign reversed)

$\underline{3e^- + 3Ag^+ \rightarrow 3Ag}$    $E° = +0.8$

Sum: $Al + 3Ag^+ \rightarrow Al^{+3} + 3Ag$    $\Delta E° = +2.5$ volts

*Question #37* (Answer: c) The Nernst equation for the balanced reaction is:

$$\Delta E = \Delta E° - \frac{0.059}{n} \log \frac{[Al^{+3}]}{[Ag^+]^3} \approx 2.5 - \frac{0.06}{3} \log \frac{0.1}{(0.1)^3} \approx 2.5 - 0.02 \log \frac{10^{-1}}{(10^{-1})^3}$$

$$\approx 2.5 - 0.02 \log \frac{10^{-1}}{10^{-3}} \approx 2.5 - 0.02 \log 10^2$$

$$\approx 2.5 - 0.02(2) \approx 2.5 - 0.04 \approx 2.46 \text{ volts.}$$

*Question #38* (Answer: b) The equation for $\Delta G$ is,

$$\Delta G = -nF\Delta E = -(3)(23,000)(2.46) \approx (-3)(2.5)(23,000) \approx -(7.5)(23,000)$$

$$\approx -(7)(23,000) - (\tfrac{1}{2})(23,000) \approx -161,000 - 11,500 = -172,500 \text{ cals}$$

$$= -172.5 \text{ kcals}$$

Exact answer by calculator $= -169,740$ cals.

*Question #39* (Answer: b) The voltage in this cell is generated by a chemical reaction. The difference in concentrations reflect that the conditions are not standard. The classic concentration cell would have either $Al^{+3}/Al$ or $Ag^+/Ag$ in both beakers but in different concentrations in each.

*Question #40* (Answer: c) If a substance (X) oxidizes Mn, it must take electrons from it and be reduced. The half-reactions are

oxidation:    $Mn \rightarrow Mn^{+2} + 2e^-$    $E° = +1.2$

reduction:    $X^{+n} + ne \rightarrow X$.

Therefore any substance will oxidize Mn if its reduction potential is greater than $-1.2$ volts (more positive than). Since the reduction potentials for $Ca^{+2}$ ($-2.9$) and $Al^{+3}$ ($-1.7$) are too negative and Na cannot be reduced normally, $Zn^{+2}$ ($-0.8$) is the best answer. Or any substance on the left side of the arrows below Mn will oxidize Mn.

*Question #41* (Answer: d) If a substance (X) reduces $I_2(s)$, it must be oxidized in the process. The half-reactions are:

reduction:    $I_2(s) + 2e^- \rightarrow 2I$    $E° = +0.5$

oxidation:    $X \rightarrow X^{+n} + ne^-$.

Therefore, any substance will reduce $I_2(s)$ if its oxidation potential (reverse of that found in table) is more positive than $-0.5$ volts. This makes Zn, with an oxidation potential $= +0.8$ volts, the only possibility given.

*Question #42* (Answer: b) Since oxidizing agents are reduced, another way of asking the problem is which substance has a more positive reduction potential. Referring to the table, $MnO_4^-$ is the only possibility.

*Question #43* (Answer: c) This question can be rephrased to ask which substance has a more positive oxidation potential than Zn. This is because reducing agents are oxidized. Remembering that the signs of the $\Delta E°$ and the directions of the equations are reversed to get oxidation potentials, the table shows that Al is the only possibility.

*Question #44* (Answer: a) This is an electrolysis problem. First, moles of electrons are determined:

$$\text{moles of electrons} = \frac{\text{charge passed}}{96{,}500 \text{ coulombs/mole of elec.}} = \frac{36{,}000}{96{,}500} = \frac{360}{965}$$

$$\text{charged passed} = (\text{current})(\text{time in secs}) = \text{coulombs}$$
$$= (10)(60 \times 60) = (10)(3600) = 36{,}000$$

Since $Ag^+ + e^+ \rightarrow Ag$, the moles of electrons correspond to the moles of Ag plated out. (If, e.g., one had $Ni^{+2} + 2e^- \rightarrow Ni$, then each mole of electrons would plate out only ½ mole of Ni). Then,

$$\text{moles of electrons} = \text{moles of AG} = \text{weight of AG/GAW of Ag}$$

and,

$$\text{weight of Ag} = (\text{moles of Ag})(\text{GAW of Ag})$$
$$= (360/965)(108) \approx (360/970)(110) \approx (3/8)(110)$$
$$\approx (3/4)(55) \approx 165/4 \approx 41.25.$$

Exact answer by calculator = 40.29.

### 3.12.5 Vocabulary Checklist for Electrochemistry

_____ reduction half-cell potential
_____ oxidation
_____ reduction
_____ oxidizing agent
_____ reducing agent
_____ half-reactions
_____ anode
_____ cathode
_____ reference half-reaction
_____ oxidation state

_____ Galvanic cells
_____ concentration cells
_____ electrolysis
_____ Faraday
_____ Coulomb
_____ amperes
_____ current
_____ standard half-cell
_____ potential

### 3.12.6 Concepts, Principles, etc. Checklist for Electrochemistry

_____ terminology of electrochemistry
_____ writing and balancing half-reactions and electrochemical equations
_____ determination of cell potentials
_____ reactions at electrodes
_____ Faraday's relation and its application

## 3.13 REFERENCES FOR REVIEW OF GENERAL CHEMISTRY

Kennan, C.W., D. C. Kleinfelter, and J. H. Wood. *General College Chemistry*. Harper & Row Publishers, Inc.

> A descriptive text with coverage of theoretical concepts. It goes beyond requirements of the MCAT.

Mahan, B. *University Chemistry*. Addison-Wesley Publishing Co., Inc.

> Excellent introductory general chemistry text, but which goes beyond what is required for the MCAT.

Masterson, W. L., and E. J. Slowinski. *Chemical Principles*. Saunders College Publishing.

A good introductory text with very good problems. Might be one of the best texts for review, especially in problem solving, for the MCAT.

Murphy, D. B., and V. Rousseau. *Foundations of College Chemistry*. John Wiley & Sons, Inc.

A very good introductory text. More commensurate with the expectations of the MCAT.

Whitten, K. W., and K. D. Gailey. *General Chemistry with Qualitative Analysis*. Saunders College Publishing.

A systematic and conceptual approach to chemistry. Largely compatible with MCAT requirements in general chemistry.

# Chapter 4

# Review

## of

# Organic Chemistry

## 4.1 COVALENT BONDING

### 4.1.1 Review of Covalent Bonding

The *major elements* involved in organic compounds are carbon (C), hydrogen (H), oxygen (O), nitrogen (N) and halides (fluorine-F, chlorine-Cl, bromine-Br, iodine-I). Sulfur (S) and phosphorus (P) are also in many organic compounds. Carbon forms 4 bonds, N forms 3 and has one unshared pair of electrons, O forms 2 and has 2 unshared pairs of electrons. H forms one bond and each halogen forms one bond and has 3 unshared pairs of electrons—all of the above are assumed to be neutral. The possible bonds are *single bonds* (SB, one shared pair of electrons), *double bonds* (DB, two shared pairs of electrons) and *triple bonds* (TB, three shared pairs of electrons). C and N form all three types, O forms DB and SB and H and the halides (in organic compounds) form SB's only.

The C atom has one s orbital and three p orbitals in its outer bonding electron shells. (See Section 3.1.1). In organic molecules, these original atomic orbitals are recombined into *hybrid orbitals* made of part s and part p. If one s and three p's are mixed, there result four hybrid $sp^3$ *orbitals* (each consisting of one part s and three parts p) on the carbon atom. If one s orbital and two p orbitals mix, there result three $sp^2$ orbitals and one original p orbital on each carbon atom. If one s and one p mix, there result two *sp orbitals* and two original p orbitals on each carbon. The geometry of each of the orbitals is: sp³-tetrahedral, sp²-triangular and sp-linear (Fig. 4.1).

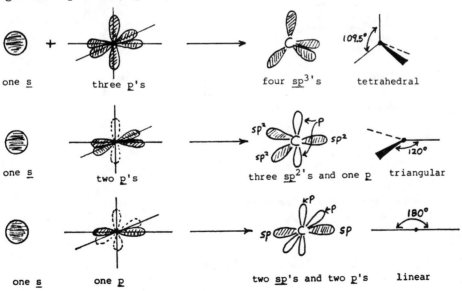

**Fig. 4.1—Hybrid Bonding Orbitals**

*Sigma (σ) bonds* have electron density between the nuclei. Sigma bonds are formed when hybrid orbitals (sp, sp², sp³) overlap directly. *Pi (π) bonds* have electron density (overlap) above and below the axis (and plane) of the atoms. They are formed by "sideways" overlap of the p orbitals. *Single bonds* are σ bonds. *Double bonds* are made of one σ bond and one π bond, *triple bonds* include one σ and two π bonds. Note that σ bonds are symmetric about the axis and can rotate freely. *Multiple bonds* (DB, TB), with π components, are not symmetric about the axis and are not free to rotate about it (Fig. 4.2).

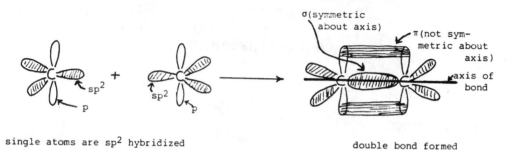

single atoms are sp² hybridized        double bond formed

Note: the sp²'s overlap between the nuclei to form the σ bond

the p's overlap above and below the axis between the C's to form a π bond

**Fig. 4.2—Sigma and Pi Bonds**

When adjacent atoms are sp² or sp hybridized, there is the possibility of side to side overlap of the leftover p orbitals over all of these atoms. This is called delocalization of the electrons in the π bonds of the molecule. Two ways of depicting these molecules are by the molecular orbital (MO) or the valence bond (resonance) approach. The MO approach takes a linear combination of atomic orbitals (LCAO) to form molecular orbitals which electrons go into to form bonds. These molecular orbitals cover the whole molecule, and, hence, the delocalization of electrons is depicted. In the *valence bond (resonance) approach*, there is a linear combination of different structures with localized π bonds (and unpaired electrons), which together depict the true molecule (the resonance hybrid). There is no one structure that is representative of the molecule (Fig. 4.3).

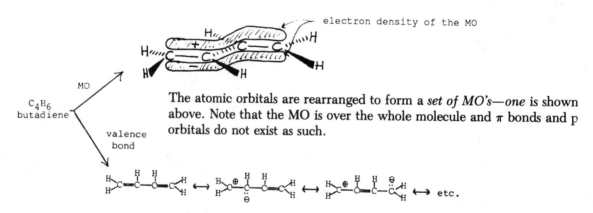

The atomic orbitals are rearranged to form a *set of MO's—one* is shown above. Note that the MO is over the whole molecule and π bonds and p orbitals do not exist as such.

Note that no one structure represents the molecule which is a composite of all of them. The π bonds and p orbitals do exist in each structure above.

**Fig. 4.3—Comparison of MO and Valence Bond Approaches**

It is the *valence electrons* (outer shell electrons) that enter into the formation of chemical bonds. (See sections 3.1.1 and 3.2.1). *Electron dot structures* are a means of illustrating the valence electrons and how they enter into bond formation. They are used in conjunction with the octet rule that states that a maximum of eight electrons is possible in the outermost shell of atoms. This rule holds only for the second row elements (C, N, O, F). Third row elements (Si, P, S, Cl) can use d orbitals and, hence, can have more. Examples of the use of the electron dot formulas:

(1) $CO_2$    C-4 valence electrons   $\cdot\ddot{c}\cdot$

           O-6 valence electrons     $:\ddot{o}:$

           combine single electrons (may have to make double or triple bonds)   $\ddot{o}::c::\ddot{o}$

(2) $CO_3{}^{-2}$ (an example of resonance)

           C-4 valence electrons

           O-6 valence electrons

        -2 means two extra electrons to place on the atoms

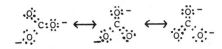

Each element, in the final structure, counts one half the electrons in a bond as its own and counts all unpaired electrons as its own. The sum of these two numbers should equal the number of valence electrons the element began with.

When atoms of differing electronegativity form the chemical bond, a situation of charge separation exists. For example,

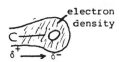

There is a slight pulling of electron density by the oxygen (the more electronegative) from the carbon (the less electronegative) as shown. This results in the C-O bond having *partial ionic character*. The separation of charge also causes an electrical dipole to be set up in the direction of the arrow as shown. A dipole has a positive end (the C above) and a negative end (the O above). A dipole will line up in an electric field (see Section 5.7.1). The most electronegative elements are: fluorine (4.0) > oxygen (3.5) > nitrogen (3.0) = chlorine (3.0). These are often combined with hydrogen (2.1) and carbon (2.5) and, hence result in bonds with partial ionic character. The numbers in parenthesis show eletronegativities. The *dipole moment* is a measure of the charge separation and, hence, the electronegativities of the elements that make up the bond. The larger the dipole moment, the larger the charge separation.

See Section 3.11.1.1 for a discussion of Lewis acids and bases.

### 4.1.2     Questions to Review Covalent Bonding

(1)     Which type of bond has electron density directly between the nuclei?

    (a) pi ($\pi$)
    (b) sigma ($\sigma$)
    (c) both
    (d) neither

(2) Which type of bond is formed by overlap of p orbitals perpendicular to the 2 nuclei?

(a) pi ($\pi$)
(b) sigma ($\sigma$)
(c) both
(d) neither

(3) Single bonds are composed of _____ bonds.

(a) pi ($\pi$)
(b) sigma ($\sigma$)
(c) both
(d) neither

(4) Double bonds are composed of _____ bonds.

(a) pi ($\pi$)
(b) sigma ($\sigma$)
(c) both
(d) neither

(5) Rotation about the bonding axis can occur with:

(a) pi ($\pi$) bonds
(b) double bonds
(c) both
(d) neither

(6) Delocalization of electrons (i.e., resonance) occurs over

(a) sigma bonds between separated atoms
(b) sigma bonds on adjacent atoms
(c) pi bonds on adjacent atoms
(d) pi bonds between separated atoms

(7) The resonance approach implies that

(a) one structure cannot be drawn which accurately depicts the electrons in the true molecule
(b) one structure can be drawn which accurately depicts the electrons in the true molecule

(8) The octet rule does not have to hold for which of the following elements?

(a) C
(b) O
(c) F
(d) P

(9) An acceptable resonance form of the following ion is:

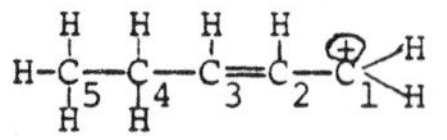

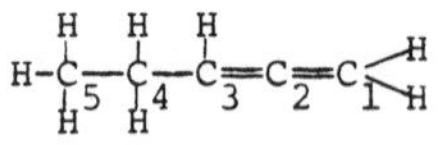

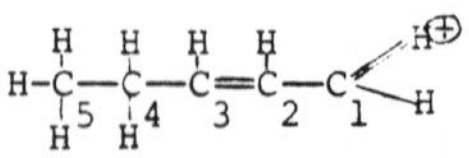

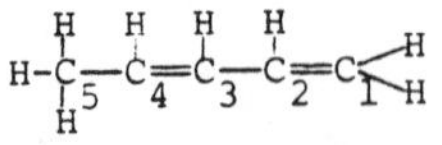

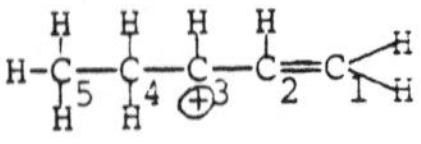

(10) All of the following are acceptable resonance forms of the following ion except:

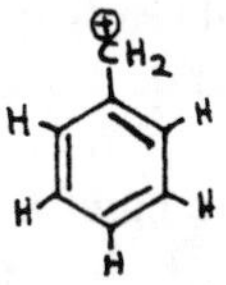

(a) 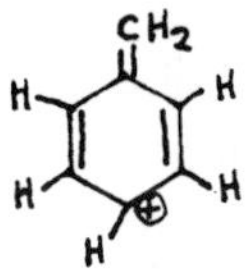 (b) 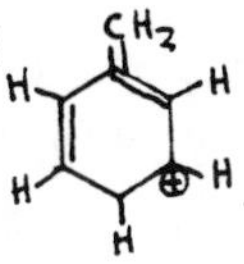 (c) 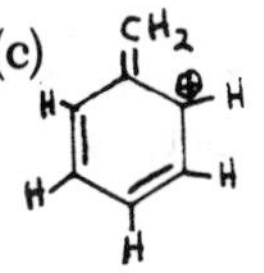 (d)

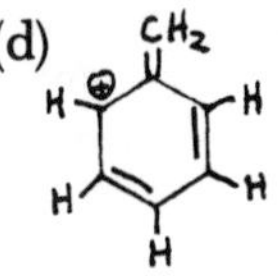

(11) What is the electron dot formula of $H_2O$?
(Atomic numbers: H = 1, O = 8)

(a) H:H:Ö:    (b) H:Ö:H    (c) ·H:Ö:H·    (d) Ḣ:Ḣ:Ö:

(12) What is the electron dot formula for $SO_4^{-2}$?
(Atomic numbers: O = 8, S = 16)

(a) 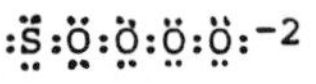 :S̈:Ö:Ö:Ö:Ö:⁻²    (b) 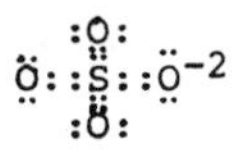 Ö::S̈::Ö⁻²    (c) 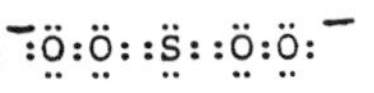 ⁻:Ö:Ö::S̈::Ö:Ö:⁻    (d) 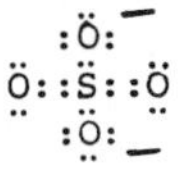 Ö::S̈::Ö

For the following questions use the electronegativities given in the section.

(13) In which compound does the starred carbon have the largest partial positive charge?

(a) 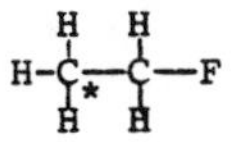 H-C*-C—F    (b) H-C*-Cl

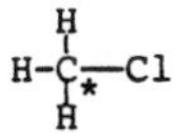

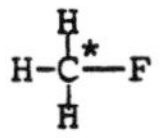

(c) H-C*—F    (d) 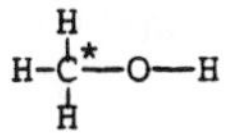 H-C*-O—H

(14) Select the following compound with the largest dipole moment:

(a) $CH_3$-$CH_2$-$CH_3$
(b) $CH_3$-$CH_2$-Cl
(c) $CH_3$-$CH_2$-OH
(d) $CH_3$-$CH_2$-H

(15) Select the compound with the largest dipole moment:

(a) $CCl_4$    (b)

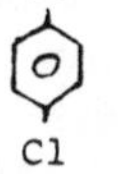

(c) 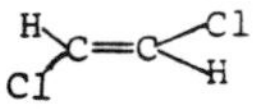    (d)

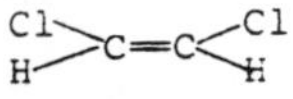

## 4.1.3    Answers to Questions in Section 4.1.2

( 1) b  ( 2) a  ( 3) b  ( 4) c  ( 5) d  ( 6) c  ( 7) a  ( 8) d  ( 9) d  (10) b  (11) b
(12) d  (13) c  (14) c  (15) d

## 4.1.4    Discussion of Answers to Questions in Section 4.1.2

*Questions #1 to #8 Adequately discussed in the Section.*

*Question #9* (Answer: d) Pi ($\pi$) electrons can be delocalized over charges ( + or − ) and over radicals. So, view the plus charge as if it were an adjacent p orbital ready to overlap. Option (a) is not acceptable because an atom is displaced (the H)—resonance forms are of the same molecule, so no atoms can move. This is also true of option (c). Option (c) also places a p orbital on C where none existed. Hydrogens have no p orbitals and can form only one bond so option (b) is incorrect. Option (d) is correct which shows a simple 'shift' of the bond from $C_3$-$C_2$ to $C_2$-$C_1$.

*Question #10* (Answer: b) Options (a), (c) and (d) are arrived at by simple 'shifts' of the $\pi$ bonds around the ring. There is no way to get the structure in option (b)—also, one carbon has five bonds.

*Question #11* (Answer: b) Oxygen has an electron configuration of $1s^2\, 2s^2\, 2p^4$, so there are 6 valence electrons (see sections 3.1.1 and 3.2.1). The hydrogen's is $1s^1$, and it has one valence electron. These are symbolized and combined as:

$$\text{H}\bullet + \bullet\ddot{\underset{\bullet\bullet}{\text{O}}}\bullet + \bullet\text{H} \longrightarrow \text{H}\!:\!\ddot{\underset{\bullet\bullet}{\text{O}}}\!:\!\text{H}.$$

Note: (1) that the single element is usually the central element, (2) single electrons are paired up, (3) the octet rule is followed for oxygen, and (4) the number of electrons that belong to each element is the same as the number of valence electrons it started with (see section discussion).

*Question #12* (Answer: d) If you thought that none of the structures accurately depicts the true $SO_4^{-2}$ ion, you are correct because resonance is possible with this structure. The electron configurations are:

$$O = 1s^2\, 2s^2\, 2p^4 \qquad S = 1s^2\, 2s^2\, 2p^6\, 3s^2\, 3p^4.$$

The valence electrons (in the outer shell only) are:

$$O = 6 \quad \text{and } S = 6 \text{ plus two electrons for charge } (-2).$$

The electron dot formula is:

Note: (1) The electron "pairs" on S (I → II) broken up to accommodate the free electron pairs of O (esp. #1 and #3). Hence, sulfur does not follow the octet rule (II, III). (2) The O's in II (i.e., #2 and #4) have one unpaired electron each; these are paired with the two extra electrons (II → III) to make the O's follow the octet rule. (3) An equivalent structure is,

(4) In counting up the valence electrons for each atom, remember the two extra electrons are spread out among the O's (actually the O's and S). See Question #11 for other points.

*Question #13* (Answer: c) The element with the highest electronegativity is F, so this pulls the most electron density away from the C making it slightly positive. The F is more effective when attached directly to the C as in (c) than when another atom (the other C) intervenes as in (a).

*Question #14* (Answer: c) The reasoning is the same as in #13. The O is the most electronegative and causes the largest charge separation,

$$C - O$$
$$\delta+ \quad \delta-$$
$$\longrightarrow$$

and, hence, the largest dipole moment.

*Question #15* (Answer: d) This is to point out that dipole moments are vectors (directions and magnitude) and are additive as such. The molecules in (a), (b) and (c) are all symmetric and the dipoles are opposite and equal and, hence, cancel. This is not true for (d):

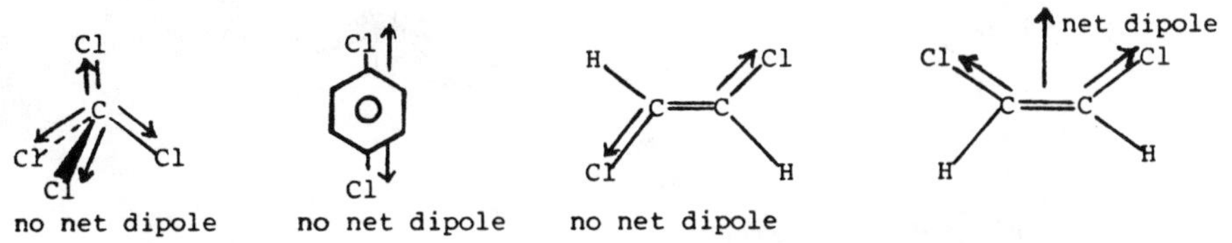

## 4.1.5 Vocabulary, Concepts, etc. Checklist for Covalent Bonding

_____ sigma bonds                    _____ dipole moment
_____ pi bonds                       _____ electron dot structures
_____ resonance                      _____ partial ionic character

## 4.2 STEREOCHEMISTRY

### 4.2.1 Review of Stereochemistry

If two molecules have the same number and type of atoms, they are called *isomers*. *Structural isomers* have different atoms and/or bonding patterns in relation to each other. *Stereoisomers* differ by virtue of different spatial orientations of isomers even though the same atoms are attached to each other and the bonding patterns (i.e., location and number of single bonds, double bonds, etc., and to the same atoms) are the same. *Geometric isomers* are stereoisomers that differ by virtue of orientation about a double bond or ring, i.e., cis or trans isomers. *Optical isomers* are stereoisomers that differ by different spatial orientations about an asymmetric carbon atom (all four substituents are different) (Fig. 4.4).

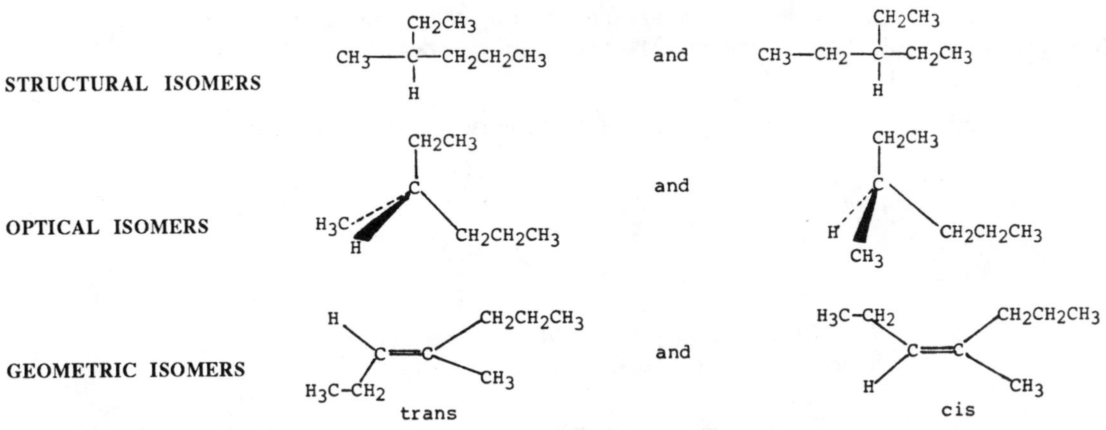

*Fig. 4.4(a)—Isomers*

4-7

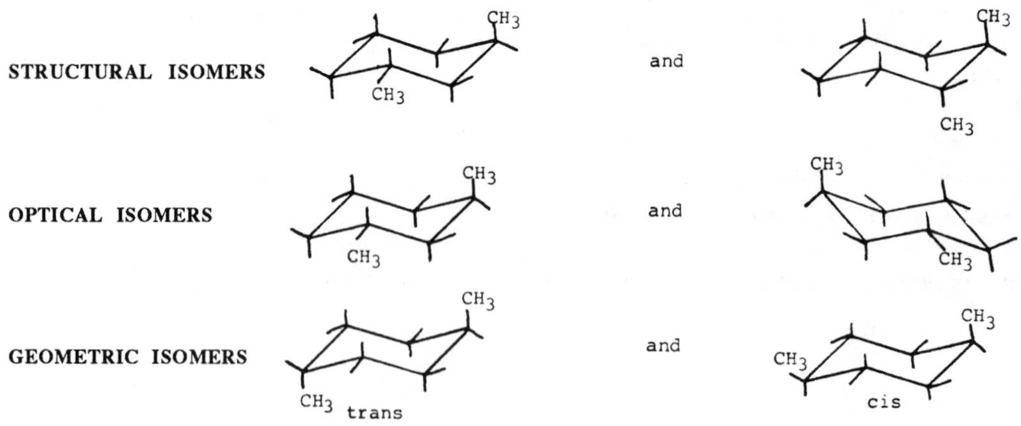

**STRUCTURAL ISOMERS** ... and ...

**OPTICAL ISOMERS** ... and ...

**GEOMETRIC ISOMERS** ... trans ... and ... cis

*Fig. 4.4(b)—Isomers*

*Cis-Trans isomers* can be distinguished by differences in dipole moments, melting and boiling points, chemical reactivity and spectra (UV, NMR). The number of possible geometric isomers in a molecule is $2^n$, where n = 1, 2, 3, etc., and is the number of double bonds in a molecule.

*Structural and geometric isomers* in general, differ in most chemical and physical properties. *Optical isomers* differ from each other only in the rotation of *plane polarized light*. Light travels as waves in all planes. Certain substances can select out one of these planes to yield plane polarized light. When this polarized light passes through an optical isomer it will be rotated in a given direction. If it is rotated clockwise, the direction is called *dextrorotatory* and symbolized by a *d* or a +. When rotation is counterclockwise, it is called *levorotatory* and is symbolized by an *l* or a −. Equal amounts of d and l together is a *racemic mixture*, the rotation is zero degrees. The *specific rotation* ($\alpha$) is:

$$\alpha = \frac{\text{observed rotation in degrees}}{(\text{length of sample in decimeters})(\text{concentration in gm/ml})}$$

Since the rotation depends upon the temperature, the wavelength of light used, concentration of substance, the solvent and the structure (d or l) of the molecule, these should all be specified.

Optical isomers are called *enantiomers* when they are nonsuperimposable mirror images of each other. This occurs when the absolute configuration at each asymmetric carbon is the inverse of the other. Optical isomers which are not mirror images (at one or more asymmetric carbons) are called *diastereomers*. The maximum number of possible optical isomers in a compound is given by,

$2^n$ where n = 1, 2, 3 = the number of asymmetric carbons (Fig. 4.5)

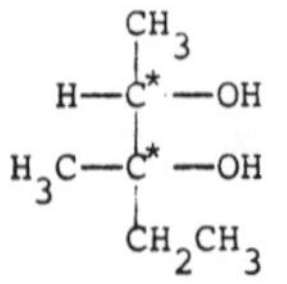

*the starred carbons are asymmetric
there are $2^2 = 4$ optical isomers

*Fig. 4.5(a)—Stereoisomers*

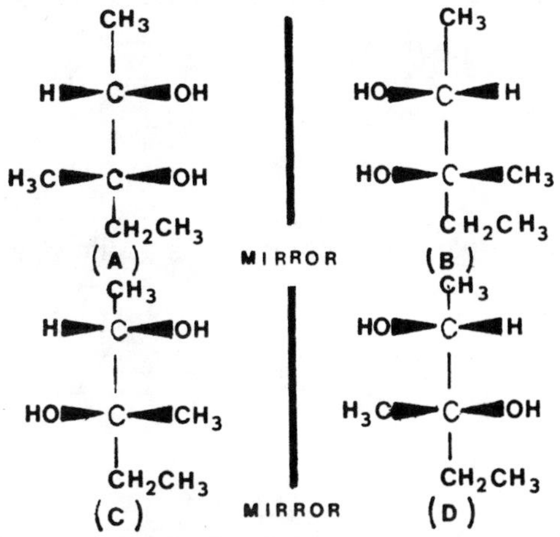

```
        CH₃                          CH₃
         |                            |
   H ►─C─◄ OH              HO ►─C─◄ H
         |                            |
  H₃C ►─C─◄ OH             HO ►─C─◄ CH₃
         |                            |
       CH₂CH₃                      CH₂CH₃
        (A)        MIRROR           (B)
        CH₃                          CH₃
         |                            |
   H ►─C─◄ OH              HO ►─C─◄ H
         |                            |
  HO ►─C─◄ CH₃             H₃C ►─C─◄ OH
         |                            |
       CH₂CH₃                      CH₂CH₃
        (C)        MIRROR           (D)
```

enantiomers: A & B; C & D
diastereomers: (A) & (D); (A) & (C); (B) & (C); (B) & (D).

*Fig. 4.5(b)—Stereoisomers*

A racemic mixture contains both *d* and *l* forms of an enantiomer. Since these differ only in rotation of light, it is impossible to separate them unchanged. One way of separating enantiomers is by reacting them with a second optically active compound. For example,

> A(d) and A(l) are original enantiomers
> react with B(d) to get
> A(d)-B(d) and A(l)-B(d)
> now the compounds A(d)-B(d) and A(l)-B(d) are no
> longer optical isomers and can be separated by
> chemical or physical means.

### 4.2.2    Questions to Review Stereochemistry

(1)    Stereoisomers, in contrast to structural isomers, have

(a) the same number and types of atoms
(b) different numbers of single, double and triple bonds
(c) the same atoms bonded to each other
(d) none of the above

(2)    Asymmetric carbons are key features of:

(a) optical isomers
(b) geometric isomers
(c) structural isomers
(d) all of the above

(3)    Cis-trans isomers can be distinguished by:

(a) dipole moments
(b) chemical reactivity
(c) melting points
(d) all of the above

(4)    Optical isomers can be best distinguished from each other by:

(a) chemical reactivity
(b) rotation of polarized light
(c) melting points
(d) all of the above

(5) A symbol of + or _____ indicates that a molecule causes _____ rotation of polarized light.

(a) d, counterclockwise
(b) d, clockwise
(c) l, counterclockwise
(d) l, clockwise

(6) The specific rotation of light by a substance depends upon all the following except:

(a) concentration of substance
(b) length of sample
(c) wavelength of light used
(d) refractive index of substance

(7) Enantiomers are:

(a) geometric isomers
(b) racemic
(c) optically inactive
(d) nonsuperimposable mirror images

(8) If n is the number of asymmetric carbons in a compound, the number of optical isomers possible is:

(a) $n^2$
(b) $2n$
(c) 2n
(d) 4n

(9) A racemic mixture

(a) is composed of geometric isomers
(b) rotates plane polarized light
(c) contains equal amounts of enantiomers
(d) contains equal amounts of diastereomers

(10) The components of a racemic mixture may be separated (resolved) by:

(a) precipitation
(b) distillation
(c) hydrolysis
(d) none of the above

(11) How many structural isomers does $C_5H_{12}$ have?

(a) 1
(b) 2
(c) 3
(d) 4

(12) Select the structural isomer of the following compound:

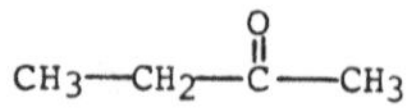

$$CH_3-CH_2-\overset{\overset{O}{\|}}{C}-CH_3$$

(a) 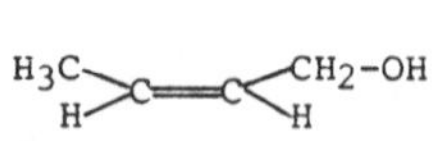 $H_3C$—$\overset{H}{\underset{}{C}}$=$\overset{CH_2-OH}{\underset{H}{C}}$

(b) 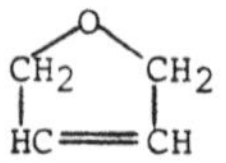 CH$_2$ CH$_2$ / O \ HC=CH

(c) $CH_3-CH_2-CH_2-O-CH_3$

(d) 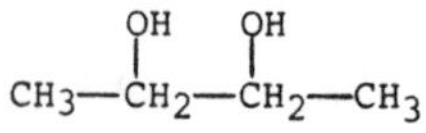 $CH_3-\overset{OH}{\underset{}{CH_2}}-\overset{OH}{\underset{}{CH_2}}-CH_3$

(13) Select the geometric isomer of the following compound:

H3C–CH2
CH2–Cl
C═C
CH3
Cl

(a) 
H3C–CH2
Cl
C═C
CH3
CH2–Cl

(b) 
H3C–CH2
CH2Cl
C═C
Cl
CH3

(c) 
H3C–CH2
Cl
C═C
ClCH2
CH3

(d) 
CH3
Cl
C═C
CH3–CH2
CH2Cl

(14) Select the geometric isomer of the following compound:

O
OH
OH

(a) 
O
OH
OH

(b) 
O
HO
OH

(c) 
O
OH
OH

(d) 
OH
O
OH

(15) In #14 select the compound(s) that is(are) optical isomer(s) of the given compound:

(a)
(b)
(c)
(d)

(16) In #14 select the compound(s) that is(are) structural isomer(s) of the given compound:

(a)
(b)
(c)
(d)

(17) Ten gms of a compound are placed in 2 mls of $H_2O$ in a sample cylinder 10 cms long. The observed rotation of light is – 15°, the specific rotation (for Na light and 25°C) is:

(a) – 3°
(b) – 0.3°
(c) + 5°
(d) none of these

(18) The substance in #17 is:

(a) dextrorotatory
(b) levorotatory

(19) Which of the labeled carbon(s) in the following compound is(are) asymmetric?

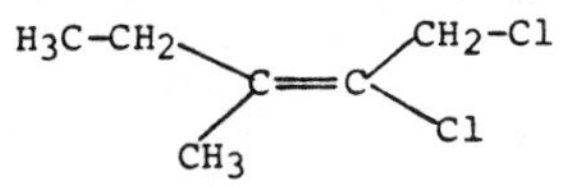

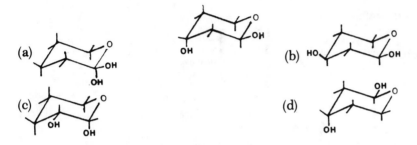

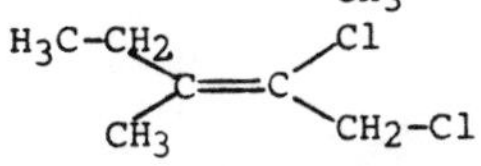

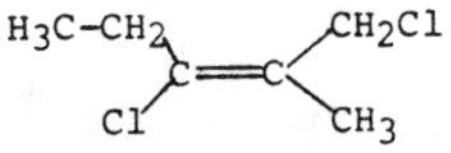

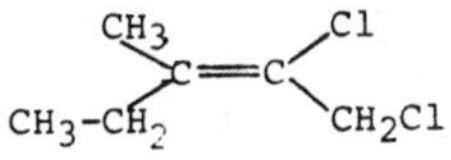

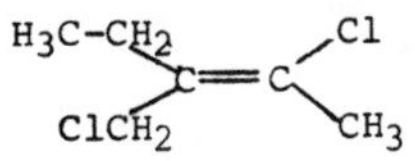

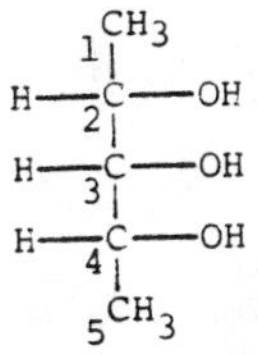

1 CH3
H—2C—OH
H—3C—OH
H—4C—OH
5 CH3

(a) 1,5
(b) 2,4
(c) 2,3,4
(d) 3 only

(20)   How many optical isomers does the compound in #19 have?

   (a) 2
   (b) 4
   (c) 6
   (d) 8

(21)   An enantiomer of the following compound is

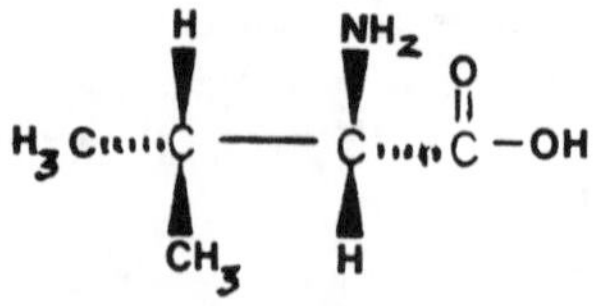

valine (an amino acid)

(a)

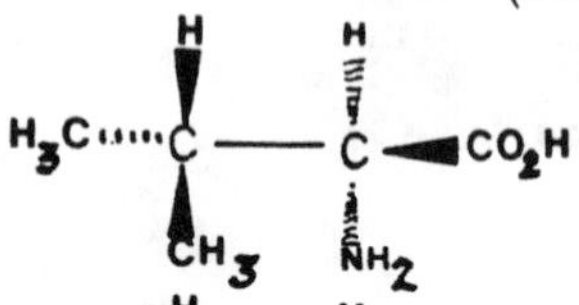

(b)

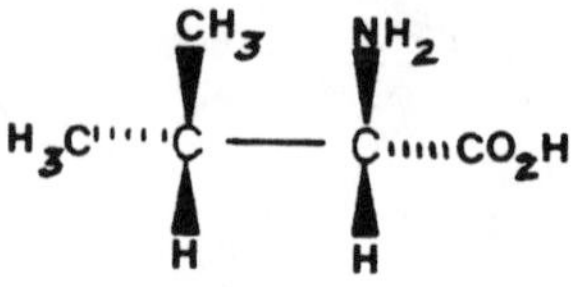

(c)

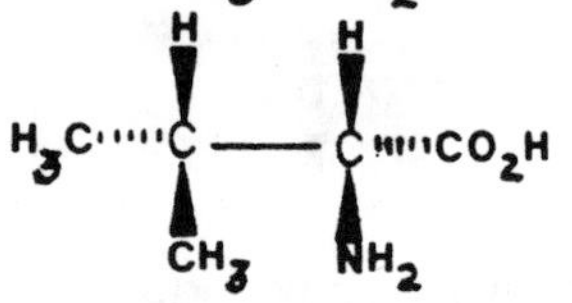

(d)  none of the above


## 4.2.3     Answers to Questions in Section 4.2.2

( 1) c   ( 2) a   ( 3) d   ( 4) b   ( 5) b   ( 6) d   ( 7) d   ( 8) b   ( 9) c   (10) d   (11) c
(12) a   (13) a   (14) b   (15) d   (16) a,c (17) a   (18) b   (19) b   (20) b   (21) c


## 4.2.4     Discussion of Answers to Questions in Section 4.2.2

*Questions #1 to #10* Adequately discussed in Section.

*Question #11* (Answer: c) The H's can be neglected and use only the carbon skeleton. Work systematically, starting with $C_5$ then $C_4$ then $C_3$ and place the extra carbons onto these systematically:

$C_5$:        C—C—C—C—C          only possible one

$C_4$:        $\underset{1}{C}$—$\underset{2}{C}$—$\underset{3}{C}$—$\underset{4}{C}$          only possible one

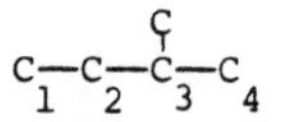

> note that the last C cannot go on $C_1$ or $C_4$ (the *end* carbons) because this gives $C_5$ again.
> and $C_2 \equiv C_3$ so only one compound is possible.

$C_3$:              $\underset{1}{C}$—$\underset{2}{C}$—$\underset{3}{C}$

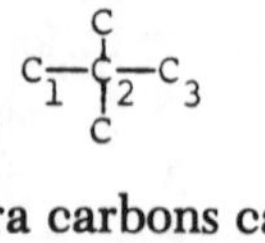

> the extra carbons can be C,C or C-C, but C-C will give either $C_4$ or $C_5$ and just duplicate prior structures.
> the C,C cannot go on $C_1$ or $C_3$.

Since the formula was $C_5H_{12}$, which is a $C_nH_{2n+2}$, there were no double bonds or rings (see Sections 4.3.1 and 4.4.1).

*Question #12* (Answer: a) The other options (b, c and d) either contain too few or too many H's or O's.

*Question #13* (Answer: a) Options (b) and (c) have atoms or groups of atoms bonded to different atoms. Option (d) is just the original compound flipped over. Note: (b) and (c) are structural isomers of the original compound.

*Question #14* (Answer: b) Option (b) is the CIS isomer of the compound.

*Question #15* (Answer: d) Option (d) is the mirror image of the compound:

*Question #16* (Answer: a,c) Both (a) and (c) have atoms which are attached to different atoms in contrast to (b) and (d) which are stereoisomers.

*Question #17* (Answer: a)

$$\text{specific rotation} = \frac{-15°}{(1)(5)} = \frac{-15°}{5} = -3°/\text{dm} \cdot \text{gm/ml}$$

observed rotation $= -15°$

length of sample in decimeters (dm) $= (10 \text{ cms}) \left(\frac{1 \text{ dm}}{10 \text{ cms}}\right) = 1 \text{ dm}$

conc. in gms/ml $= \dfrac{10 \text{ gms}}{2 \text{ mls}} = 5 \text{ gms/ml}.$

*Question #18* (Answer: b) Negative observed rotation is levorotatory.

*Question #19* (Answer: b) Only (2) and (4) are asymmetric, (1) and (5) have 3 hydrogens each; (3) has two identical groups attached:

$$H-\overset{\displaystyle |}{\underset{\displaystyle CH_3}{C}}-OH$$

*Question #20* (Answer: b) $2^n = 2^2 = 4$.

*Question #21* (Answer: c) Only the carbon containing the $-NH_2$ is asymmetric, the rest are not asymmetric. Then,

Mirror image = option (C)

Options (a) and (b) are rotations about the bond labelled (1) above.

## 4.2.5  Vocabulary, Concepts, etc. Checklist for Stereochemistry

| | | |
|---|---|---|
| _____ isomers | _____ cis-trans isomers | _____ enantiomers |
| _____ structural isomers | _____ polarized light | _____ diastereomers |
| _____ stereoisomers | _____ dextrorotatory | _____ racemic mixtures |
| _____ geometric isomers | _____ levorotatory | _____ separation of racemers |
| _____ optical isomers | _____ specific rotation | |

## 4.3 ALKANES

### 4.3.1 Review of Alkanes

The basic ideas of *nomenclature* for alkanes will hold for more complex molecules also. Alkanes are simple because they contain only carbon and hydrogen (also called hydrocarbons) and contain no aromatic rings. The longest straight carbon chain is determined and is named depending upon the number of carbons:

$C_1$-meth-, $C_2$-eth-, $C_3$-prop-, $C_4$-but(a), $C_5$-pent(a), $C_6$-hex(a), $C_7$-hept(a), $C_8$-oct(a), $C_9$-non(a), $C_{10}$-dec(a).

If these carbons contain only C and H the suffix -yl is added:

$CH_3-$ = methyl, $CH_3CH_2-$ = ethyl, $CH_3CH_2CH_2-$ = propyl, etc.

There are special names for some branched chain alkanes:

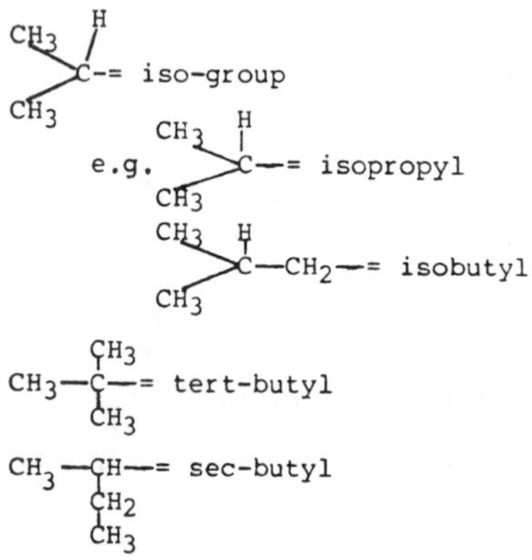

Once the longest chain is determined, the groups attached to it are numbered such that the lowest set of numbers is obtained. The side groups are placed in the molecule name in alphabetical order or in order of increasing size. The prefixes di-(two), tri-(three), tetra-(four), etc., are used when a particular group is present more than once. The suffix indicating alkanes is -ane. For example:

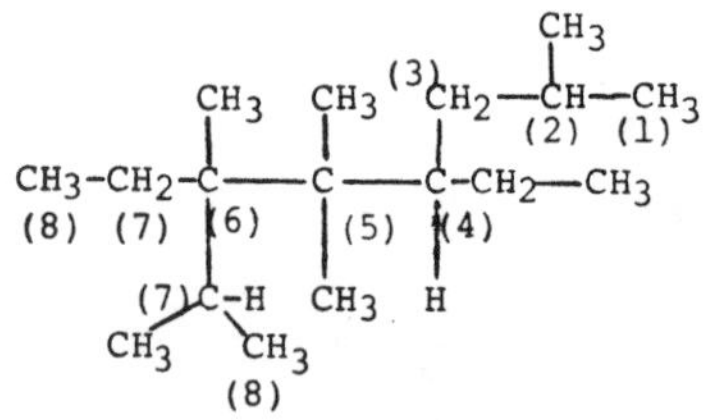

2,5,5,6-Tetra methyl-4-ethyl-6-isopropyl octane or 2,5,5,6,7-Pentamethyl-4, 6-diethyl octane.

*Alkanes* (if no rings, $C_nH_{2n+2}$; and lose 2 hydrogens for each ring) may be open chains or rings. The rings are named for the number of carbons that make them up:

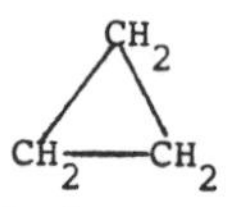

cyclo-propane

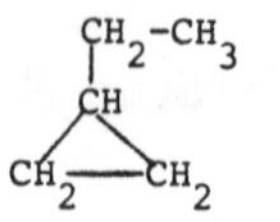

ethylcyclopropane

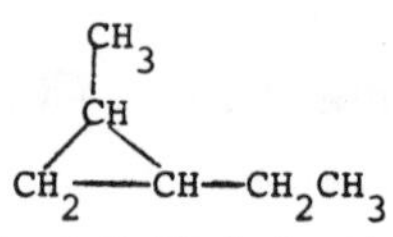

cis-1,Methyl-2-ethyl cyclopropane

cyclobutane    cyclopentane    cyclohexane

The main *chemical features* are the lack of functional groupings (e.g., $-OH$, Br) and full saturation (no double or triple bonds). These factors cause them to be chemically unreactive except when induced by heat or light.

*Physical properties* of alkanes are fairly straightforward. Because they are nonpolar and have weak intermolecular forces, they have low boiling points and are not soluble in water. Branching makes the molecules more symmetrical and this lowers the boiling points even more, which is true for other classes of compounds as well. With increasing molecular weights, the intermolecular forces increase and the boiling point increases; this is also observed in other classes of molecules. Melting points increase as molecular weights increase. Solubility is in nonpolar solvents and not in aqueous solvents.

The main reactions of alkanes are combustion and substitution (radical) reactions:

(1) Combustion

$$C_n + H_{2n+2} + O_2 \text{ (excess)} \xrightarrow{\text{flame}} nCO_2 + (n+1)H_2O$$

(2) Substitution (radical)

$$CH_3CH_3 + Cl_2 \xrightarrow{\text{light}} CH_3CH_2Cl + HCl$$

also get di, tri, etc. substitutions.

The mechanism is:

(a) *initiation* - production of radicals de novo, e.g., from heat or ultraviolet light
$$Cl_2 \rightarrow 2Cl-$$

(b) *propagation* - generation of radicals by radicals
$$Cl- + CH_3 - CH_3 \rightarrow CH_3 - CH_2 + HCl$$
$$CH_3 - CH_2 + Cl_2 \rightarrow CH_3 - CH_2Cl + Cl-$$

(c) *termination* - reaction of radicals with radicals
$$Cl- + CH_3 - CH_2 \rightarrow CH_3 - CH_2 - Cl$$
$$CH_3 - CH_2 + CH_3 - CH_2 \rightarrow CH_3 - CH_2 - CH_2 - CH_3$$

*Chain reactions* will result when one intermediate adds to a molecule producing another radical which can react further, and then this repeats itself:

$$CH_3 - CH_2 + H_2C = CH_2 \rightarrow CH_3 - CH_2 - CH_2 - CH_2 + H_2C = CH_2 \rightarrow CH_3 - CH_2 - CH_2 - CH_2 - CH_2 - CH_2, \text{ etc.}$$

Radicals result from homolytic cleavage of chemical bonds:

$$X\text{-}Y \rightarrow X\cdot + Y\cdot$$

Note that each species is neutral (if begun neutral), and that each has a free unpaired electron. Because of the free unpaired electron, radicals are paramagnetic. Most radicals are very unstable and react rapidly. The stability of radicals depends on the ability to delocalize the free electron. Remember that benzene rings and allylic double bonds can delocalize electrons readily:

benzyl    allylic    tertiary($3°$) secondary($2°$) primary($1°$) methyl.

4-15

The smaller the number of carbons in a ring, the less stable the ring is. This is due to *ring strain* of the bonding orbitals. The usual angle between bonds is 109.5° in the sp³ hybridized carbon. The expected bond angles in the following ring compounds are:

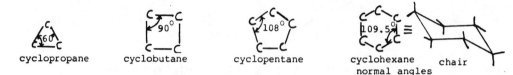

cyclopropane          cyclobutane          cyclopentane          cyclohexane          chair
                                                                  normal angles

The ring strain is very high in cyclopropane. This makes cyclopropane as reactive with $H_2, Br_2$ as alkenes are (see 4.4.1). Cyclobutane relieves some of the ring strain by assuming a bent conformation,

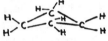

Cyclopentane is puckered to relieve the strain,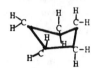

Cyclohexane has no strain in the chair form as shown. Cyclobutane is fairly reactive, but cyclopentane or cyclohexane are not.


## 4.3.2     Questions to Review Alkanes

(1)  Alkanes tend to have _____ boiling points because they are _____ and, hence, have _____ intermolecular forces.

    (a) low, nonpolar, weak
    (b) high, polar, strong
    (c) low, polar, weak
    (d) high, nonpolar, strong

(2)  Alkanes are _____ in water because they are _____.

    (a) soluble, polar
    (b) insoluble, polar
    (c) soluble, nonpolar
    (d) insoluble, nonpolar

(3)  Branching tends to make an alkane more _____ and this _____ the boiling point.

    (a) symmetric, lowers
    (b) symmetric, raises
    (c) asymmetric, lowers
    (d) asymmetric, raises

(4)  The step in which radicals react with radicals is:

    (a) termination
    (b) propagation
    (c) initiation
    (d) none of these

(5)  Of the following radicals, in general, the most stable is:

    (a) allylic
    (b) primary
    (c) secondary
    (d) tertiary

(6)     Which ring has the greatest ring strain?

(a) cyclohexane
(b) cyclopentane
(c) cyclobutane
(d) cyclopropane

(7)     Which of the following rings has no ring strain?

(a) cyclohexane
(b) cyclobutane
(c) cyclopropane
(d) none of the above

(8)     Name the following compound:

$$CH_3-\overset{\overset{\displaystyle CH_3}{|}}{CH}-\underset{\underset{\displaystyle CH_3}{|}}{CH}-CH_2-CH_3$$

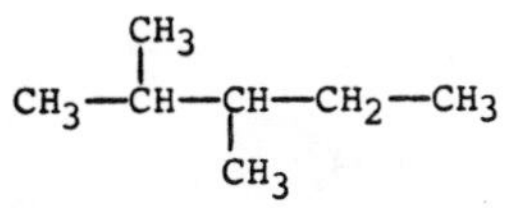

(a) 2-Isopropyl pentane
(b) 2,3 Dimethylpentane
(c) 3,4-Dimethyl pentane
(d) none of the above

(9)     Name the following compound:

$$CH_3-\overset{\overset{\displaystyle CH_2CH_3}{|}}{\underset{\underset{\displaystyle CH_3}{|}}{C}}-CH_2-\overset{\overset{\displaystyle CH_3}{|}}{CH}-\overset{}{CH}-CH_2CH_2-CH\overset{\diagup CH_3}{\diagdown CH_3}$$

with $\overset{|}{CH}-CH_3$ and $\overset{|}{CH_3}$

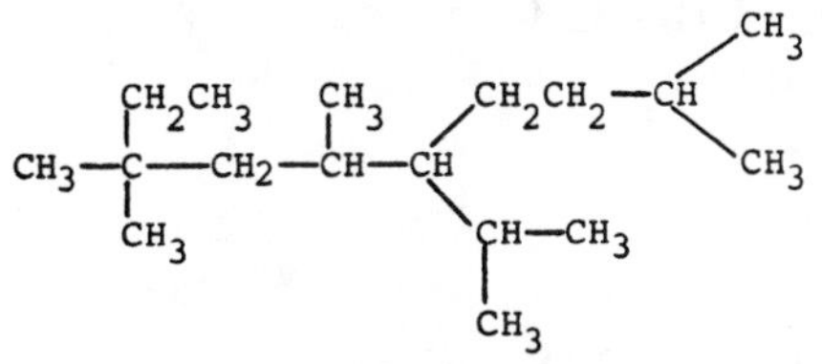

(a) 2,4,8-Trimethyl-2-ethyl-5-isopropylnonane
(b) diisoprene
(c) 3,3,5,9-Tetramethyl-6-isopropyldecane
(d) none of the above

(10)    Give the structure of 2,6-Dimethyl-4-ethyloctane:

(a) 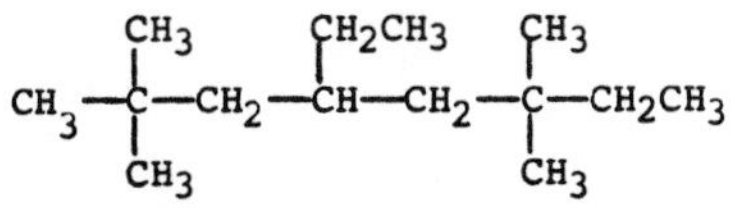 $CH_3-\overset{\overset{\displaystyle CH_3}{|}}{\underset{\underset{\displaystyle CH_3}{|}}{C}}-CH_2-\overset{\overset{\displaystyle CH_2CH_3}{|}}{CH}-CH_2-\overset{\overset{\displaystyle CH_3}{|}}{\underset{\underset{\displaystyle CH_3}{|}}{C}}-CH_2CH_3$     (b) $CH_3-\overset{\overset{\displaystyle CH_3}{|}}{CH}-CH_2-\overset{\overset{\displaystyle CH_2CH_3}{|}}{CH}-CH_2-\overset{\overset{\displaystyle CH_3}{|}}{CH}-CH_2CH_3$

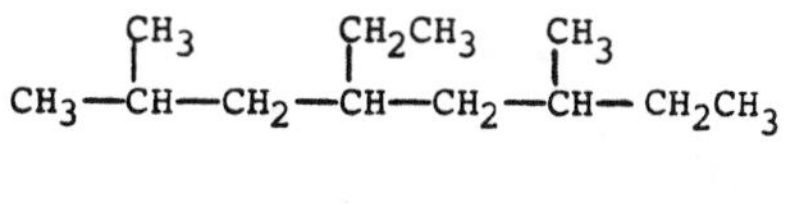

(c) $CH_3-\overset{\overset{\displaystyle CH_2CH_3}{|}}{CH}-CH_2-\overset{\overset{\displaystyle CH_3}{|}}{CH}-CH_2-\overset{\overset{\displaystyle CH_2CH_3}{|}}{CH}-CH_2CH_3$     (d) none of the above

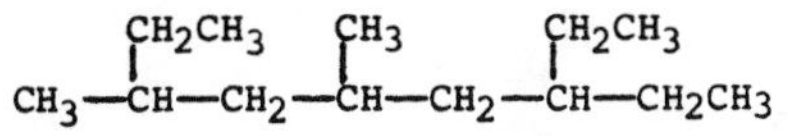

(11)    Name the following compound:

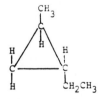

(a) cis-1-Methyl-2-ethylcyclopropane
(b) 2,3-Methylpentane
(c) trans-Dimethylcyclopropane
(d) none of the above

4-17

(12)    What is the structure of trans-1-Ethyl-4-t-butylcyclohexane?

(a)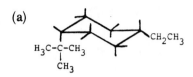

(b)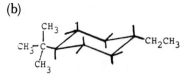

(c)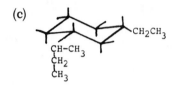

(d) none of the above

(13)    Which compound probably has the higher boiling point?

$$CH_3—CH_2—CH_2—CH_2—CH_3 \qquad\qquad CH_3—\overset{\overset{\displaystyle CH_3}{|}}{CH}—CH_2—CH_3$$
$$\text{(I)} \qquad\qquad\qquad\qquad \text{(II)}$$

(a) I
(b) II
(c) both equal

(14)    Which compound probably has the higher boiling point?

$$CH_3—CH_2—CH_3 \qquad\qquad CH_3—CH_2—CH_2—CH_2—CH_3$$
$$\text{(I)} \qquad\qquad\qquad\qquad \text{(II)}$$

(a) I
(b) II
(c) both equal

(15)    How many $CO_2$'s are produced by the complete combustion of 3,3-Diethylhexane?

(a) 10
(b) 8
(c) 6
(d) 4

(16)    Which of the following radicals is the most stable?

(a)

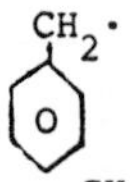

(b) 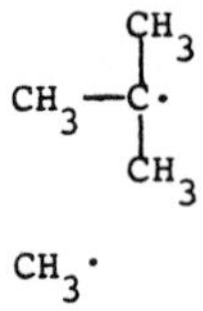 $CH_3—\overset{\overset{\displaystyle CH_3}{|}}{\underset{\underset{\displaystyle CH_3}{|}}{C}}\cdot$

(c) $CH_3—\overset{\overset{\displaystyle CH_3}{|}}{CH}\cdot$

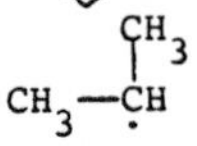

(d) $CH_3\cdot$

(17)    The removal of which H will result in the most stable radical in the following compound?

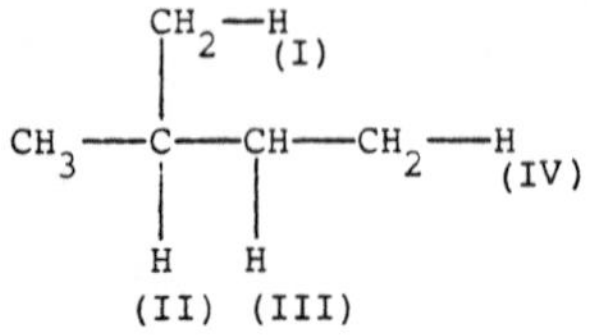

$$CH_3—\overset{\overset{\displaystyle CH_2—H\ (I)}{|}}{\underset{\underset{\displaystyle H}{|}}{C}}—\overset{\overset{}{}}{\underset{\underset{\displaystyle H}{|}}{CH}}—CH_2—H\ (IV)$$
$$\text{(II)} \quad \text{(III)}$$

(a) I
(b) II
(c) III
(d) IV

(18) The formula for an *alkane* is $C_4H_8$. Therefore, this compound:

    (a) is a straight chain
    (b) is branched
    (c) contains a ring
    (d) none of these

### 4.3.3 Answers to Questions in Section 4.3.2

( 1) a  ( 2) d  ( 3) a  ( 4) a  ( 5) a  ( 6) d  ( 7) a  ( 8) b  ( 9) c  (10) b  (11) d
(12) b  (13) a  (14) b  (15) a  (16) a  (17) b  (18) c

### 4.3.4 Discussion of Answers to Questions in Section 4.3.2

*Questions #1 to #7* Adequately discussed in Section.

*Question #8* (Answer: b) The numbering is:

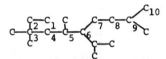

*Question #9* (Answer: c) The numbering is:

*Question #10* (Answer: b) Study answer and options given.

*Question #11* (Answer: d) The correct answer is trans-1-Methyl-2-ethylcyclopropane.

*Question #12* (Answer: b) Study the answer and options given.

*Question #13* (Answer: a) Compound (II) is more branched than (I) and has a lower predicted boiling point.

*Question #14* (Answer: b) Compound (II) has the higher molecular weight and the higher predicted boiling point.

*Question #15* (Answer: a) The structure is,

$$CH_3-CH_2-\overset{\overset{\displaystyle CH_2-CH_3}{|}}{\underset{\underset{\displaystyle CH_2CH_3}{|}}{C}}-CH_2-CH_2-CH_3$$

The formula is: $C_{10}H_{22}$.

The equation is: $C_{10}H_{22} + 3\frac{1}{2} O_2 \rightarrow 10\ CO_2 + 11\ H_2O$

*Question #16* (Answer: a) Given in Section.

*Question #17* (Answer: b) The resulting radicals would be:

$$CH_3-\overset{\overset{\displaystyle \cdot CH_2}{|}}{\underset{\underset{\displaystyle H}{|}}{C}}-CH_2-CH_3 \quad (1°) \qquad CH_3-\overset{\overset{\displaystyle CH_3}{|}}{\underset{}{\overset{\cdot}{C}}}-CH_2-CH_3 \quad (3°)$$
$$(I) \qquad\qquad\qquad (II)$$

$$CH_3-\overset{\overset{\displaystyle CH_3}{|}}{CH}-\overset{\cdot}{C}H-CH_3 \quad (2°) \qquad CH_3-\overset{\overset{\displaystyle CH_3}{|}}{CH}-CH_2-\overset{\cdot}{C}H_2 \quad (1°)$$
$$(III) \qquad\qquad\qquad (IV)$$

Then the 3° radical (II) is the most stable.

*Question #18* (Answer: c) Since the compound is an alkane, there are no double or triple bonds. One would expect $C_4H_{10}$ for a fully saturated alkane without rings. The two missing H's ($C_4H_8$) suggest the presence of one ring.

## 4.3.5    Vocabulary, Concepts, etc. Checklist for Alkanes

_____ nomenclature of alkanes                    _____ isobutyl
_____ meth-, methyl                              _____ sec-butyl
_____ eth-, ethyl                                _____ tert-butyl
_____ prop-, propyl                              _____ cyclopropane
_____ but(a)-, butyl                             _____ cyclobutane
_____ pent(a)-, pentyl                           _____ cyclopentane
_____ hex(a)-, hexyl                             _____ cyclohexane
_____ hept(a)-, heptyl                           _____ combustion reactions
_____ oct(a)-, octyl                             _____ physical properties of alkanes
_____ non(a)-, nonyl                             _____ radical reactions
_____ dec(a)-, decyl                             _____ isopropyl
_____ stability of radicals                      _____ ring strain

## 4.4    ALKENES

### 4.4.1    Review of Alkenes

See Section 4.2.1 for cis-trans isomerism. See Section 4.3.1 for basic points on nomenclature. See Section 4.1.1 for composition of the double bond.

*Alkenes* (if no ring, $C_nH_{2n}$) have the double bond as the functional group. For each double bond, the molecule loses two hydrogens from the alkane formula of $C_nH_{2n+2}$. The only addition to the nomenclature as discussed in 4.3.1 is that the double bond(s) is(are) numbered in the molecule. Again try to get the smallest possible number(s) for the double bonds:

$$CH_3\!\!-\!\!CH\!\!=\!\!CH\!\!-\!\!CH_3$$
2-Butene

$$CH_3\!\!-\!\!CH\!\!=\!\!\overset{\overset{\displaystyle CH_3}{|}}{CH}\!\!-\!\!CH\!\!=\!\!CH\!\!-\!\!CH_3$$
3-Methyl-2,4-hexadiene

Nearly all of the *chemistry of alkenes* can be understood in terms of the double bond and its key feature of attack by electrophiles (partial or complete positively charged substances seeking out electron rich substances) with the resulting *carbonium ions* (positive charges on carbon):

E = electrophile          carbonium          Nu = nucleophile
                          ion                (see below)

The other key feature of the double bond is its ability to stabilize carbonium ions, or radicals which are on adjacent carbons:

All are resonance stabilized (Section 4.1.1)

The *stability of the intermediate carbonium ion* as shown in (I) above depends on the groups (G) attached which can stabilize or destabilize it. In general, groups which can share electrons by $\pi$ orbital overlap (resonance) stabilize the carbonium ion (as the double bond in (II) above). In general, groups which place a positive (partial or total) charge adjacent to the carbonium ion withdraw electrons inductively (by sigma bonds) to destabilize it (see electronegativity in Section 4.1.1). (Fig. 4.6).

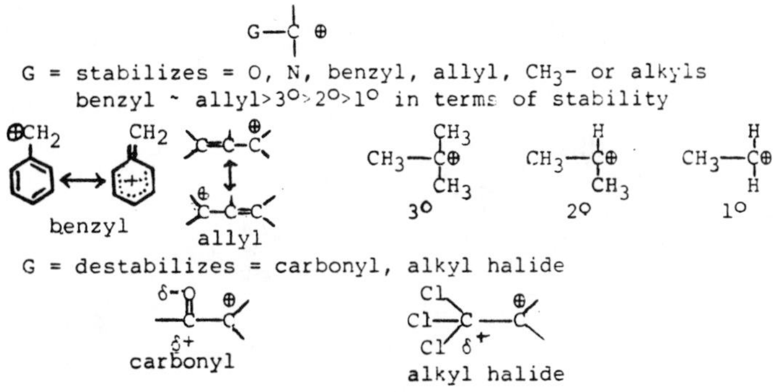

G = stabilizes = O, N, benzyl, allyl, CH₃- or alkyls
benzyl ~ allyl>3°>2°>1° in terms of stability

benzyl    allyl    3°    2°    1°

G = destabilizes = carbonyl, alkyl halide

carbonyl    alkyl halide

**Fig. 4.6—Stability of Carbonium Ions**

The above points are useful in predicting which carbon (1 or 2 in (I) above) will become the carbonium ion and which one the E and Nu will bond to. The intermediate carbonium ion formed must be the most stable. Markownikoff's rule is a sequel to this: the nucleophile (a molecule with a free pair of electrons and sometimes a negative charge that seeks out partially or completely positive charge species) will be bonded to the most substituted carbon (fewest hydrogens attached) in the product, or equivalently, the electrophile will be bonded to the least substituted (most hydrogens attached) carbon in the product. An example:

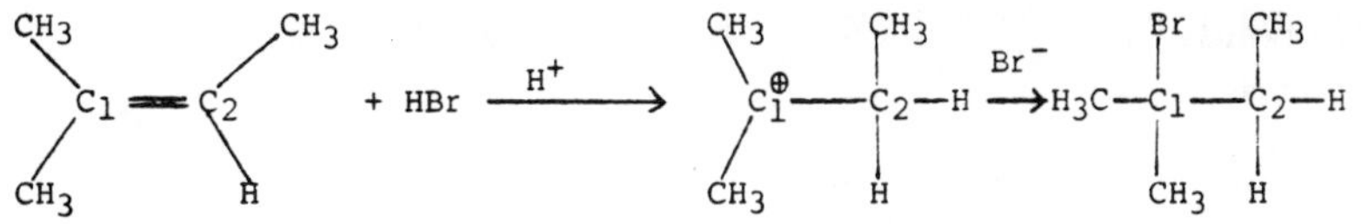

$H^+$ = electrophile        $Br^-$ = nucleophile
$C_1$ = most substituted C,    $C_2$ = least substituted C
$C_1$ forms the most stable carbonium ion.

The *physical properties* of alkenes are similar to the alkanes (Section 4.3.1). One difference is that alkenes may be polar due to cis-trans isomers and to the nature of the double bond itself (an electron withdrawer):

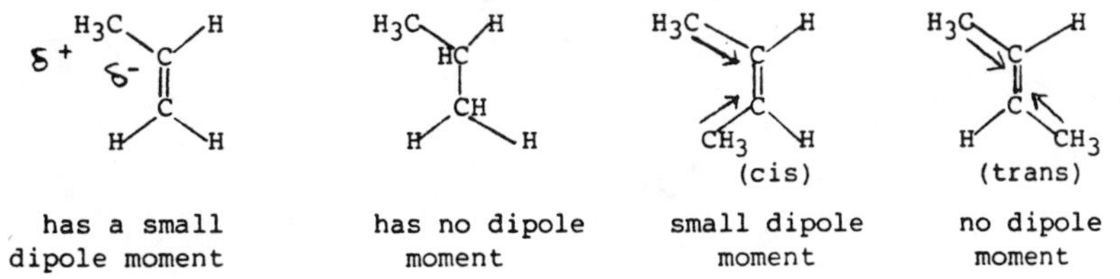

has a small       has no dipole      small dipole       no dipole
dipole moment       moment            moment            moment

Also trans compounds tend to have higher melting points (due to better symmetry) but lower boiling points (due to less polarity) than the corresponding cis compounds (see Sections 3.4.1 and 3.5).

## 4.4.2 Questions to Review Alkenes

(1) The general formula for an alkene with one double bond and no rings is:

(a) $C_nH_{2n-2}$
(b) $C_nH_{2n+2}$
(c) $C_nH_n$
(d) $C_nH_{2n}$

(2) Select the most stable carbonium ion:

(a) 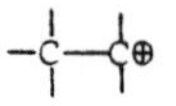 ![structure] (b) 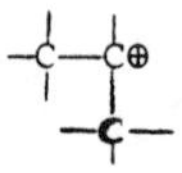 ![structure]

(c) 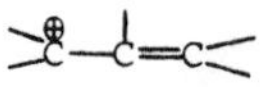 ![structure] (d) 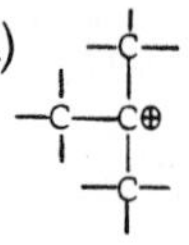 ![structure]

(3) Select the most unstable carbonium ion:

(a) 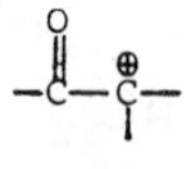 ![structure] (b) 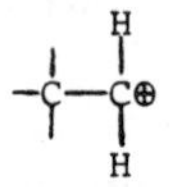 ![structure]

(c) 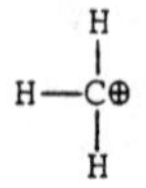 ![structure] (d) 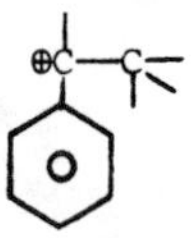 ![structure]

(4) Although alkanes and alkenes are both composed of carbon and hydrogen, alkenes may show _____ due to _____.

(a) hydrogen bonding, the double bond
(b) less reactivity, double bond
(c) polarity, cis-trans isomerism
(d) none of the above

(5) Name the following compound:

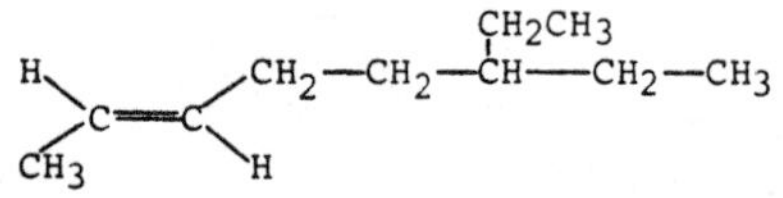

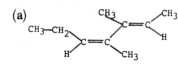

(a) 2-Ethyl-trans-6-octene
(b) 6-Ethyl-trans-2-octene
(c) 2-Ethyl-cis-6-octene
(d) 6-Ethyl-cis-2-octene

(6) Give the structure for 3,4 Dimethyl-cis-2-trans-4-heptadiene:

(a) ![structure] (b) ![structure]

(c)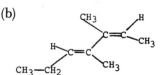

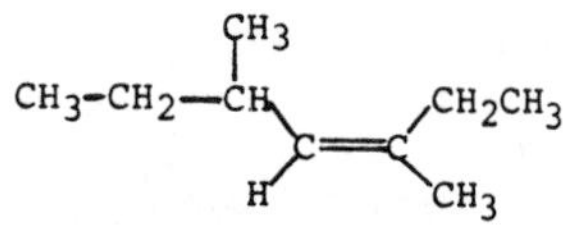

(d) none of the above

(7)     A double bond can stabilize an adjacent carbonium ion by _____ (of) the positive charge with its _____-bond.

(a) neutralizing, $\pi$
(b) neutralizing, $\sigma$
(c) delocalization, $\pi$
(d) delocalization, $\sigma$

(8)     The reaction of H+ with the following compound will form which carbonium ion:

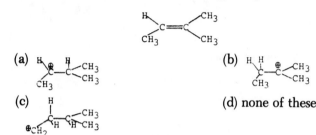

(a)

(b)

(c)

(d) none of these

(9)     The product of the following reaction is:

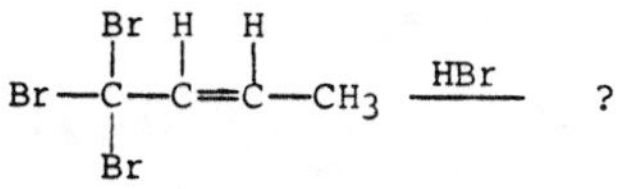

(a)

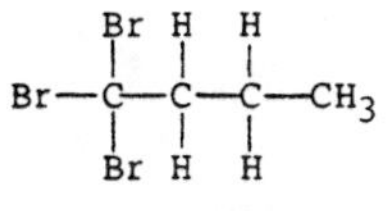

(b)

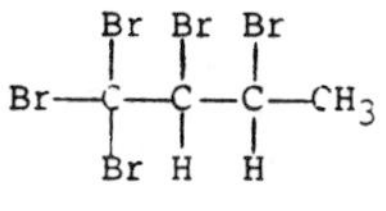

(c)

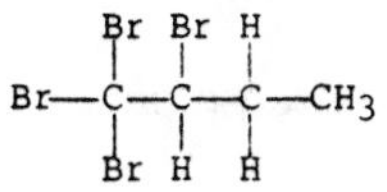

(d)

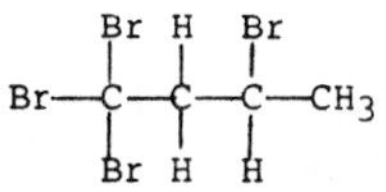

(10)    Which compound has the higher boiling point?

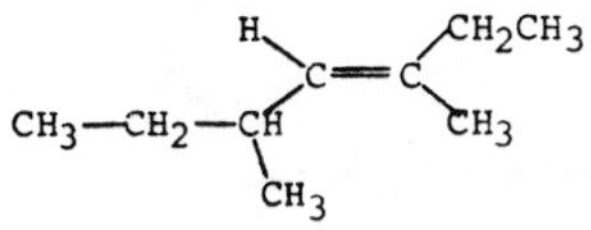

(I) 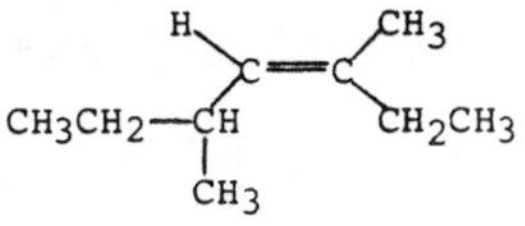                              (II)

(a) I
(b) II
(c) both equal

(11)    Which compound has the higher dipole moment?

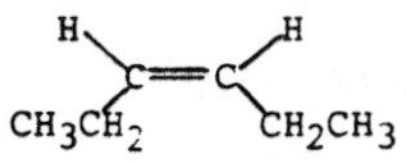

(I) 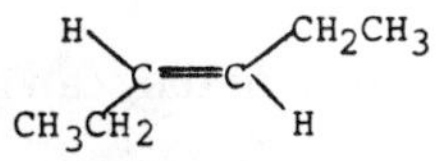                              (II)

(a) I
(b) II
(c) both equal

### 4.4.3     Answers to Questions in Section 4.4.2

( 1) d   ( 2) c   ( 3) a   ( 4) c   ( 5) b   ( 6) b   ( 7) c   ( 8) b   ( 9) d   (10) b   (11) a

**4.4.4     Discussion of Answers to Questions in Section 4.4.2**

*Questions #1 to #4, #7* Adequately discussed in Section.

*Question #5* (Answer: b) The numbering is,

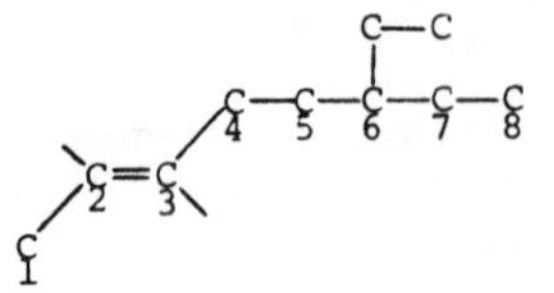

*Question #6* (Answer: b) Study correct answer vs. other options.

*Question #8* (Answer: b) The only possible cations from this double bond are (a) which is 2° and (b) which is 3°. Tertiary (3°) is more stable than secondary (2°).

*Question #9* (Answer: d) The mechanism is,

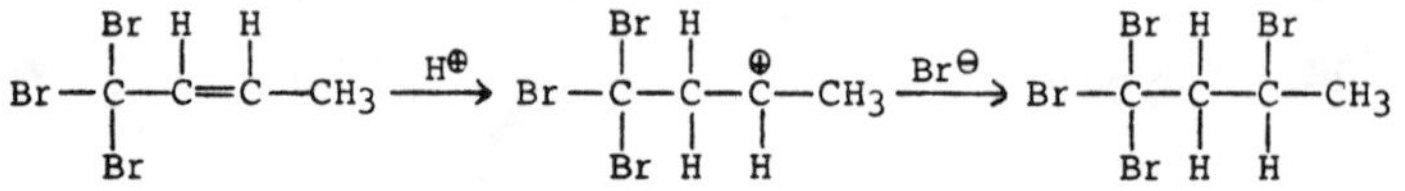

This carbonium ion is more stable than the alternate because of the adjacent brominated carbons,

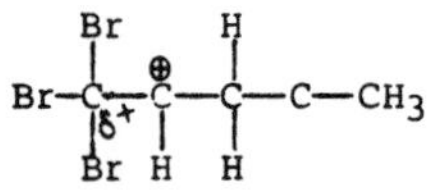

(alternate; less stable)

*Question #10* (Answer: b) Cis-compounds tend to have higher boiling points because of higher polarity than the corresponding trans compound.

*Question #11* (Answer: a) See #10 and discussion in Section.


**4.4.5     Vocabulary, Concepts, etc. Checklist for Alkenes**

_____ carbonium ions
_____ stability of carbonium ions
_____ dipole moments of alkenes

_____ nomenclature of alkenes
_____ physical properties of alkenes


**4.5     BENZENE**

**4.5.1     Review of Benzene**

Many *monosubstituted benzenes* have special names or they can be named by the substituent attached:

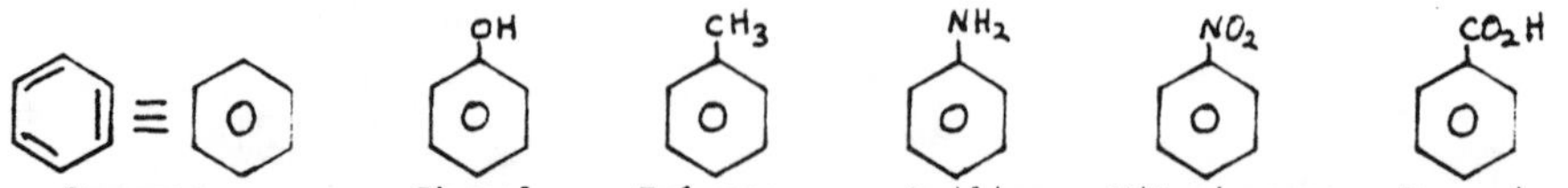

Benzene     Phenol     Toluene     Aniline     Nitrobenzene     Benzoic Acid

*Disubstituted benzenes* can be named as a derivative of the primary substituent with numbers or the o-p-m system:

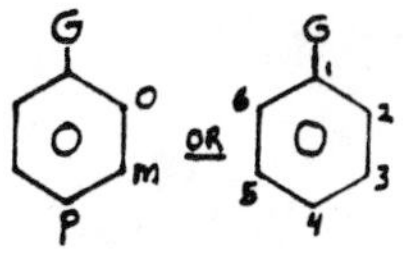

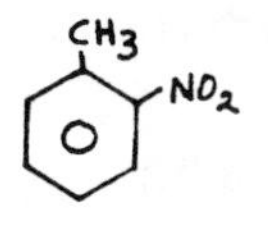

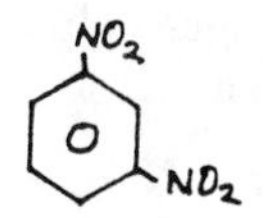

o=ortho
m=meta
p=para

o-Nitrotoulene

m-Dinitrobenzene

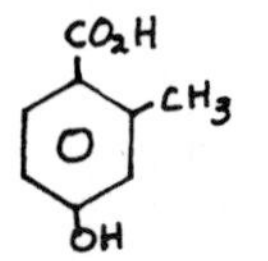

2-methyl-4-Hydroxybenzoic acid

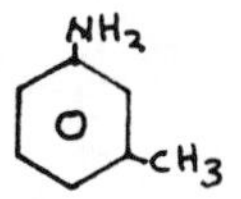

m-Methylaniline, or m-Aminotoluene

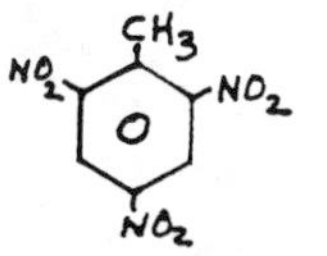

2,4,6-Trinitro-toluene

*Tri and higher substituted* benzenes require the numbering system as above.

The benzene ring is a set-up for resonance delocalization of charges (Section 4.1.1):

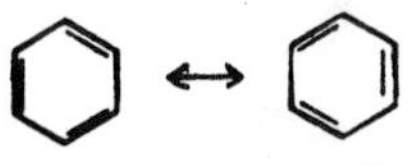

The key reaction of the benzene ring is the addition and eventual substitution of an electrophile (E$^+$, see Section 4.4.1) for a hydrogen (H) which requires stabilization of the intermediate positive charge:

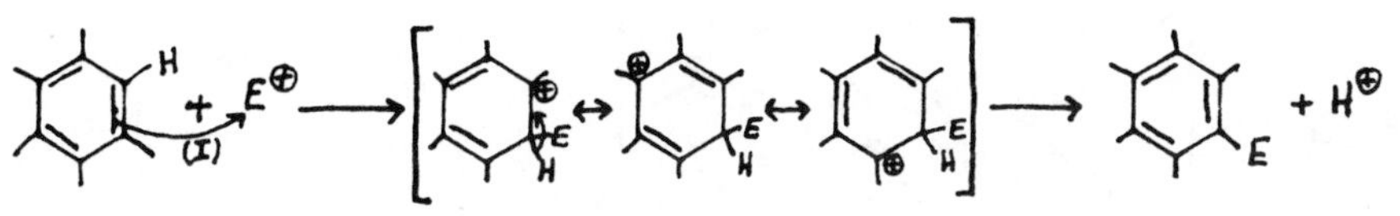

This stabilization of the intermediate positive charge is affected greatly by the substituents attached to the ring. Two types of substituents are identified. One group directs substituents to the ortho-para positions (o-p directors), and the other type directs substituents to the meta positions (meta directors):

*o-p directors* (e.g., $-OH$, $-NH_2$, $-OR$, $-NR_2$, alkyls)

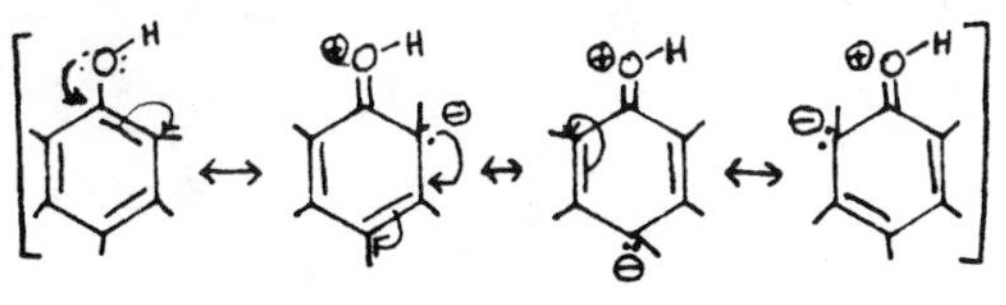

—note the electron density is at the o-p positions so the E$^+$ favors attack at o-p positions,

—with a substituent (E$^+$) at ortho or para get good stabilization:

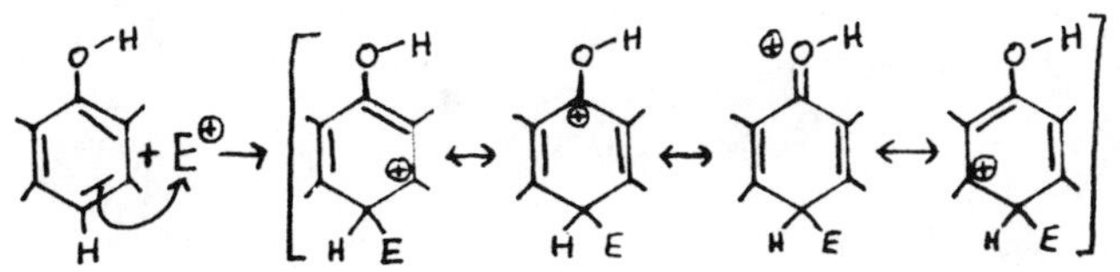

—with a substituent at meta:

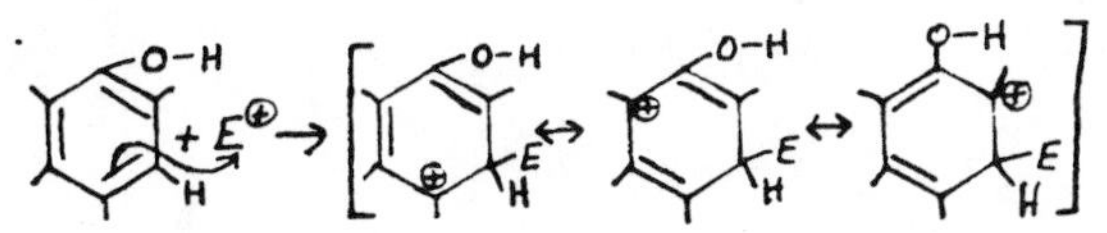

the − OH can no longer help delocalize the positive charge so the o-p is favored over the meta.

*meta directors* (e.g., − NO₂, − SO₂ −, − CN)

—without a substituent:

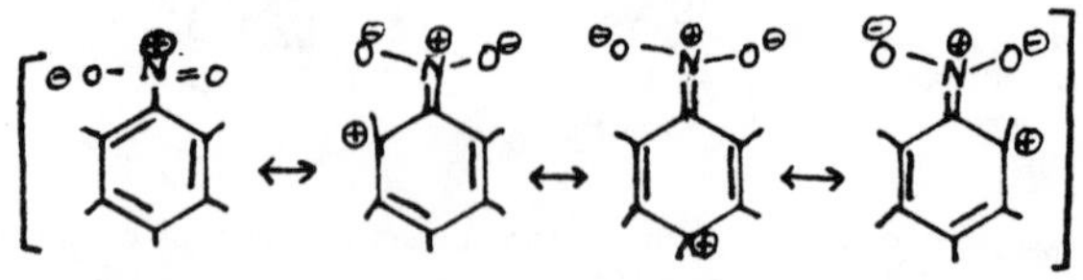

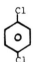

notice that + charge is put at the o-p positions so the E + favors attack at meta position

—with a substituent at meta positions:

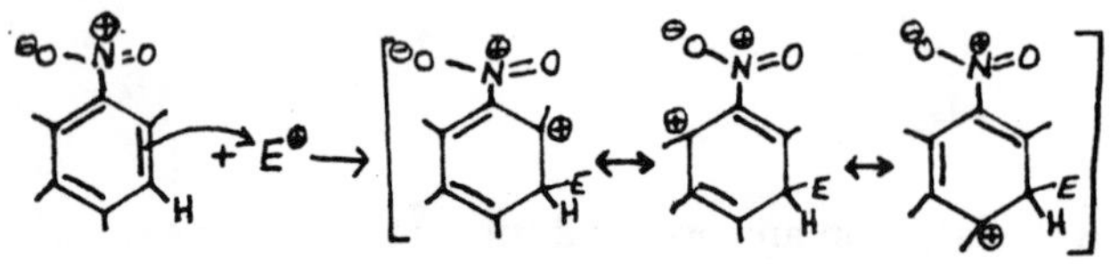

—with a substituent at o-p position:

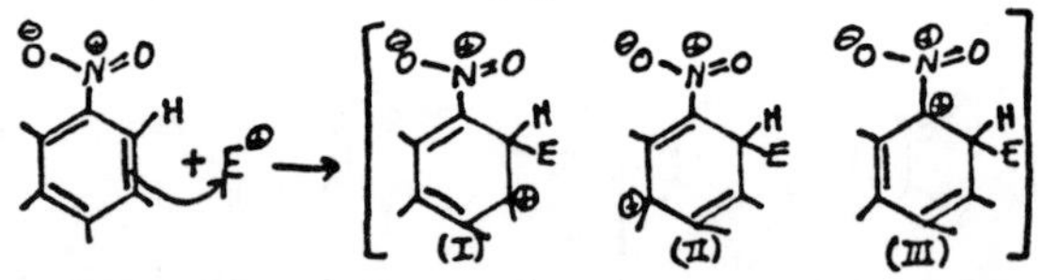

resonance form III is useless because of the adjacent positive charge; analogous situations exist with the other meta directors also; so, meta substitution is favored.

### 4.5.2  Questions to Review Benzene

(1)  Name the following compound:

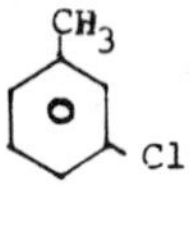

(a) o-Chlorotoluene
(b) p-Chloromethylbenzene
(c) 1-Methyl-2-chlorobenzene
(d) none of the above

(2)  Name the following compound:

(a) p-Dichlorobenzene
(b) m-Dichlorobenzene
(c) 1,3-Dichlorobenzene
(d) none of the above

(3)  Give the structure of 2-Chloro-4-Iodonitrobenzene:

(a)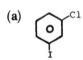

(b)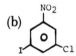

(d) none of the above

(c)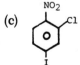

(4) Given the following compound, give the positions which will have the most electron density due to delocalization:

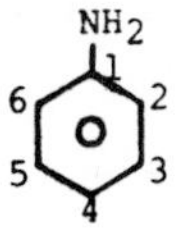

(a) 1,3,5
(b) 3,4,5
(c) 2,5
(d) none of these

(5) Given the following compound, give the positions which will have the most electron density due to delocalization:

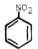

(a) 3,5
(b) 2,4,6
(c) 3,4,5
(d) none of these

(6) If $Br^+$ is an electrophile (e.g., from $Br_2$ + $AlCl_3$), the most likely product of its reaction with the following compound is:

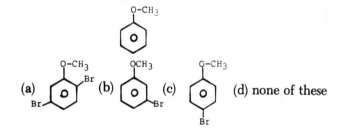

(d) none of these

(7) Assume the $Br^+$ from #6 reacts with the following compound, the most likely product is:

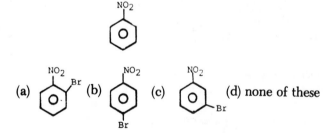

(d) none of these

## 4.5.3    Answers to Questions in Section 4.5.2

(1) d    (2) a    (3) c    (4) d    (5) a    (6) c    (7) c

## 4.5.4    Discussion of Answers to Questions in Section 4.5.2

*Question #1* (Answer: d) The correct name is m-Chlorotoluene (others also possible).

*Questions #2 - #5* Are adequately discussed in the Section.

*Question #6* (Answer: c) The $-O-CH_3$ is an o-p director. Of the products given (c) is the most likely. This para-product is also favored over the ortho product because of steric (bulk) consideration.

*Question #7* (Answer: c) The $-NO_2$ is a meta director.

## 4.5.5    Vocabulary, Concepts, etc. Checklist for Benzene

_____ nomenclature
_____ resonance of benzene
_____ reactions of benzene

## 4.6    ALCOHOLS

### 4.6.1    Review of Alcohols

See Section 4.3.1 for the basics of *nomenclature*. Alcohols are named by replacing the -e of the corresponding alkane with -ol for simple alcohols:

| $CH_4$ | $CH_3OH$ | $CH_3CH_2CH_3$ | $CH_3CH_2CH_2OH$ |
|--------|----------|----------------|------------------|
| methane | methanol | propane | propanol |
| | (methyl alcohol) | | (propyl alcohol) |

The use of sec-, iso-, and tert- are also appropriate:

$$\underset{\text{OH}}{CH_3-\overset{|}{C}H-CH_3} \qquad\qquad CH_3-\overset{CH_3}{\underset{CH_3}{\overset{|}{\underset{|}{C}}}}-OH$$

| isopropanol | tert-butyl alcohol |
|-------------|--------------------|
| (isopropyl alcohol) | (tert-butanol) |

For more complex alcohols, the numbering system is used and the carbon with the $-OH$ should, in general, have the lowest number (if the compound is named as an alcohol):

$$CH_3-CH_2-CH_2-\overset{CH_3}{\overset{|}{C}H}-CH_2-\overset{OH}{\overset{|}{C}H}-CH_2-C\overset{CH_3}{\underset{CH_3}{<}}$$

2,6-Dimethyl-4-nonanol

$$CH_3CH_2\overset{OH}{\overset{|}{C}H}CH_2CH_3$$

3-Pentanol

Alcohols are acidic because of the $-OH$ group:

$$>\overset{|}{C}-\underset{\delta^-}{O}-\underset{\delta^+}{H} \rightleftharpoons -\overset{|}{\underset{|}{C}}-O^{\ominus} + H^{\oplus}$$

They are very weakly acidic, being less strong than water. As the number of carbon groups attached to the C increases, the acidity decreases:

$$CH_3OH > CH_3CH_2OH \text{ in acidity}$$

$$\underset{1^\circ}{CH_3CH_2OH} > \underset{2^\circ}{CH_3-\overset{H}{\underset{CH_3}{\overset{|}{\underset{|}{C}}}}-OH} > \underset{3^\circ}{CH_3-\overset{CH_3}{\underset{CH_3}{\overset{|}{\underset{|}{C}}}}-OH} \text{ in acidity}$$

See Section 4.3.1 for general comments on *physical properties* of organic compounds. The greater polarity (dipole moment) and, especially, hydrogen bonding account for the greater solubility of alcohols in water, and the higher boiling points than comparable alkanes, alkenes, aldehydes, ketones and alkyl halides. As the carbon chain gets longer this nonpolar hydrocarbon chain overshadows the $-OH$ group and alcohols become less soluble in water.

The three major types of reactions of alcohols are dehydration, oxidation and substitution.

The *dehydration reaction* is,

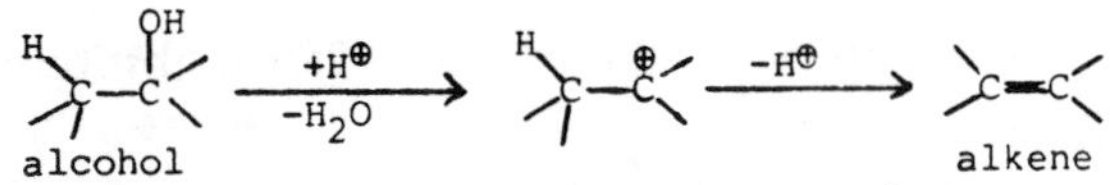

An intermediate carbonium ion is formed, and the faster reactions occur with the molecules that form the most stable carbonium ions (Section 4.4.1). The alkene formed is the most stable. Note that a phenyl group ( 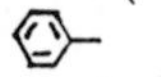 ) takes preference over 1 or 2 alkyl groups. Otherwise, the most substituted (i.e., most alkyl groups) double bond is the most stable:

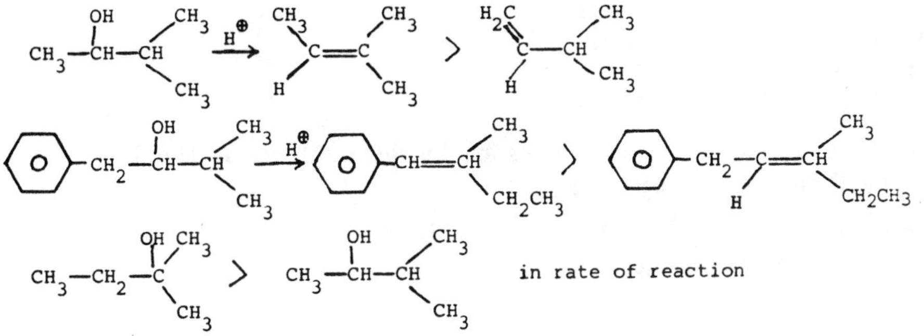

The *substitution reactions* are usually the replacement of the $-OH$ by a halide (usually Cl or Br) using a variety of reagents (HCl, HBr, $PCl_3$). In the most common mechanism, an intermediate carbonium ion is formed; so, the fastest reacting molecules are there with the most stable carbonium ion (Section 4.4.1). The 1° alcohols, especially, require vigorous conditions and/or the addition of extra reagents such as $ZnCl_2$ or $H_2SO_4$ to make the reaction go. Examples:

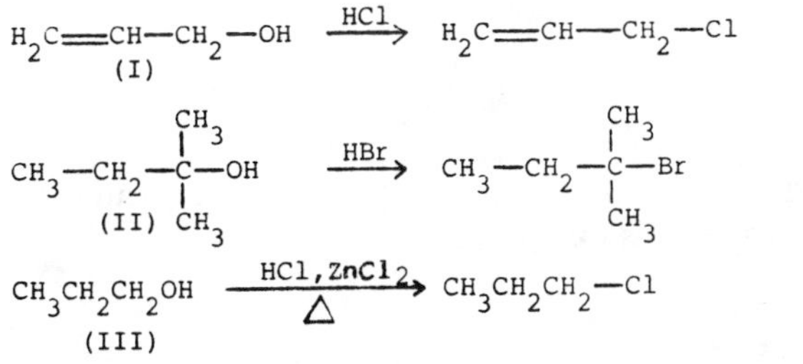

$$(I) > (II) > (III) \quad \text{in rate of reaction.}$$

*Oxidation reactions* can convert alcohols to aldehydes, ketones or carboxylic acids depending upon the structure of the alcohol (1° or 2°) and upon the reaction conditions. Primary (1°) alcohols may be converted to carboxylic acids (Section 4.10.1) or aldehydes (Section 4.7.1):

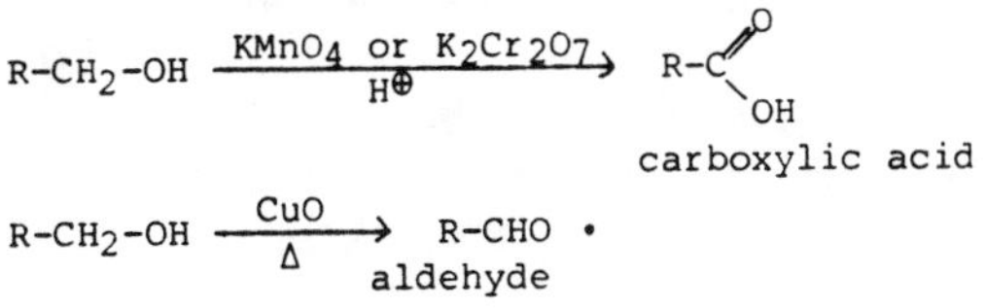

A secondary (2°) alcohol is converted to a ketone (Section 4.7.1):

$$R-\underset{\underset{R'}{|}}{\overset{\overset{H}{|}}{C}}-OH \xrightarrow{\text{any of the above}} R-\underset{\underset{R'}{|}}{C}=O \quad \text{Ketone}$$

Note that tertiary (3°) alcohols are not oxidized under basic conditions but may be oxidized under acidic conditions by being dehydrated first and then by the double bond being oxidized.

*Substitution reactions* may be further separated into $S_N1$ and $S_N2$. The $S_N1$ (Substitution Nucleophilic Monomolecular) mechanism is:

$$R\text{-}L \xrightarrow{\text{slow}} R^\oplus + L^\ominus$$

$$Nu^\ominus + R^\ominus \xrightarrow{\text{fast}} Nu\text{-}R$$

for reactions above: R = carbon group, L = $-OH$, $Nu^-$ = Cl, e.g.

The key features of the $S_N1$ are

(1) the rate depends on $[R-L]$,
(2) there is racemization of configuration (4.2.1),
(3) a stable carbonium ion should be formed,
    benzyl $\approx$ allyl > 3° > 2° > 1° in terms of rate.

Note the benzyl, allyl, 3° and 2° alcohol substitutions are by this mechanism. The $S_N2$ (Substitution Nucleophilic Bimolecular) mechanism is:

$$Nu^\ominus + R-L \rightarrow [Nu\ldots R\ldots L] \rightarrow NuR + L^\ominus$$
$$\text{(symbolism as before).}$$

The key features of $S_N2$ are:

(1) rate depends on $[R-L]$ and $[Nu^-]$.
(2) there is inversion of configuration (the opposite enantiomer is formed) (Section 4.2.1) if the alcohol was optically active to begin with,
(3) steric factors are important and not carbonium ions:

$$CH_3 - > 1° > 2° \ggg 3° \text{ in terms of rate.}$$

So, the substitutions for $CH_3OH$ and 1° alcohols are by the $S_N2$ mechanism.


## 4.6.2 Questions to Review Alcohols

(1) Alcohols have _____ boiling points and _____ solubility in water than corresponding alkanes and alkenes which is due to _____.

(a) lower, lesser, hydrogen bonding
(b) higher, greater, hydrogen bonding
(c) lower, lesser, polarity
(d) none of these

(2) In the dehydration reaction of alcohols, the _____ stable double bond is formed.

(a) most
(b) least

(3) Which of the following alcohols undergoes a substitution reaction the fastest?

(a) primary
(b) secondary
(c) allyl
(d) tertiary

(4) Which of the following types of alcohols is not normally oxidizable?

(a) primary
(b) secondary
(c) tertiary
(d) all of these are oxidizable

(5) Which type of alcohol probably undergoes substitution by an $S_N2$ mechanism?

(a) primary
(b) tertiary
(c) allyl
(d) none of these

(6) Name the following alcohol:

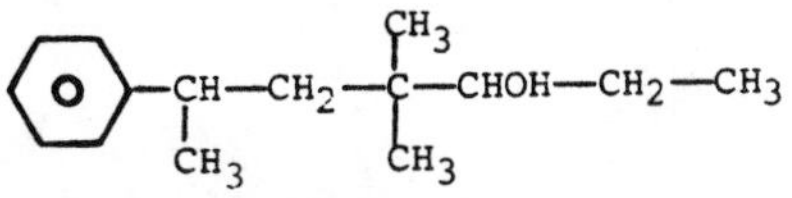

(a) 2-Phenyl-4, 4-dimethyl heptanol
(b) 4,4 Dimethyl-6-phenyl-3-heptanol
(c) Phenyl-2-heptanol
(d) none of these

(7) Select the strongest acid of the following:

(a) $CH_3—CH(CH_3)—OH$

(b) $CH_3—CH_2—CH(CH_3)—OH$

(c) $CH_3—CH_2—C(CH_3)_2—OH$

(d) $CH_3—CH_2—CH_2—OH$

(8) Which alcohol is least soluble in water?

(a) $CH_3—CH(CH_3)—CH_2—OH$

(b) $CH_3—CH_2—CH_2—CH_2—CH_2—CH_2—OH$

(c) $CH_3—CH_2—OH$

(d) $CH_3OH$

(9) Which alcohol will be dehydrated the fastest?

(a) 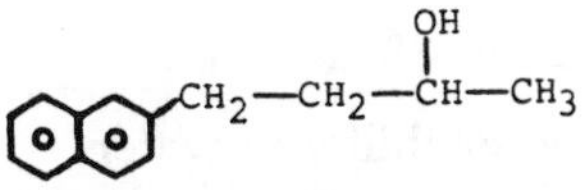

(b) $CH_3—CH_2—CH_2—CH_2—C(CH_3)_2—CH_2OH$

(c) $CH_3—CH(CH_3)—CH_2—C(CH_3)_2—OH$

(d) all at the same rate

(10) What is the most likely (or greatest) product of the following reaction?

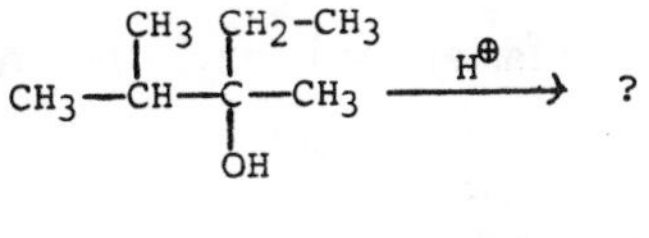

(a) 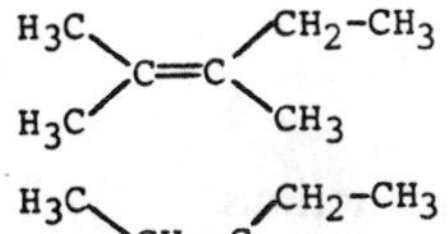

(b) 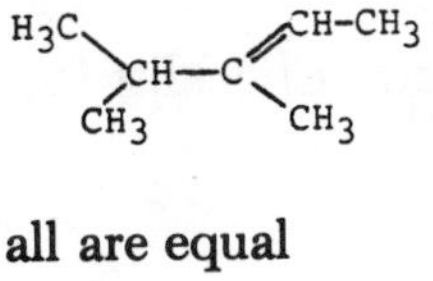

(c) 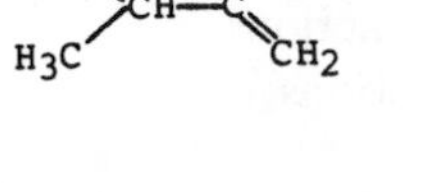

(d) all are equal

(11)  What is the most likely product of the following reaction:

(a)

(b)

(c)

(d) all are equal

(12)  Which alcohol will undergo the fastest reaction with HBr?

(a)

(b) $CH_3CH_2OH$

(c)

(d)

## 4.6.3    Answers to Questions in Section 4.6.2

( 1) b   ( 2) a   ( 3) c   ( 4) c   ( 5) a   ( 6) b   ( 7) d   ( 8) b   ( 9) c   (10) a   (11) c
(12) d

## 4.6.4    Discussion of Answers to Questions in Section 4.6.2

*Questions #1 to #5* Adequately discussed in Section.

*Question #6* (Answer: b) The numbering is,

*Question #7* (Answer: d) Primary alcohols are stronger than similar 2° or 3° alcohols.

*Question #8* (Answer: b) The longer the carbon chain, the smaller the solubility in water.

*Question #9* (Answer: c) Tertiary alcohols undergo dehydration faster than the 1° or 2° alcohols shown.

*Question #10* (Answer: a) The most substituted double bond will be the one that is formed.

*Question #11* (Answer: c) The double bond will be most stable when conjugated with the benzene ring even though it is not the most substituted.

*Question #12* (Answer: d) Substitution reactions are faster for benzyl (shown) or allyl type alcohols.

## 4.6.5    Vocabulary, Concepts, etc. Checklist for Alcohols

_____ nomenclature of alcohols
_____ acidity of alcohols
_____ physical properties of alcohols

_____ dehydration reactions
_____ substitution reactions
_____ oxidation reactions

## 4.7 ALDEHYDES AND KETONES

### 4.7.1 Review of Aldehydes and Ketones

See Section 4.3.1 for the basics of nomenclature. *Aldehydes* are generally symbolized as

$$R\overset{\overset{\displaystyle O}{\|}}{-C}-H,$$

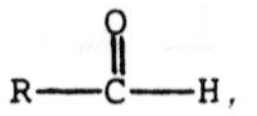

and the suffix -al replaces the -e of alkanes:

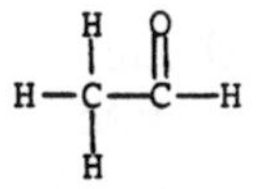

$$H-\overset{\overset{\displaystyle H}{|}}{\underset{\underset{\displaystyle H}{|}}{C}}-\overset{\overset{\displaystyle O}{\|}}{C}-H$$

ethanal
(acetaldehyde)

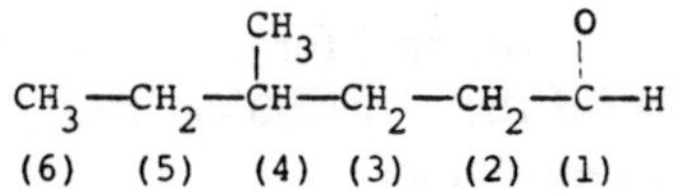

$$CH_3-CH_2-\overset{\overset{\displaystyle CH_3}{|}}{CH}-CH_2-CH_2-\overset{\overset{\displaystyle O}{\|}}{C}-H$$
(6)  (5)  (4)  (3)  (2)  (1)
4-Methylhexanal
the aldehyde carbon is always #1

Ketones are generally symbolized as

$$R-\overset{\overset{\displaystyle O}{\|}}{C}-R'$$

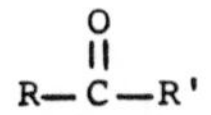

and the suffix -one replaces the -e of alkanes:

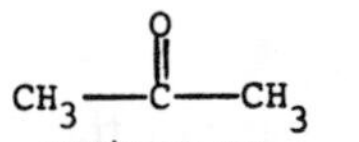

$$CH_3-\overset{\overset{\displaystyle O}{\|}}{C}-CH_3$$
acetone <u>or</u>
2-Propanone
(the location of the $\left(\overset{\overset{\displaystyle O}{\|}}{\underset{}{C}}\right)$
is always shown)

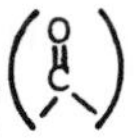

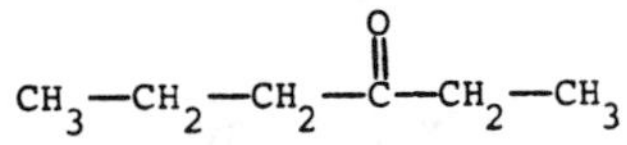

$$CH_3-CH_2-CH_2-\overset{\overset{\displaystyle O}{\|}}{C}-CH_2-CH_3$$
3-Hexanone <u>or</u>
Ethyl propyl ketone

The *carbonyl group* $\left(\overset{\overset{\displaystyle O}{\|}}{\underset{}{C}}\right)$ is the basis for the chemistry of aldehydes and ketones. The key features are:

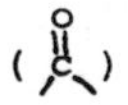

(1) Polarity of C = O bond. The oxygen is attacked by electrophiles ($E\oplus$), and the carbon by nucleophiles (Nu: $\ominus$).

Both of these disrupt the double bond:

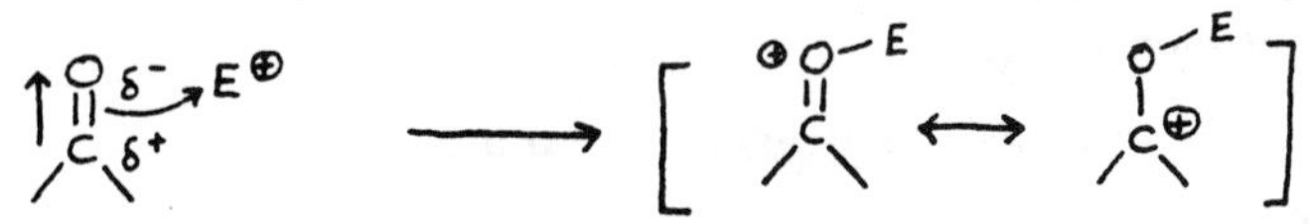

large dipole moment

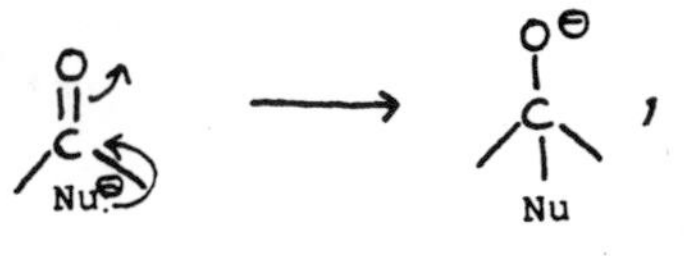

(2) The $\alpha$-hydrogen is acidic and can be abstracted by bases. It is even more acidic if between two carbonyls:

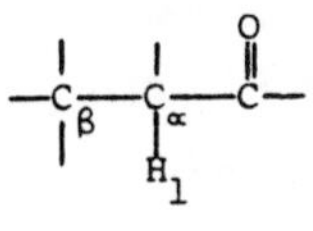

$H_2 > H_1$ in acidity

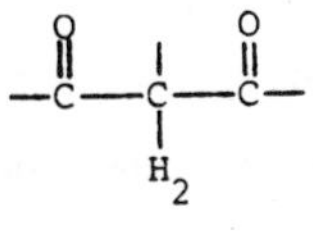

(3) The main reason for the acidity of the $\alpha$-H is that the resulting $\alpha$-carbanion is stabilized by resonance. This stabilization also allows for nucleophilic addition at the $\beta$-carbon in

$\alpha$-$\beta$ unsaturated carbonyls:

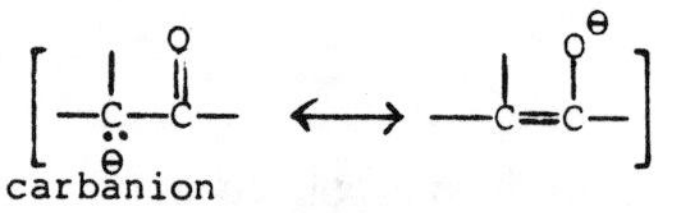

resonance stabilization

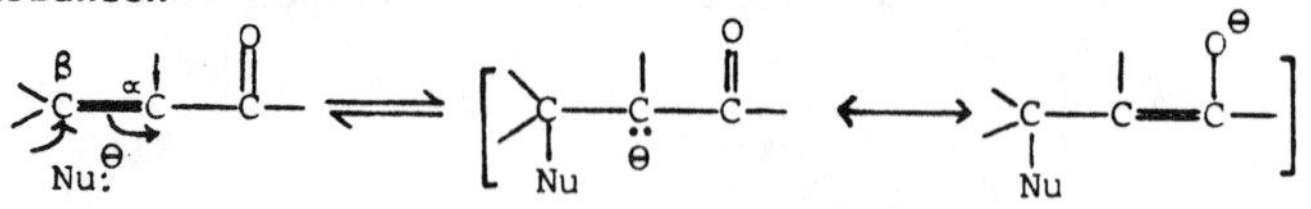

carbanion

$\alpha$,$\beta$ unsaturated carbonyl

(4) The carbonyl exists in equilibrium with the enol form; this is tautomerization. Usually the carbonyl form predominates, but if the enol double bond can be conjugated with other double bonds, it can become very stable:

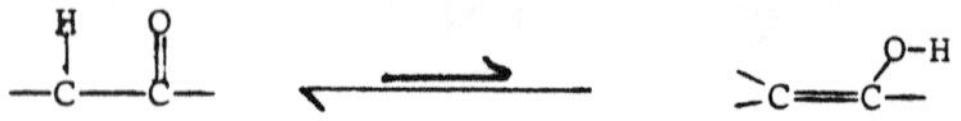

carbonyl

enol (undergoes reactions of the double bond)

(5) The O of the carbonyl forms hydrogen bonds with Hs attached to other O's or N's:

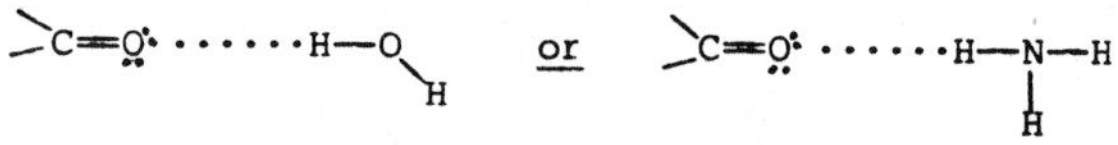

or

Most of the reactions and properties of carbonyls may be understood on the basis of the above features. In general, aldehydes oxidize easier and undergo nucleophilic addition easier than ketones.

The *boiling point* of carbonyls is higher than most other polar organic molecules but less than that of alcohols and acids (each can hydrogen bond to molecules of itself). The low molecular weight carbonyls are soluble in water because they can form hydrogen bonds with it—as the molecular weights increase, the hydrocarbon part dominates and solubility decreases.

*Oxidation reactions* of aldehydes are:

(1) $\underset{\text{(Ar)}}{\text{RCHO}} \xrightarrow[\text{(Tollen's Reagent)}]{\text{Ag(NH}_3\text{)}2^\oplus} \underset{\text{(Ar)}}{\text{R-CO}_2\text{H}} + \text{Ag(mirror)}$

Ar = Aromatic        Benedict's Reagent is also used

(2) $\underset{\text{(Ar)}}{\text{RCHO}} \xrightarrow[\text{(2)}\,\text{K}_2\text{Cr}_2\text{O}_7]{\underset{\text{or}}{\text{(1)}\,\text{KMnO}_4}} \underset{\text{(Ar)}}{\text{RCO}_2\text{H}}$

(3) Ketones are rarely oxidized.

*Reduction reactions* of carbonyls

(1)

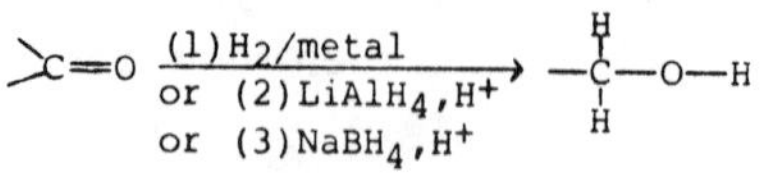

*Nucleophilic addition reactions* (See #1 and #3 of second paragraph):

(1) Addition of nitrogen bases to carbonyls. The N needs two H's to add:

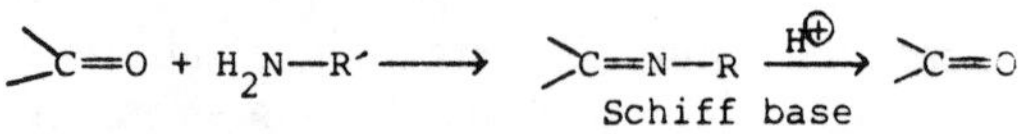

Schiff base

e.g., of R'-NH$_2$

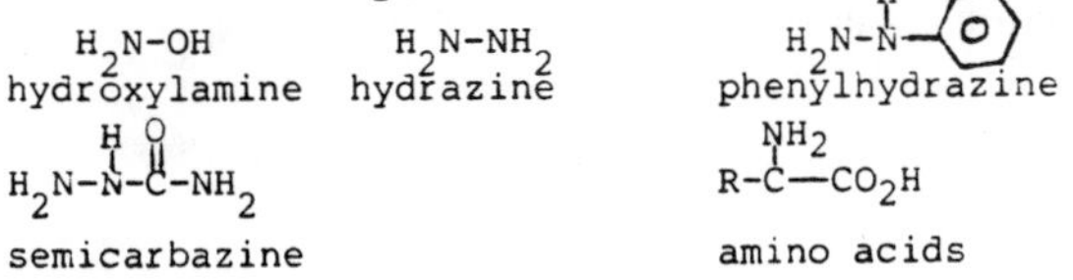

H$_2$N-OH    H$_2$N-NH$_2$
hydroxylamine  hydrazine

H O
| ||
H$_2$N-N-C-NH$_2$
semicarbazine

H$_2$N-N-⬡
phenylhydrazine

NH$_2$
|
R-C—CO$_2$H
amino acids

## (2) Acetal (Ketal) and hemiacetal (hemiketal) formation

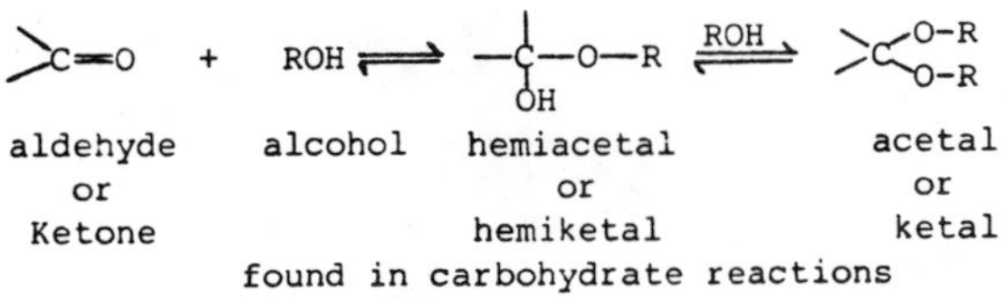

>C=O  +  ROH ⇌  —C—O—R  $\xrightarrow{ROH}$  >C$\begin{smallmatrix}O-R\\O-R\end{smallmatrix}$
       |
       OH

aldehyde    alcohol    hemiacetal    acetal
  or                      or           or
Ketone                  hemiketal     ketal
           found in carbohydrate reactions

## (3) The Aldol condensation of carbonyls. The α-H is important:

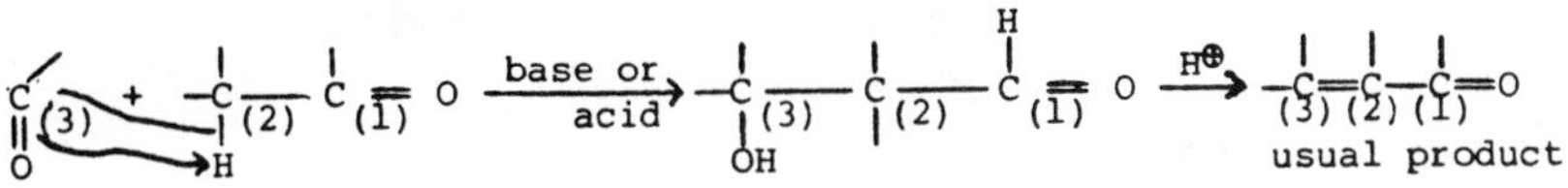

base or acid → ... $\xrightarrow{H^\oplus}$ usual product

## (4) Nucleophilic addition to α, β-unsaturated carbonyls:

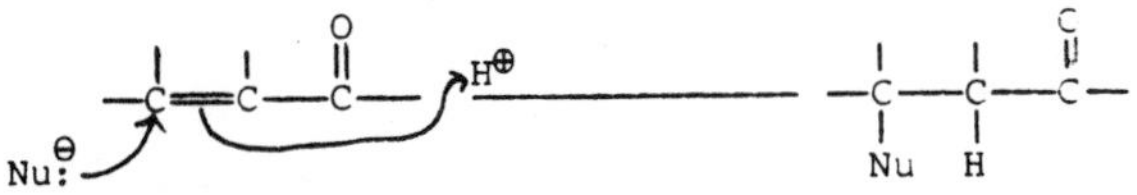

e.g., Nu:'s (do not have to be negative; need pair of electrons)

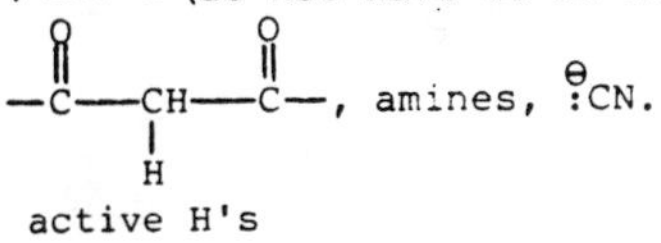

O       O
||      ||
—C—CH—C—, amines, $^\ominus$:CN.
   |
   H
active H's

## 4.7.2    Questions to Review Aldehydes and Ketones

(1)   The carbonyl group is _____ with the carbon being slightly _____ and the oxygen being slightly _____.

(a) polarized, negative, positive
(b) polarized, positive, negative
(c) neither (a) nor (b)

(2)   Which hydrogen is the most acidic?

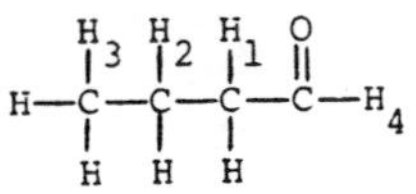

H$_3$ H$_2$ H$_1$ O
|   |   |  ||
H—C—C—C—C—H$_4$
|   |   |
H   H   H

(a) H$_1$
(b) H$_2$
(c) H$_3$
(d) H$_4$

(3)   Generally undergo nucleophilic addition more easily:

(a) aldehydes
(b) ketones
(c) both equally

(4)    Aldehydes and ketones have higher boiling points than corresponding compounds (similar carbon structures) of all the following except:

(a) alkanes
(b) alkenes
(c) ethers
(d) alcohols

(5)    Rarely oxidized:

(a) aldehydes
(b) ketones
(c) neither

(6)    Name the following compound:

$$CH_3-\underset{\underset{Cl}{|}}{\overset{\overset{CH_3}{|}}{C}}-CH_2CHO$$

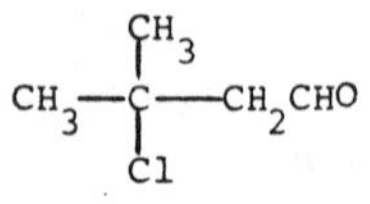

(a) tert-chlorobutanal
(b) tert-chlorobutyl ketone
(c) hydrogen chloro-tert-butyl ketone
(d) 3-chloro-3-methyl-butanal

(7)    Name the following compound:

$$\underset{CH_3}{\overset{CH_3}{>}}CH-\overset{\overset{O}{||}}{C}-CH_2CH_3$$

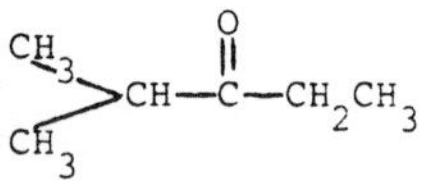

(a) 2-methyl-3-pentanone
(b) diethyl methyl ketone
(c) 2-methyl-3-butanal
(d) isobutyl ethyl ketone

(8)    Select the product of the following reaction:

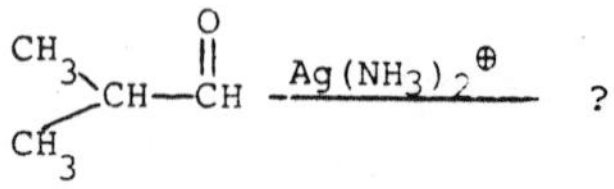

$$\underset{CH_3}{\overset{CH_3}{>}}CH-\overset{\overset{O}{||}}{CH} \xrightarrow{Ag(NH_3)_2^{\oplus}} ?$$

(a)
$$\underset{CH_3}{\overset{CH_3}{>}}CH-\underset{\underset{OH}{|}}{CH}-\underset{\underset{OH}{|}}{CH}-CH\overset{CH_3}{\underset{CH_3}{<}}$$

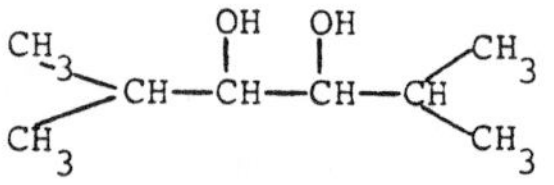

(b)
$$\underset{CH_3}{\overset{CH_3}{>}}CH-\underset{\underset{H}{|}}{\overset{\overset{O-H}{|}}{C}}-H$$

(c)
$$\underset{CH_3}{\overset{CH_3}{>}}C=CH_2$$

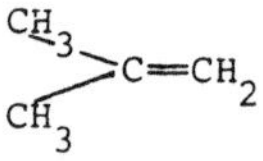

(d)
$$\underset{CH_3}{\overset{CH_3}{>}}CH-\overset{\overset{O}{||}}{C}-OH$$

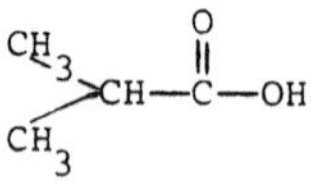

(9)    Select the product of the following reaction:

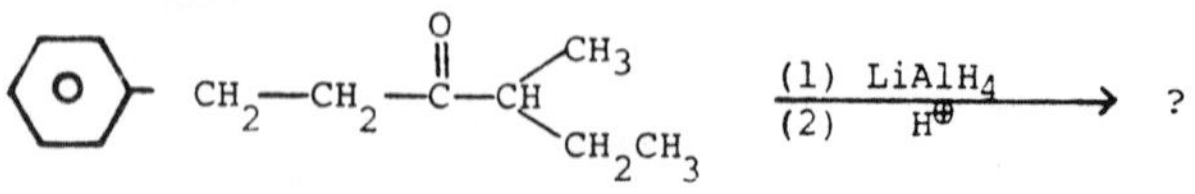

$$\langle O \rangle-CH_2-CH_2-\overset{\overset{O}{||}}{C}-CH\overset{CH_3}{\underset{CH_2CH_3}{<}} \xrightarrow[\text{(2)  } H^{\oplus}]{\text{(1)  LiAlH}_4} ?$$

(a)
$$\langle O \rangle-CH_2-CH_2-\overset{\overset{O}{\diagup}}{C}\underset{OH}{} + \underset{OH}{\overset{\overset{O}{||}}{C}}-CH\overset{CH_3}{\underset{CH_2CH_3}{<}}$$

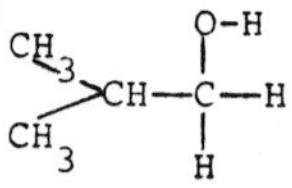

(b)
$$\langle O \rangle-CH_2-CH_2-\underset{\underset{H}{|}}{\overset{\overset{OH}{|}}{C}}-CH\overset{CH_3}{\underset{CH_2-CH_3}{<}}$$

(c)
$$\langle O \rangle-CH_2-CH_2-\overset{\overset{O}{||}}{\underset{H}{C}}-H + \overset{\overset{O}{||}}{\underset{H}{C}}-CH\overset{CH_3}{\underset{CH_2-CH_3}{<}}$$

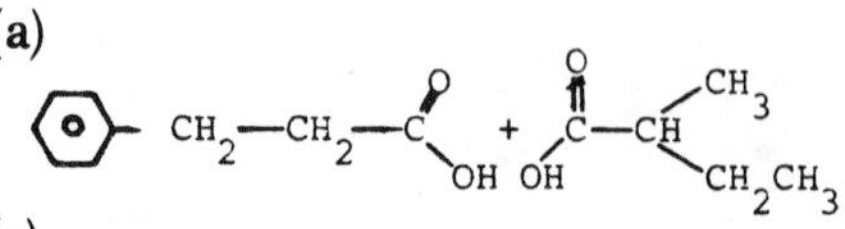

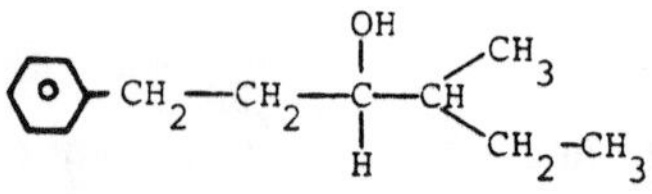

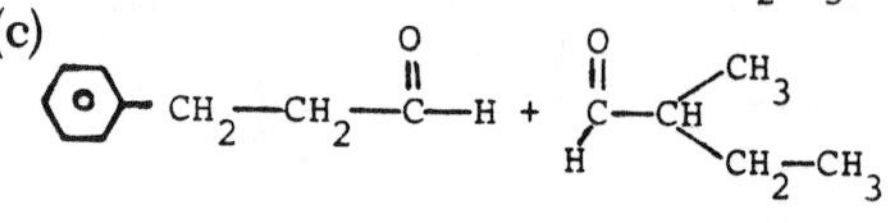

(d) none of the above

4-36

(10) Select the product of the following reaction:

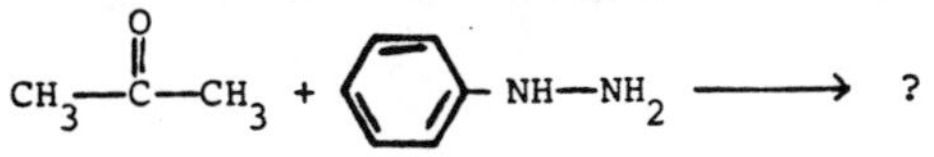

$$CH_3-\overset{\overset{\displaystyle O}{\|}}{C}-CH_3 \ + \ \langle\!\!\bigcirc\!\!\rangle - NH-NH_2 \ \longrightarrow \ ?$$

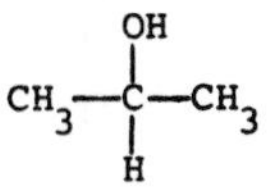

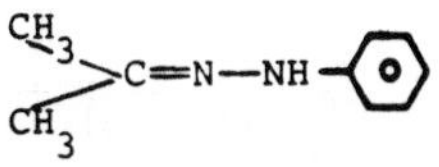

(a)

$$CH_3-\overset{\overset{\displaystyle OH}{|}}{\underset{\underset{\displaystyle H}{|}}{C}}-CH_3$$

(b)

$$\overset{\displaystyle CH_3}{\underset{\displaystyle CH_3}{>}}C=N-NH-\langle\!\!\bigcirc\!\!\rangle$$

(c)

$$\overset{\displaystyle CH_3}{\underset{\displaystyle H_3C}{>}}C=N\overset{\langle\!\!\bigcirc\!\!\rangle}{\underset{\displaystyle NH_2}{}}$$

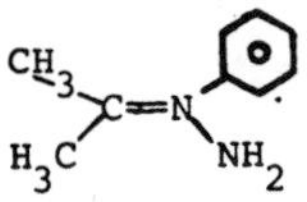

(d) none of the above

(11) Select the product of the following reaction:

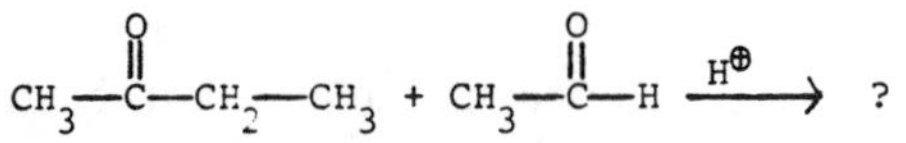

$$CH_3-\overset{\overset{\displaystyle O}{\|}}{C}-CH_2-CH_3 \ + \ CH_3-\overset{\overset{\displaystyle O}{\|}}{C}-H \ \overset{H^{\oplus}}{\longrightarrow} \ ?$$

(a) no reaction

(b)

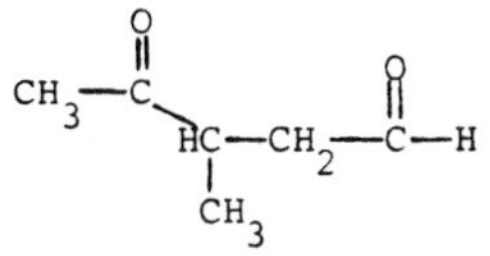

$$CH_3-\overset{\overset{\displaystyle O}{\|}}{C}\underset{\underset{\underset{\displaystyle CH_3}{|}}{HC}-CH_2-\overset{\overset{\displaystyle O}{\|}}{C}-H}{}$$

(c)

$$\overset{\displaystyle CH_3}{\underset{\displaystyle H_3C-CH_2}{>}}C=CH-\overset{\overset{\displaystyle O}{\|}}{C}-H$$

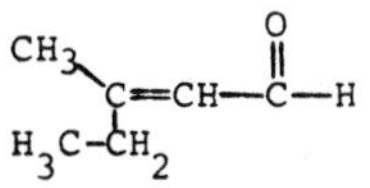

(d) none of the above

## 4.7.3  Answers to Questions in Section 4.7.2

( 1) b  ( 2) a  ( 3) a  ( 4) d  ( 5) b  ( 6) d  ( 7) a  ( 8) d  ( 9) b  (10) b  (11) c

## 4.7.4  Discussion of Answers to Questions in Section 4.7.2

*Questions #1 to #5* Adequately discussed in Section.

*Question #6* (Answer: d) This is an aldehyde numbered as

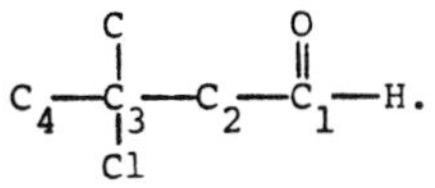

$$C_4-\overset{\overset{\displaystyle C}{|}}{\underset{\underset{\displaystyle Cl}{|}}{C_3}}-C_2-\overset{\overset{\displaystyle O}{\|}}{C_1}-H.$$

*Question #7* (Answer: a) The numbering of this ketone is

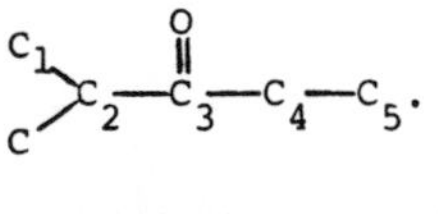

$$\overset{\displaystyle C_1}{\underset{\displaystyle C}{>}}C_2-\overset{\overset{\displaystyle O}{\|}}{C_3}-C_4-C_5.$$

An alternate name is: Ethyl isopropyl ketone

*Question #8* (Answer: d) This is an oxidation reaction as shown in the Section.

*Question #9* (Answer: b) This is a reduction reaction as shown in the Section.

*Question #10* (Answer: b) To add to the carbonyl, the N must have two H's (i.e., $-NH_2$). The N attached to the benzene ring does not complete the reaction.

*Question #11* (Answer: c) There are many possible products of this reaction. The key is that the α-carbon of one carbonyl attacks the carbonyl of the other. Other possible products are:

$$CH_3-CH_2-\underset{O}{\overset{\|}{C}}-CH_3 \qquad CH_3-\underset{O}{\overset{\|}{C}}-H$$

(1)   (2)   (3)   (4)          (5)   (6)

(the answer given)

## 4.7.5   Vocabulary, Concepts, etc. Checklist for Aldehydes and Ketones

_____ nomenclature of aldehydes and ketones      _____ nucleophilic addition reactions
_____ physical properties of aldehydes and ketones   _____ oxidation reactions
_____ acidity of α-hydrogens                      _____ carbonyl group
_____ carbanions

## 4.8   ETHERS

### 4.8.1   Review of Ethers

Ethers have the *general structure:* R—O—R'

R, R' are aliphatic or aromatic but not H. Ethers are named by naming the R and R' and following these by 'ether':

$$CH_3-CH_2-O-CH_2-CH_3 \qquad CH_3-O-CH\overset{CH_3}{\underset{CH_3}{<}}$$

Diethyl ether          Methyl isopropyl ether
(or 'ether')

The *physical properties* of ethers reflect the polar oxygen and the nonpolar hydrocarbon component. There is some solubility in water due to the O hydrogen bonding with $H_2O$. The boiling points are less than alcohols and about the same as alkanes because there is no hydrogen bonding between the molecules of ether.

### 4.8.2   Study the brief section above. No questions, etc.

## 4.9   PHENOLS

### 4.9.1   Review of Phenols

A phenol consists of a hydroxyl group attached to an aromatic ring. The *nomenclature* is as given in Section 4.5.1. Some phenols which have counterparts in biochemistry and medicine are:

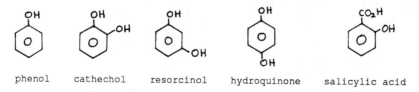

phenol   cathechol   resorcinol   hydroquinone   salicylic acid

Important features of the chemistry of phenols are:

(1) Phenols are acidic due to the dissociable hydrogen on the oxygen. Phenols are more acidic than alcohols because of the electron withdrawing and resonance stabilization effects of the aromatic ring:

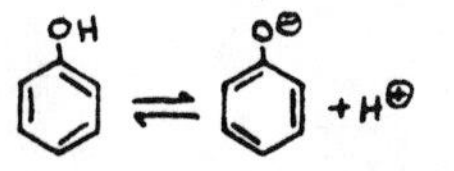

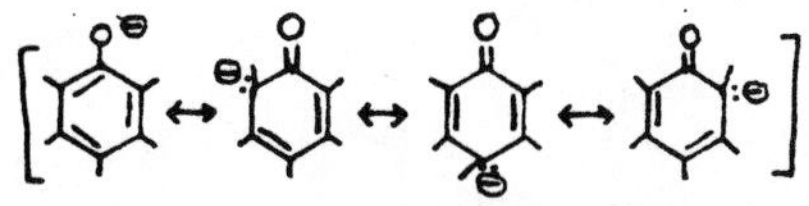

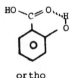

The resonance forms show that groups which stabilize electrons when placed at o-p positions should make the phenol more acidic. Groups which can stabilize the negative charge are $-NO_2$, $-CN$, $-CO_2H$. Groups which might tend to destabilize (and make less acidic) are alkyl groups or other o-p directors (see Section 4.5.1).

(2) Phenols form intramolecular and intermoleculr hydrogen bonds (see boiling point discussion below).

(3) Phenols are powerful o-p directors.

*Physical properties* are understood by considering the hydrogen bond forming capacity and the hydrophobic nature of aromatic rings. Even phenol itself is only slightly soluble in water (due to hydrogen bonding), but most other phenols are insoluble due to the aromatic ring. Most phenols will have high boiling points, primarily due to hydrogen bonding between molecules. Within the disubstituted phenols, the ortho compounds tend to have lower boiling points because they have the potential for intramolecular hydrogen bonding whereas meta and para have intermolecular hydrogen bonding (and higher boiling points):

intramolecular
hydrogen bonding

ortho

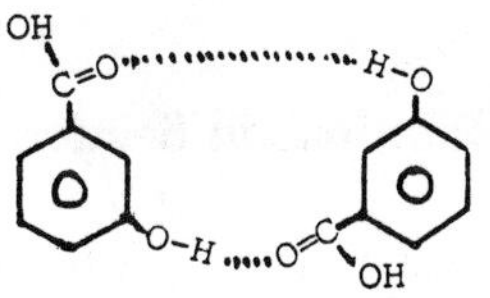

meta (or para)
intermolecular
hydrogen bonding

### 4.9.2 Questions to Review Phenols

(1) Name the following compound:

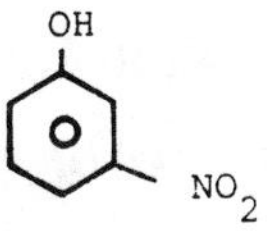

(a) o,m-Hydroxynitrobenzene
(b) 2-Nitrophenol
(c) o-Nitrophenol
(d) m-Nitrophenol

(2) Which of the following is most acidic?

(a) CH₃CH₂-OH

(b) 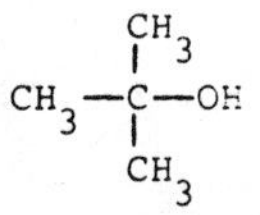 $CH_3 - \overset{\overset{\displaystyle CH_3}{|}}{\underset{\underset{\displaystyle CH_3}{|}}{C}} - OH$

(c)

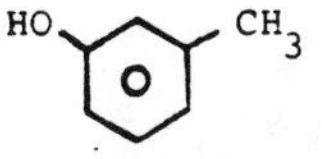

(d) all are probably equal

(3) Which of the following is most acidic?

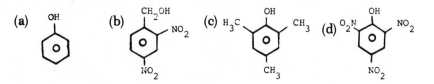

(a)  (b)  (c)  (d)

(4)    Which of the following compounds probably has the highest boiling point?

(a) $CH_3(CH_2)_2 - CH = CH_2$

(b) $CH_3 - O - CH_3$

(c) 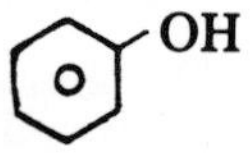 ![phenol structure with OH]

(d) $CH_3 - CH_3$

(5)    Given the following two compounds

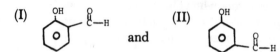

compound ____ probably has the lower boiling point because there is _____ hydrogen bonding possible.

(a) I, intramolecular

(b) II, intramolecular

(c) II, intermolecular

(d) none of these


### 4.9.3    Answers to Questions in Section 4.9.2

(1) d    (2) c    (3) d    (4) c    (5) a


### 4.9.4    Discussion of Answers to Questions in Section 4.9.2

*Question #1* (Answer: d) Name compound as a phenol with o-m-p as:

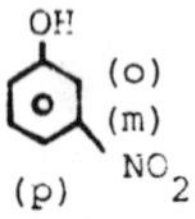

![phenol structure with OH, (o), (m), NO2, (p)]

*Question #2* (Answer: c) Phenols are more acidic than alcohols.

*Question #3* (Answer: d) Electron withdrawing groups ($-NO_2$) at o-p positions increase the acidity of phenols.

*Question #4* (Answer: c) The phenol can hydrogen bond to itself which increases the boiling point; the others cannot.

*Question #5* (Answer: a) Intramolecular H-bonding is possible if the compound is ortho and this decreases the boiling point.


### 4.9.5    Vocabulary, Concepts, etc. Checklist for Phenols

_____ nomenclature of phenols
_____ physical properties of phenols
_____ acidity of phenols
_____ hydrogen bonding of phenols

## 4.10    CARBOXYLIC ACIDS

### 4.10.1    Review of Carboxylic Acids

See Section 4.3.1 on general nomenclature. The -e of alkanes is replaced by -oic acid for carboxylic acids:

$$CH_3\text{-}CH_2\text{-}CH_2\text{-}CH_3$$

Butane

$$\underset{(4)\ \ (3)\ \ (2)\ \ (1)}{CH_3\text{-}CH_2\text{-}CH_2\text{-}CO_2H}$$

Butanoic acid

The $-CO_2H$ carbon is always numbered #1 as above. Other rules are as before. For example:

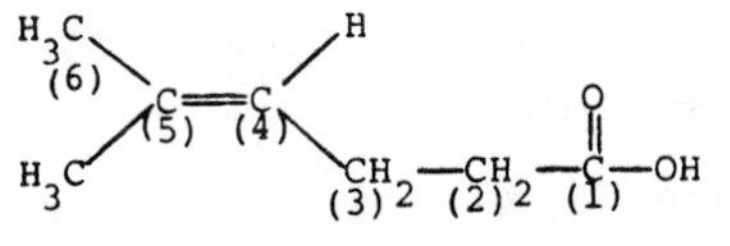

5-Methyl-4-hexenoic acid

Some common carboxylic acids are (with trivial names)

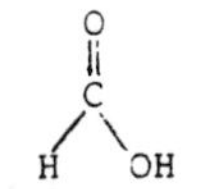

Formic acid 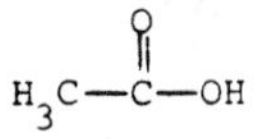        Acetic acid 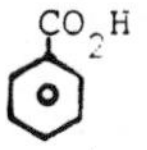        Benzoic acid

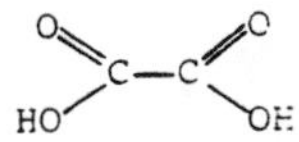

Oxalic acid 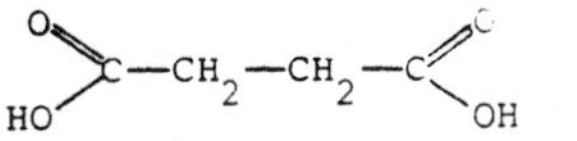        Succinic acid

The key functional group of these compounds is the carboxyl,

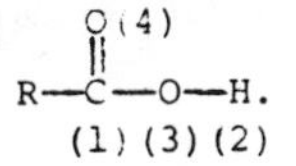

$$\underset{(1)\ (3)\ (2)}{R\text{—}\overset{\overset{O\,(4)}{\|}}{C}\text{—}O\text{—}H.}$$

Reactions of the carboxylic acids center around the four central features of the carboxyl group:

(1) The H(2) is acidic because it is weakly attached to the O(3) and because the resulting carboxylate anion is stabilized by resonance

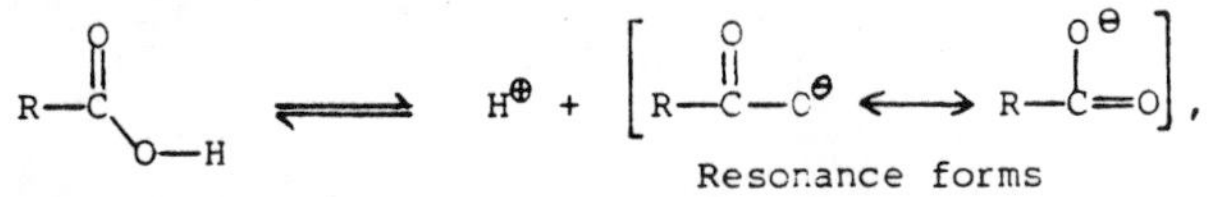

Resonance forms

(2) The carboxyl carbon (1) is very susceptible to attack by nucleophilic agents (Nu; see Section 4.4.1) because of the attached electronegative oxygens and the carbonyl oxygen (4):

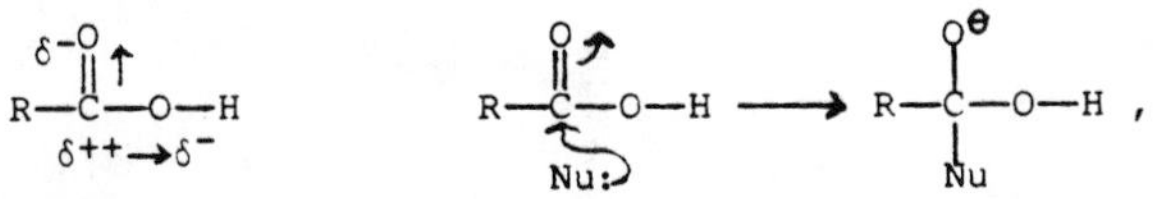

(3) The hydroxyl can become a good leaving group by appropriate solvent conditions (e.g., if basic) and/or by protonating, if acidic solution, and hence, this also promotes nucleophilic substitution,

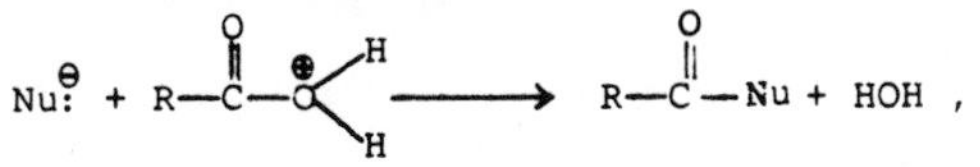

$$Nu\!:^{\ominus} + R\text{—}\overset{\overset{O}{\|}}{C}\text{—}\overset{\oplus}{O}\overset{H}{\underset{H}{\diagup}} \longrightarrow R\text{—}\overset{\overset{O}{\|}}{C}\text{—}Nu + HOH\ ,$$

(4) Hydrogen bonding is possible between molecules (intermolecular) and/or within the same molecule (intramolecular) because of the carbonyl and hydroxyl moieties,

$$R-C \underset{O-H \cdots\cdots O}{\overset{O \cdots\cdots H-O}{\phantom{xx}}} C-R$$

Intermolecular (dimerization)

Intramolecular

Low molecular weight aliphatic carboxylic acids tend to be *soluble* in water due to hydrogen bonding with water; aromatic acids are not, in general, soluble. The acids are also soluble in dilute bases, NaOH or $NaHCO_3$, e.g., because of their acid properties. The *boiling points* are high because of the hydrogen bonding possible between molecules.

Carboxylic acids are the *acids* of organic chemistry. The only other compounds which approach their acid strength are substituted phenols (see Section 4.9.1). Organic classes of molecules by decreasing acid strength are:

$$RCO_2H > HOH > ROH > HC = CH > NH_3 > RH$$

(substituted phenols may be stronger acids than $H_2O$).

The relative base strength is just the reverse. In order of decreasing base strength:

$$R^{\ominus} > NH_2^{\ominus} > HC = C^{\ominus} > RO^{\ominus} > HO^{\ominus} > RCO_2^{\ominus}$$

The *relative acid strength* of carboxylic acids depends primarily on the groups attached and the distance of these groups from the carboxyl:

$$CH_3CH_2 \underset{\underset{Cl}{|}}{\overset{\overset{Cl}{|}}{C}} CO_2H > CH_3-CH_2 \underset{\underset{Cl}{|}}{\overset{\overset{H}{|}}{C}} CO_2H \text{ in acid strength}$$

Cl is an electron withdrawer and stabilizes the carboxylate anion

$$CH_3 \underset{\underset{Cl}{|}}{\overset{\overset{Cl}{|}}{C}} CH_2-CO_2H < CH_3-CH_2 \underset{\underset{Cl}{|}}{\overset{\overset{Cl}{|}}{C}} CO_2H \text{ in acid strength}$$

The *nucleophilic substitution* reactions can involve a variety of nucleophiles (Nu) reacting under a variety of conditions,

$$R \overset{\overset{O}{\|}}{-C}-OH + Nu^{\ominus} \longrightarrow R \overset{\overset{O}{\|}}{-C}-Nu + OH^{\ominus}$$

Nu: = − OR′   R′ = (1° > 2° > 3°), esters result
   = − NH₂, amides result
   = − Cl² from SOCl₂ or PCl₃ or PCl₅, acid chlorides result

In the ester reaction,

$$R \overset{\overset{O}{\|}}{-C}-O-H + R'-\overset{*}{O}-H \longrightarrow R \overset{\overset{O}{\|}}{-C}-\overset{*}{O}-R' + H_2O$$

acid      alcohol      ester
note the origin of the O*

The major *reduction reaction* is with LiAlH₄:

$$R \overset{\overset{O}{\|}}{-C}-OH \xrightarrow{\text{LiAlH}_4} R-CH_2-OH$$

alcohol

Acids can be converted to esters or amides and then reduced also.

The typical decarboxylation reaction involves β-diacids or β-Ketoacids:

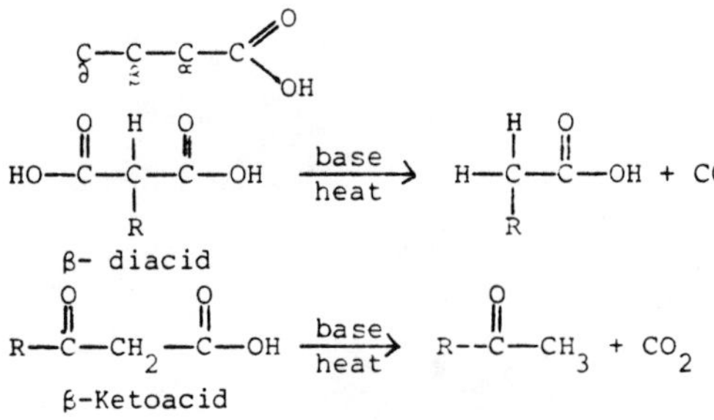

$$\underset{\beta}{C}-\underset{\gamma}{C}-\underset{\alpha}{C}-C\overset{O}{\underset{OH}{\diagup}}$$

$$HO-\overset{O}{\overset{\|}{C}}-\overset{H}{\underset{R}{\overset{|}{C}}}-\overset{O}{\overset{\|}{C}}-OH \xrightarrow[\text{heat}]{\text{base}} H-\overset{H}{\underset{R}{\overset{|}{C}}}-\overset{O}{\overset{\|}{C}}-OH + CO_2$$

β- diacid

$$R-\overset{O}{\overset{\|}{C}}-CH_2-\overset{O}{\overset{\|}{C}}-OH \xrightarrow[\text{heat}]{\text{base}} R--\overset{O}{\overset{\|}{C}}-CH_3 + CO_2$$

β-Ketoacid

## 4.10.2    Questions to Review Carboxylic Acids

(1)    Which atom below is susceptible to nucleophilic attack?

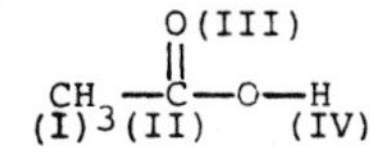

$$\underset{(I)}{CH_3}-\underset{(II)}{\overset{\overset{\textstyle O(III)}{\|}}{C}}-\underset{(IV)}{O-H}$$

(a) I
(b) II
(c) III
(d) IV

(2)    A high molecular weight carboxylic acid may be soluble in _____ but probably not in _____.

(a) dilute acid, dilute base
(b) water, dilute acid
(c) water, dilute base
(d) dilute base, water

(3)    For comparable compounds, which of the following would be most acidic?

(a) water
(b) alcohol
(c) alkene
(d) carboxylic acid

(4)    Name the following compound:

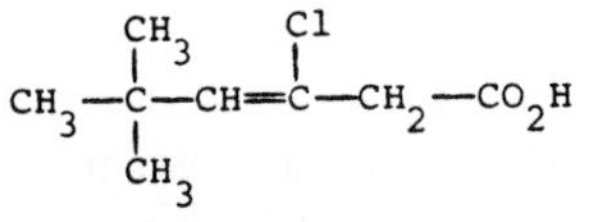

$$CH_3-\underset{\underset{\textstyle CH_3}{|}}{\overset{\overset{\textstyle CH_3}{|}}{C}}-CH=\underset{}{\overset{\overset{\textstyle Cl}{|}}{C}}-CH_2-CO_2H$$

(a) 3-Chloro-5, 5-dimethylhexanoic acid
(b) 3-Chloro-5, 5-dimethyl-3-hexenoic acid
(c) 2,2-Dimethyl-4-chloro-3-hexenoic acid
(d) none of the above

(5)    Select the compound that is most acidic:

(a) 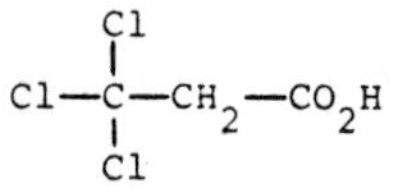 $Cl-\underset{\underset{\textstyle Cl}{|}}{\overset{\overset{\textstyle Cl}{|}}{C}}-CH_2-CO_2H$

(b) $CH_3-CH_2-CO_2H$

(c) 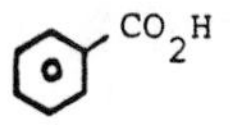 [benzene ring]$-CO_2H$

(d) all are equal

(6)    Give the product of the following reaction:

$$\bigcirc\!\!-CH_2-CH_2-\overset{O}{\overset{\|}{C}}-OH + CH_3-NH_2 \xrightarrow{\Delta} ?$$

(a) $H_3C-\overset{H}{\overset{|}{N}}-\bigcirc\!\!-CH_2-CH_2-\overset{O}{\overset{\|}{C}}-OH$    (b) $\bigcirc\!\!-CH_2-CH_2-CH_2-OH$

(c) $\bigcirc\!\!-CH_2-CH_2-CH_2-NH-CH_3$    (d) none of the above

(7)    Give the product of the following reaction:

$$CH_3-\overset{Cl}{\overset{|}{CH}}-CH_2-\overset{O}{\overset{\|}{C}}-OH + LiAlH_4 \longrightarrow ?$$

(a) $CH_3-\overset{Cl}{\overset{|}{CH}}-CH_2-CH_2-OH$    (b) $CH_3-CH=CH-\overset{O}{\overset{\|}{C}}-OH$

(c) $CH_3-\overset{Cl}{\overset{|}{CH}}-CH_2-\overset{O}{\overset{\|}{C}}-O^{\ominus}Li^{\oplus}$    (d) none of the above

(8)    Which of the following compounds has the potential for decarboxylation?

(a) $\bigcirc\!\!-\overset{O}{\overset{\|}{C}}-\overset{O}{\overset{\|}{C}}-OH$    (b) $\bigcirc\!\!-\overset{O}{\overset{\|}{C}}-CH_2-CO_2H$

(c) $CH_3-CH_2-\overset{CO_2H}{\underset{CH_2-CO_2H}{CH}}$    (d) none of these

## 4.10.3    Answers to Questions in Section 4.10.2

(1) b    (2) d    (3) d    (4) b    (5) c    (6) d    (7) a    (8) b

## 4.10.4    Discussion of Answers to Questions in Section 4.10.2

*Questions #1 to #3* Adequately discussed in Section.

*Question #4* (Answer: b) The numbering is:

$$\underset{(6)}{C}-\overset{C}{\underset{\underset{C}{|}}{\overset{|}{\underset{(5)}{C}}}}-\underset{(4)}{C}=\underset{(3)}{C}-\overset{Cl}{\underset{(2)}{\overset{|}{C}}}-\underset{(1)}{C}-CO_2H$$

Note how the double bond is handled.

*Question #5* (Answer: c) The benzene ring withdraws electrons, and, therefore, increases the acidity. The Cl's on option (a) are one carbon from the $-CO_2H$ and they are much less effective than a benzene ring attached to the carboxyl group.

*Question #6* (Answer: d) Correct product, $\bigcirc\!\!-CH_2-CH_2-\overset{O}{\overset{\|}{C}}-NHCH_3$

*Question #7* (Answer: a) Discussed in Section.

*Question #8* (Answer: b) Option (b) is the only $\beta$-Ketoacid (no $\beta$-diacids) given.

## 4.10.5    Vocabulary, Concepts, etc. Checklist for Carboxylic Acids

_____ nomenclature                     _____ key chemical features of carboxyl group
_____ physical properties              _____ strengths of organic acids
_____ reduction reactions              _____ nucleophilic substitution reactions

## 4.11    AMINES

### 4.11.1    Review of Amines

Amines are symbolized generally as:

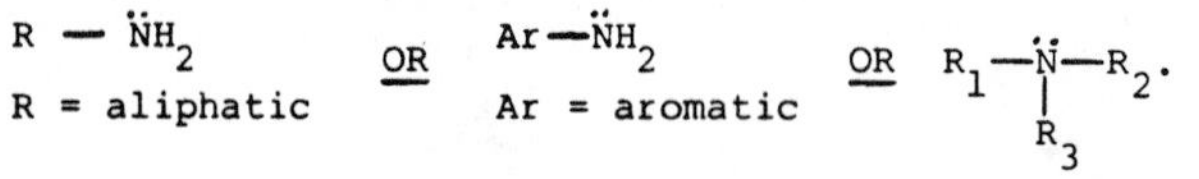

$$R — \ddot{N}H_2 \quad \text{OR} \quad Ar—\ddot{N}H_2 \quad \text{OR} \quad R_1—\underset{\underset{R_3}{|}}{\overset{\cdot\cdot}{N}}—R_2 \cdot$$

R = aliphatic        Ar = aromatic

All the R's ($R_1$, $R_2$, $R_3$) or any combination can be carbon groups or hydrogens. If R's are carbon groups,

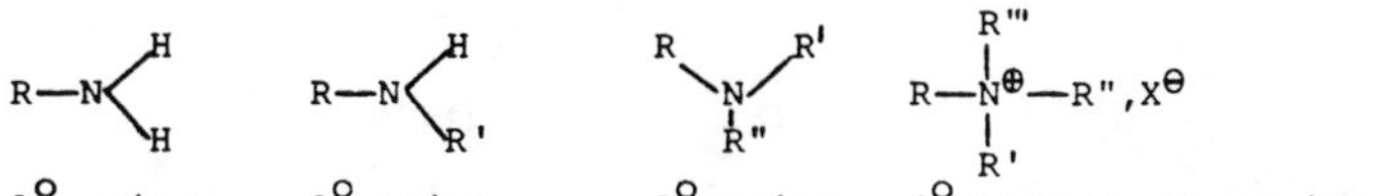

$$R—N\overset{H}{\underset{H}{\big\langle}} \qquad R—N\overset{H}{\underset{R'}{\big\langle}} \qquad \underset{R''}{\overset{R}{\big\diagdown}}N\overset{R'}{\big\diagup} \qquad R—\overset{\overset{R'''}{|}}{\underset{\underset{R'}{|}}{N^{\oplus}}}—R'', X^{\ominus}$$

1° amine       2° amine       3° amine       4° (quaternary) amine.

Amines may be named by locating the $-NR_2$ in a compound by numbers, e.g.,

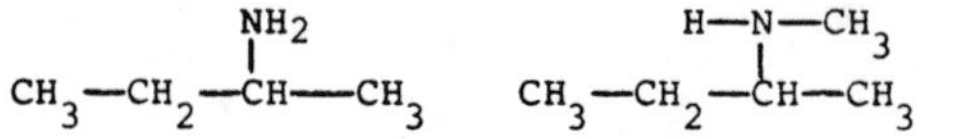

$$CH_3—CH_2—\overset{\overset{NH_2}{|}}{CH}—CH_3 \qquad CH_3—CH_2—\overset{\overset{H—N—CH_3}{|}}{CH}—CH_3$$

2-Aminobutane        N-Methyl-2-amino butane

Or by naming each group attached to the N,

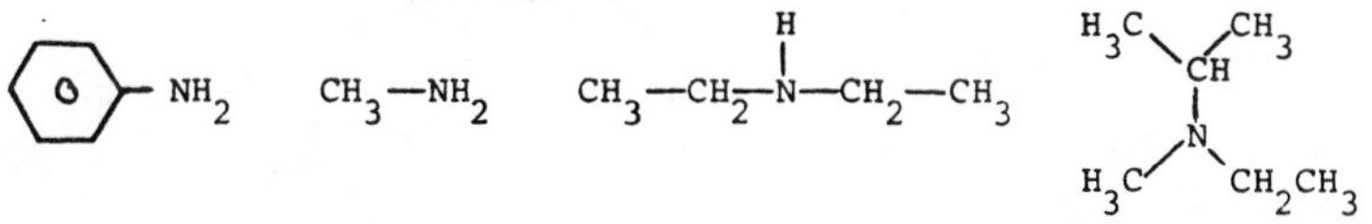

Aniline    Methylamine        Diethylamine        Methylethylisopropylamine

Nearly all the chemistry of amines depends upon the free pair of electrons upon nitrogen:

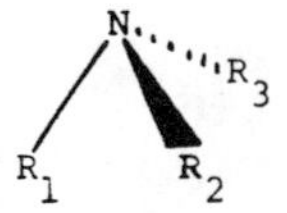

R = aliphatic, aromatic or H's.

Groups that withdraw electron density (aromatics, halides, e.g.) from nitrogen decrease the availability of this electron pair. Groups that donate electron density (especially alkyls) increase the availability. The availability of the electrons is reflected in this sequence of decreasing *base strengths*:

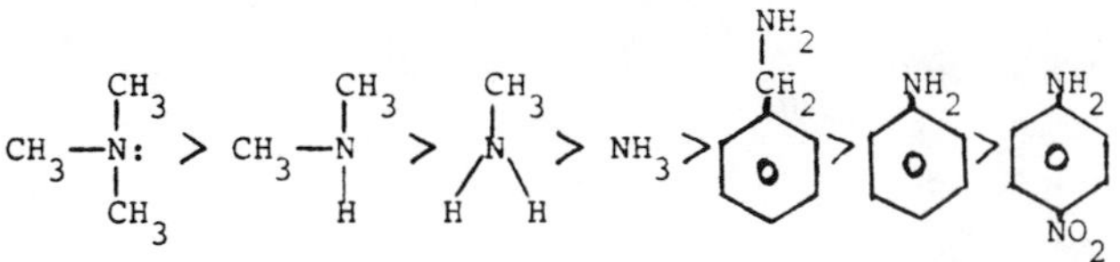

The available electron pair classifies amines as Lewis bases. Amines are also nucleophiles. Other important features of amines:

(1) The N can form hydrogen bonding via its electron pair with hydrogens attached to other N's or O's, and it can form hydrogen bonds from hydrogens attached to it with electron pairs of N, O, F or Cl:

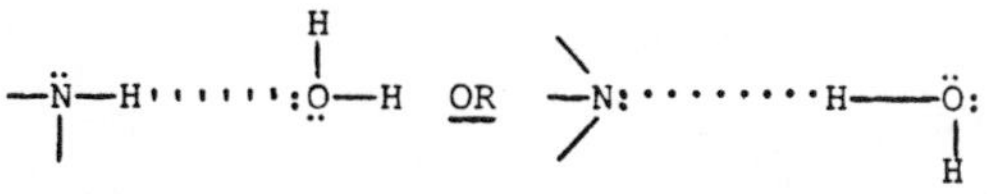

$$—\overset{\cdot\cdot}{\underset{|}{N}}—H\cdots\cdots:\overset{\overset{H}{|}}{O}—H \quad \text{OR} \quad \overset{\diagdown}{\underset{\diagup}{N}}:\cdots\cdots H—\overset{\cdot\cdot}{\underset{\underset{H}{|}}{O}}:$$

Note that 1° or 2° amines can hydrogen bond with each other (intermolecularly) but 3° amines cannot (no Hs attached to the N). For this reason 1° and 2° amines have higher than expected boiling points for compounds of similar molecular weight (but lower than similar alcohols or carboxylic acids). Low molecular weight amines are also soluble in $H_2O$ (due to H-bonding).

(2) A dipole moment is possible:

(3) Amines are ortho-para directors (Section 4.5.1).

Remember that the key reaction of amines is the nucleophilic attack (Section 4.4.1) by it upon an electron deficient carbon.

A very important reaction of 1° and 2° amines is with carboxylic acids (or usually their derivatives) to form *amides:*

$$R-\overset{\overset{O}{\|}}{C}-OH + R'-NH_2 \xrightarrow{\Delta} R-\overset{\overset{O}{\|}}{C}-\overset{\overset{H}{|}}{N}-R'$$

$$1° \text{ or } 2°$$

Carboxylic acid                 Amide
(or Acyl chloride)

This is the reaction important in protein synthesis.

Another common reaction of amines is *alkylation* of amines by alkyl halides:

$$R-CH_2-Cl + R'-NH_2 \longrightarrow R-CH_2-\overset{\overset{H}{|}}{N}-R' + HCl$$

$$1°, 2° \text{ or } 3°$$

Both amide formation and alkylation make use of the nucleophilic character of the electrons on nitrogen.


## 4.11.2     Questions to Review Amines

(1)     Name the following compound:

$$CH_3-CH_2-CH=CH-CH-\overset{\overset{NH_2}{|}}{CH}-CH\underset{CH_3}{\overset{CH_3}{<}}$$

      (a) 6-Amino 7-methyl-3-octene
      (b) Isononenyl amine
      (c) 2-Methyl-3-aminooctene
      (d) none of the above

(2)     Give the structure of Isopropyl diethyl amine:

      (a) $H-\overset{\overset{}{|}}{N}-CH_2CH_3$                   (b) $CH_3CH_2-\overset{}{N}-CH_2CH_3$

               $\underset{H_3C \quad CH_3}{\overset{|}{CH}}$                         $\underset{H_3C \quad CH_3}{\overset{|}{CH}}$

      (c)      $\overset{NH_2 \quad CH_2CH_3}{CH_3-CH_2-CH_2}$          (d) none of the above

(3) Which compound has the greatest base strength?

(a) $CH_3—NH_2$

(b) 
$$CH_3 \quad CH_3$$
$$\overset{|}{CH}—\overset{|}{C}—NH_2$$
$$H_3C \quad CH_3$$

(c) 
$$CH_2—CH_2—CH_3$$
$$\overset{|}{N}—CH_3$$
$$\overset{|}{CH_3}$$

(d) all are equal

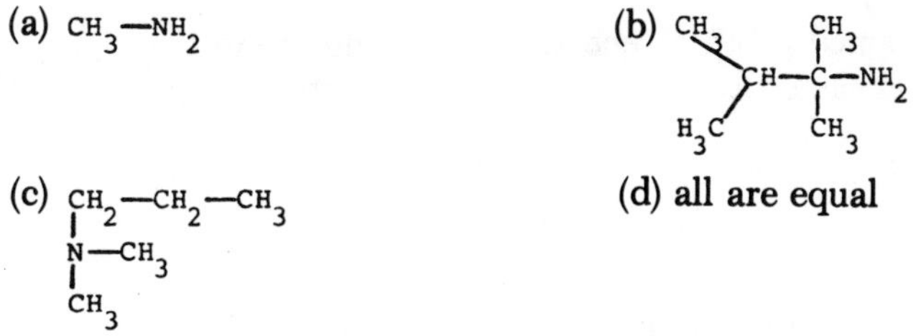

(4) Which compound has the greatest base strength?

(a) $O_2N—\langle\!\bigcirc\!\rangle—NH_2$

(b) $NC—\langle\!\bigcirc\!\rangle\!\overset{CN}{—}NH_2$

(c) $H_3C—\langle\!\bigcirc\!\rangle—NH_2$

(d) none of the above

(5) Which of the following compounds probably has the lowest boiling point?

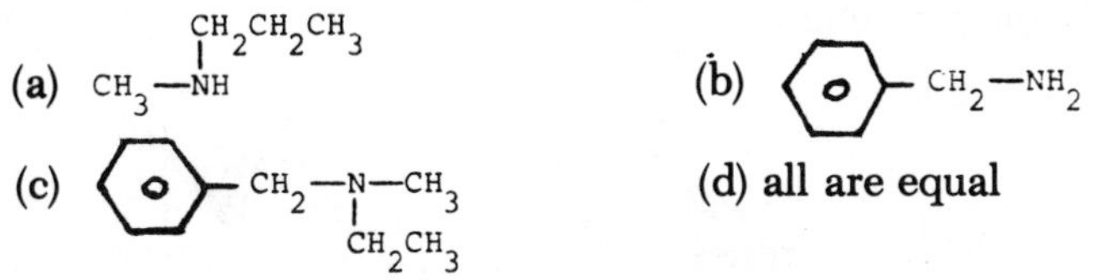

(a) 
$$\overset{CH_2CH_2CH_3}{\overset{|}{CH_3—NH}}$$

(b) $\langle\!\bigcirc\!\rangle—CH_2—NH_2$

(c) 
$$\langle\!\bigcirc\!\rangle—CH_2—\overset{|}{N}—CH_3$$
$$\overset{|}{CH_2CH_3}$$

(d) all are equal

(6) Give the product of the following reaction:

$$CH_3—\overset{CH_3}{\overset{|}{CH}}—\overset{O}{\overset{||}{C}}—OH + CH_3—CH_2—\overset{|}{\underset{CH_3}{N}}H \xrightarrow{\Delta} ?$$

(a) 
$$CH_3—\overset{CH_3}{\overset{|}{CH}}—\overset{H}{\overset{|}{C}}{=}N—CH_2CH_3$$
$$\overset{|}{CH_3}$$

(b) 
$$CH_3—\overset{CH_3}{\overset{|}{CH}}—CH_2—OH$$

(c) 
$$CH_3—\overset{CH_3}{\overset{|}{CH}}—\overset{N—CH_2CH_3}{\overset{|}{CH}}—N—CH_2CH_3$$
$$\overset{|}{CH_3}$$

(d) 
$$CH_3—\overset{CH_3}{\overset{|}{CH}}—\overset{O}{\overset{||}{C}}—N—CH_2CH_3$$
$$\overset{|}{CH_3}$$

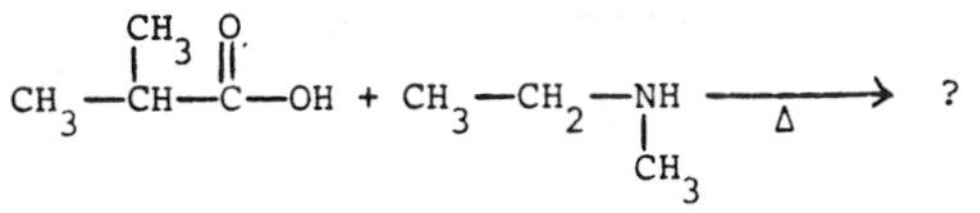

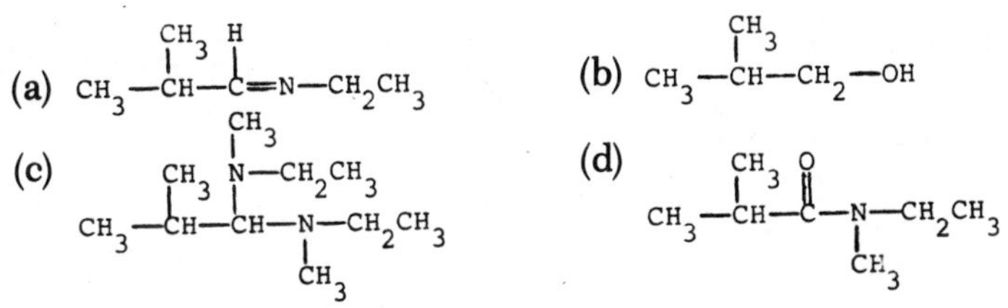

(7) Give the product of the following reaction:

$$\langle\!\bigcirc\!\rangle—CH_2—NH_2 + CH_3Cl \longrightarrow ?$$

(a) $\langle\!\bigcirc\!\rangle—CH_2—\overset{CH_3}{\overset{|}{N}}H$

(b) $\langle\!\bigcirc\!\rangle\!\overset{}{—}CH_2—NH_2 \;\;\overset{}{CH_3}$

(c) $\langle\!\bigcirc\!\rangle—CH_2—NH_2 \;\;\overset{}{Cl}$

(d) none of the above

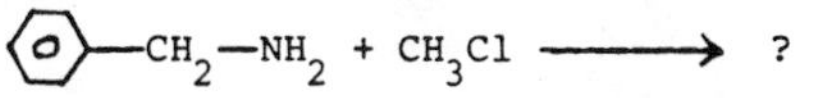

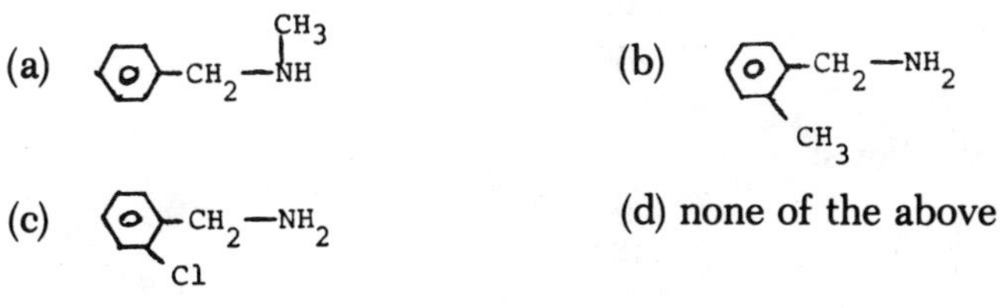

## 4.11.3    Answers to Questions in Section 4.11.2

(1) a    (2) b    (3) c    (4) c    (5) c    (6) d    (7) a

## 4.11.4 Discussion of Answers to Questions in Section 4.11.2

*Question #1* (Answer: a) The compound is named as an alkene and the amino group is considered to be a substituent (it could have been named as an amine also). The numbering is,

$$
\underset{1}{C} - \underset{2}{C} - \underset{3}{C} = \underset{4}{C} - \underset{5}{C} - \underset{6}{\overset{NH_2}{\overset{|}{C}}} - \underset{7}{C} \overset{\overset{C}{\diagup} 8}{\diagdown C}
$$

*Question #2* (Answer: b) The name is just taken literally. Study it.

*Question #3* (Answer: c) Tertiary amines (option c) have greater base strength than primary (a or b) or secondary amines.

*Question #4* (Answer: c) Aromatic amines have low base strength in general, but electron withdrawing groups ($-CN$, $-NO_2$) placed ortho/para decreases it even more. Electron donating groups ($-CH_3$) placed o/p can increase base strength.

*Question #5* (Answer: c) Tertiary amines have lower boiling points than 1° and 2° because there is no intermolecular hydrogen bonding.

*Question #6* (Answer: d) This is the amide forming reaction.

*Question #7* (Answer: a) This is the alkylation reaction.

## 4.11.5 Vocabulary, Concepts, etc. Checklist for Amines

_____ nomenclature of amines

_____ physical properties of amines

_____ amide formation

_____ alkylation of amines

_____ basicity of amines

## 4.12 CARBOXYLIC ACID DERIVATIVES

### 4.12.1 Review of Carboxylic Acid Derivatives

#### 4.12.1.1 REVIEW OF AMIDES

See *nomenclature* of carboxylic acids (Section 4.10.1). The -oic acid (or -ic acid) is changed to -amide, e.g.:

3-Methyl butanoic acid

$$
\overset{H_3C}{\underset{H_3C}{\diagdown}} CH - CH_2 - \overset{O}{\overset{\parallel}{C}} - OH
$$

$$
\overset{CH_3}{\underset{CH_3}{\diagdown}} CH - CH_2 - \overset{O}{\overset{\parallel}{C}} - NH_2 \quad \text{3-Methyl butanamide}
$$

If the N is substituted, this feature is added as follows:

$$
\overset{H_3C}{\underset{H_3C}{\diagdown}} CH - CH_2 - \overset{O}{\overset{\parallel}{C}} - N \overset{\diagup CH_3}{\diagdown CH_3}
$$

N, N - Dimethyl -3- methyl butanamide

The *boiling points* of unsubstituted and monosubstituted amides are very high due to strong intermolecular hydrogen bonds. Disubstituted amides have boiling points like ketones or aldehydes (due to the carbonyl moiety). Amides have essentially no *acidity* (as compared to carboxylic acids) and no *basicity* (as compared to amines).

Amides are *formed from* carboxylic acids (or its derivatives) by,

$$R-\overset{\overset{O}{\|}}{C}-OH + NH_3 \text{ (or } R-NH_2, \text{ etc.)} \xrightarrow{\Delta} R-\overset{\overset{O}{\|}}{C}-NH_2$$

Amides are susceptible to *nucleophilic substitution* at the carbonyl carbon,

$$R-\overset{\overset{O}{\|}}{C}-NH_2 + NuH \longrightarrow R-\overset{\overset{O}{\|}}{C}-Nu + NH_3$$

Nu = nucleophile
(see Section 4.10.1).

Amides undergo hydrolysis back to the original acid and amine under basic or acidic conditions:

$$R-\overset{\overset{O}{\|}}{C}-NHR \xrightarrow[H_2O]{H^{\oplus}} R-\overset{\overset{O}{\|}}{C}-OH + RNH_2$$
amide                     acid          amine

$$R-\overset{\overset{O}{\|}}{C}-NHR \xrightarrow{OH^{\ominus}} R-NH_2 + R-\overset{\overset{O}{\|}}{C}-O^{\ominus} \xrightarrow{H^{\oplus}} R-\overset{\overset{O}{\|}}{C}-OH.$$
amine   carboxylate        acid

## 4.12.1.2   REVIEW OF ESTERS

See *nomenclature* of carboxylic acids (Section 4.10.1). The -oic acid of carboxylic acids is replaced by -oate and the carbon fragment of the ester precedes the base name:

$$\overset{H_3C}{\underset{H_3C}{>}}CH-CH_2-\overset{\overset{O}{\|}}{C}-OH$$
3-Methyl butanoic acid

$$\overset{CH_3}{\underset{CH_3}{>}}CH-CH_2-\overset{\overset{O}{\|}}{C}-O-CH_2CH_3$$
Ethyl-3-methyl butanoate

Esters have no *acidity* (because no $-OH$) and have *boiling points* comparable to ketones and aldehydes because they have carbonyl groups but not hydrogen bonding.

Esters are formed from carboxylic acids (or derivatives) under acidic or basic conditions.

$$R-\overset{\overset{O}{\|}}{C}-OH + R'-\overset{*}{O}-H \longrightarrow R-\overset{\overset{O}{\|}}{C}-\overset{*}{O}-R.$$
acid             alcohol                        ester

Esters undergo *nucleophilic substitution* at the carbonyl carbon,

$$R-\overset{\overset{O}{\|}}{C}-O-R' + NuH \longrightarrow R-\overset{\overset{O}{\|}}{C}-Nu + R'OH \quad \text{Nu = nucleophile}$$
(Section 4.10.1)

Esters are *hydrolized* by acid or base back to the original acid and alcohol:

$$R-\overset{\overset{O}{\|}}{C}-OR' \xrightarrow{H^{\oplus}} R-\overset{\overset{O}{\|}}{C}-OH + R'-OH$$
ester                     acid        alcohol

$$R-\overset{\overset{O}{\|}}{C}-OR' \xrightarrow{NaOH} R-\overset{\overset{O}{\|}}{C}-O^{\ominus}Na^{\oplus} + R'OH \xrightarrow{H^{\oplus}} R-\overset{\overset{O}{\|}}{C}-OH.$$
ester          carboxylate ion                          acid.

*Fats* are a special class of esters of biologic importance. They are formed as follows:

$$CH_3(CH_2)_{14}CO_2H + \begin{matrix} CH_2OH \\ | \\ CH_2OH \\ | \\ CH_2OH \end{matrix} \longrightarrow \begin{matrix} CH_2-O-\overset{\overset{O}{\|}}{C}-(CH_2)_{14}-CH_3 \\ | \\ CH_2OH \\ | \\ CH_2OH \end{matrix} \longrightarrow II \longrightarrow III.$$

fatty acid    glycerol     monoglyceride
(long chain acids)       (a fat)

More fatty acids (FA) can be added to the glycerol to form di- (II) and tri-glycerides (III). Fats may be hydrolyzed back to FA's and glycerol by base (a process called *saponification*):

$$\begin{matrix} CH_2-O-\overset{\overset{O}{\|}}{C}-(CH_2)_{14}CH_3 \\ | \\ CH_2-O-\overset{\overset{O}{\|}}{C}-(CH_2)_{14}CH_3 \\ | \\ CH_2-O-\overset{\overset{O}{\|}}{C}-(CH_2)_{14}CH_3 \end{matrix} \xrightarrow{NaOH} \begin{matrix} CH_2OH \\ | \\ CH_2OH \\ | \\ CH_2OH \end{matrix} + 3\ CH_3(CH_2)_{14}CO_2^{\ominus}Na^{\oplus}$$

a triglyceride         glycerol    salt of the FA
(a fat)

### 4.12.2     Questions to Review Carboxylic Acid Derivatives

(1)  Amides have essentially no:

(a) acidity
(b) basicity
(c) hydrogen bonding
(d) both (a) and (b)

(2)  Fats are _____ and are made of _____ and _____.

(a) esters, glycerol, fatty acids
(b) amide, an amine, fatty acids
(c) ethers, glycerol, fatty acids
(d) none of the above

(3)  Saponification is the _____ of _____.

(a) alkaline hydrolysis, fats
(b) acidic hydrolysis, fats
(c) neutral hydrolysis, amides
(d) none of the above

(4)  Name the following compound:

$$\begin{matrix} H_3C \\ \phantom{H}\!\!\diagdown \\ \phantom{xx}C=C \\ \phantom{H}\!\!\diagup \phantom{xxxx}\diagdown \\ H_3C \phantom{xxxxx} CH_2-\overset{\overset{O}{\|}}{C}-\overset{\overset{H}{|}}{N}-CH_3 \end{matrix}$$

(a) N-Methyl-4-Methyl-3-pentenamide
(b) 2-Methyl-2-pentenamide
(c) Dimethyl pentenamide
(d) none of the above

(5)  Which of the following compounds probably has a boiling point similar to comparable molecular weight ketones or aldehydes?

(a) $CH_3-\overset{\overset{O}{\|}}{C}-N(CH_3)_2$             (b) $CH_3-\overset{\overset{O}{\|}}{C}-\overset{\overset{H}{|}}{N}CH_3$

(c) $CH-\overset{\overset{O}{\|}}{C}-NH_2$                (d) none of the above

(6) Give the product of the following reaction:

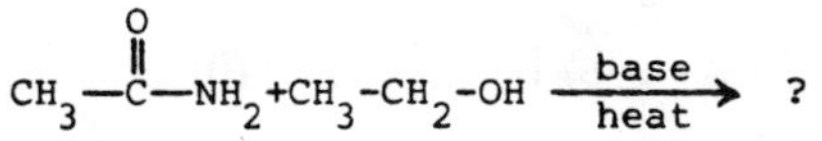

$$CH_3-\overset{O}{\overset{\|}{C}}-NH_2 + CH_3-CH_2-OH \xrightarrow[\text{heat}]{\text{base}} \quad ?$$

(a) $CH_3-CH_2-NH_2$

(b) $CH_3-\overset{O}{\overset{\|}{C}}-OCH_2-CH_3$

(c) $CH_3-\overset{O}{\overset{\|}{C}}-\overset{H}{\overset{|}{N}}-CH_2-CH_3$

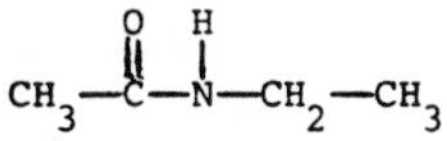

(d) none of the above

(7) Give the product of the following reaction:

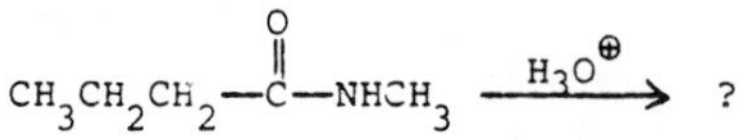

$$CH_3CH_2CH_2-\overset{O}{\overset{\|}{C}}-NHCH_3 \xrightarrow{H_3O^{\oplus}} \quad ?$$

(a) $CH_3CH_2CH_2-\overset{O}{\overset{\|}{C}}-NH_2$

(b) $CH_3-CH_2CH_2-CH_2-NH_2$

(c) $CH_3-CH_2CH_2-CH_2-OH$

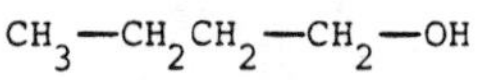

(d) none of the above

(8) Name the following compound:

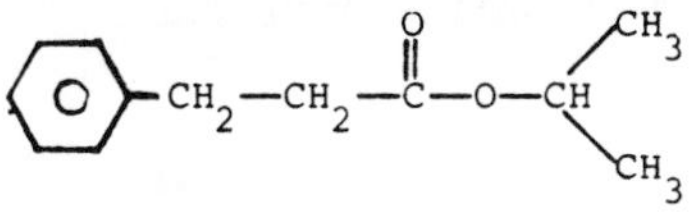

(a) Isopropyl benzoate
(b) Isopropyl-3-phenyl propanoate
(c) Phenyl isopropyl ester
(d) none of the above

(9) Give the product of the following reaction:

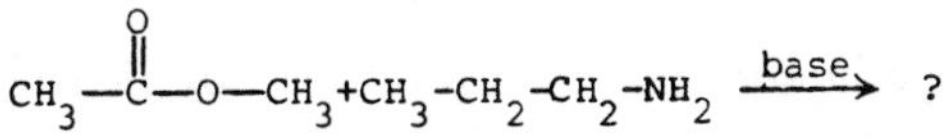

$$CH_3-\overset{O}{\overset{\|}{C}}-O-CH_3 + CH_3-CH_2-CH_2-NH_2 \xrightarrow{\text{base}} \quad ?$$

(a) $CH_3-\overset{H}{\overset{\|}{C}}=N-CH_2-CH_2-CH_3$

(b) $CH_3-\overset{O}{\overset{\|}{C}}-\overset{H}{\overset{|}{N}}-CH_2CH_2CH_3$

(c) $CH_3-CH_2-CH_2-OH$

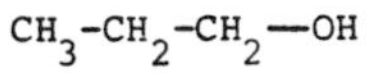

(d) none of the above

(10) Give the product of the following reaction:

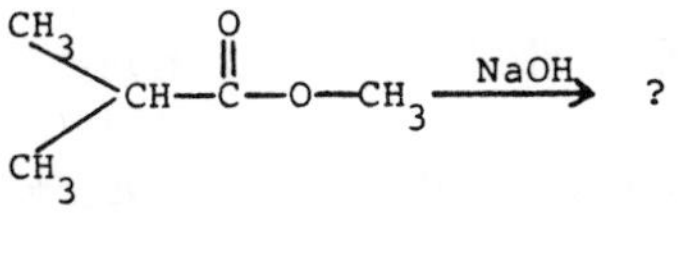

(a)

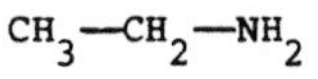

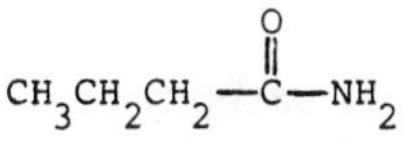

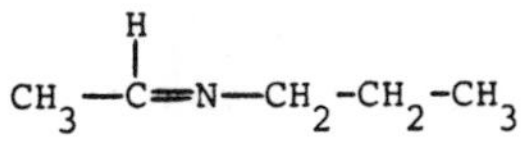

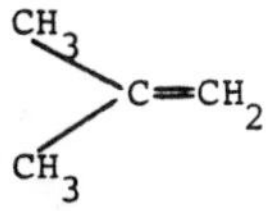

(b)

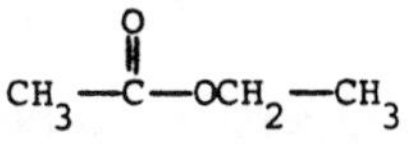

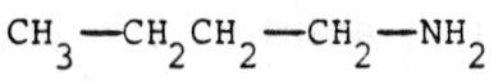

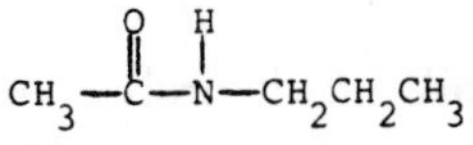

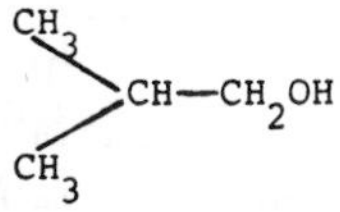

(c)

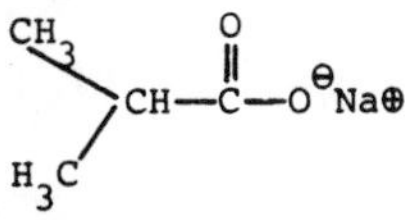

(d) none of these

(11) The following compound is a:

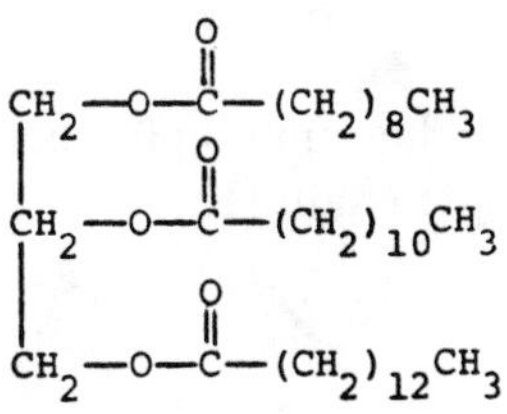

(a) nucleotide
(b) monosaccharide
(c) amino acid
(d) triglyceride

## 4.12.3  Answers to Questions in Section 4.12.2

( 1) d  ( 2) a  ( 3) a  ( 4) a  ( 5) a  ( 6) b  ( 7) d  ( 8) b  ( 9) b  (10) c  (11) d

## 4.12.4  Discussion of Answers to Questions in Section 4.12.2

*Questions #1 to #3* Adequately discussed in Section.

*Question #4* (Answer: a) The numbering is

*Question #5* (Answer: a) Disubstituted amides have boiling points similar to carbonyls because there is no intermolecular hydrogen bonding.

*Question #6* (Answer: b) Amides undergo nucleophilic substitution just like carboxylic acids. An ester is formed in this case.

*Question #7* (Answer: d) This is an hydrolysis of an amide; the products are the original acid and amine:

$$CH_3CH_2CH_2-\overset{O}{\overset{\|}{C}}-NHCH_3 \longrightarrow CH_3CH_2CH_2\overset{O}{\overset{\|}{C}}-OH + CH_3NH_2$$

*Question #8* (Answer: b) The numbering is:

*Question #9* (Answer: b) Esters undergo nucleophilic substitution just like carboxylic acids. An amide is the product in this reaction.

*Question #10* (Answer: c) This is the alkaline hydrolysis of an ester, so a carboxylate anion results.

*Question #11* (Answer: d) Refer to Section.

## 4.12.5  Vocabulary, Concepts, etc. Checklist for Carboxylic Acid Derivatives

_____ nomenclature of amides
_____ nomenclature of esters
_____ physical properties of amides
_____ physical properties of esters
_____ nucleophilic substitution of amides

_____ nucleophilic substitution of esters
_____ hydrolysis of amides
_____ hydrolysis of esters
_____ fats
_____ saponification

## 4.13  AMINO ACIDS AND PROTEINS

### 4.13.1  Review of Amino Acids and Proteins

Amino acids (AA) are organic molecules with the common features of a carboxyl group and an α(alpha) -amino group as shown and a side chain (R):

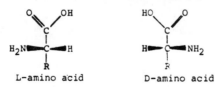

L-amino acid          D-amino acid

There are about 20 AA and all are in the *L* configuration. AA's serve primarily as the structural components of proteins. The types and sequence of AA in proteins determine their structural properties and acid-base behavior. The following AA's have R groups which are hydrocarbon in nature, are hydrophobic and are found in the interiors of proteins:

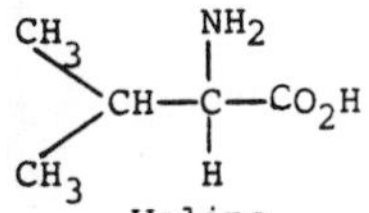

Valine 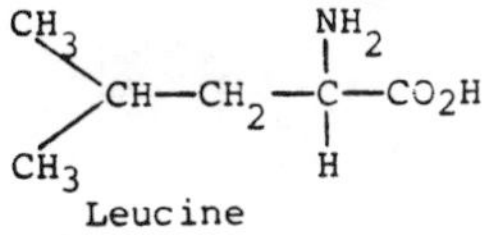          Leucine 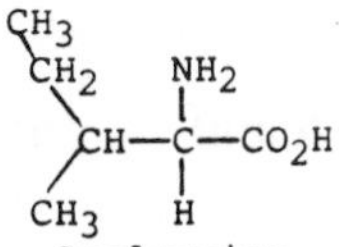          Isoleucine

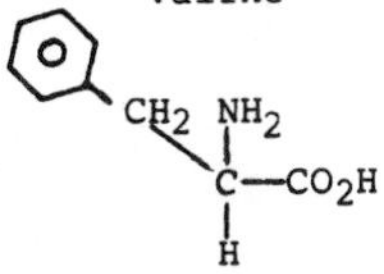

Phenylalanine 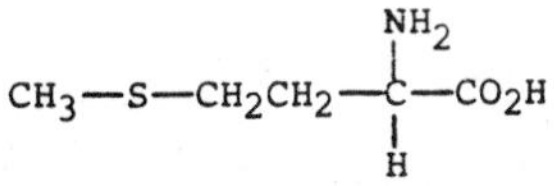          Methionine

Knowledge of these amino acids *is not* required for the MCAT.

Ionic and/or polar AA's are hydrophilic and tend to be found on the exterior of proteins:

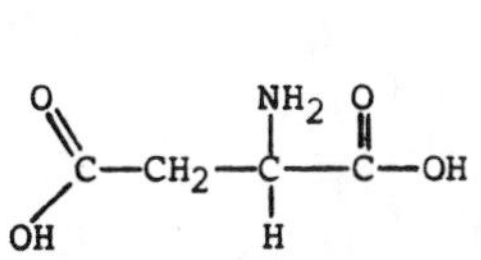

Aspartic Acid          Glutamic Acid          Lysine
(and its amide)        (and its amide)

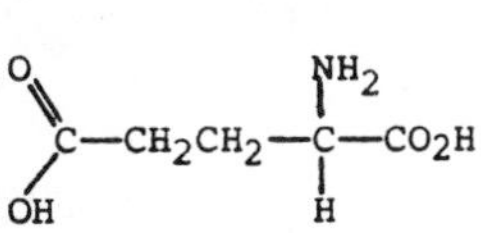

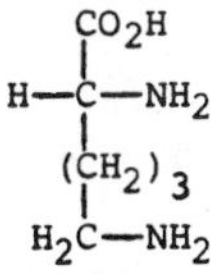

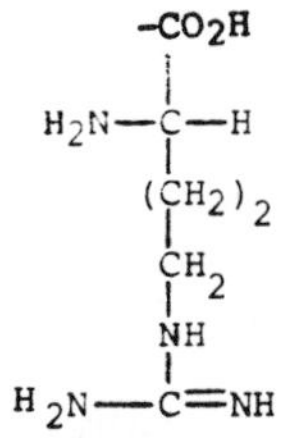

Arginine 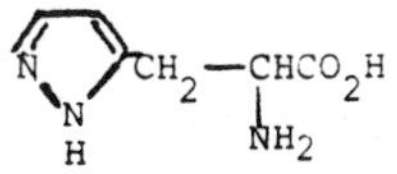          Histidine

Certain amino acids can be found on the exterior or interior of proteins (these are polar also):

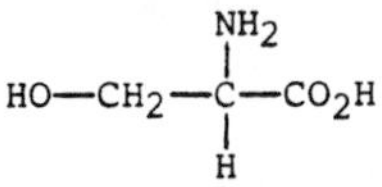

Serine 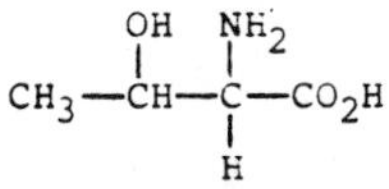          Threonine 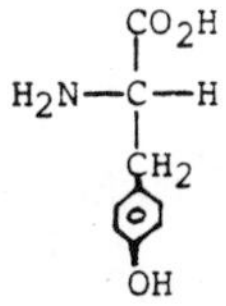          Tyrosine 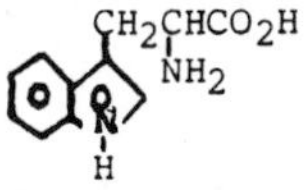          Tryptophan

Cysteine forms sulfur-sulfur covalent bonds with itself to stabilize the tertiary structure of proteins:

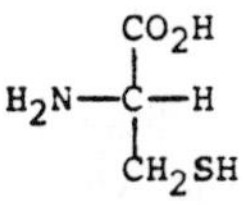

cysteine 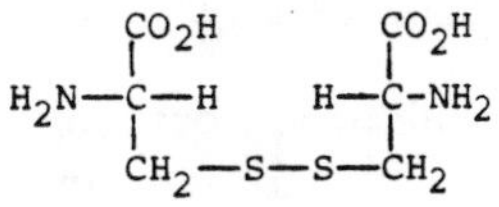          cystine

Glycine, the smallest AA and the only one that is not optically active, is often found at the 'corners' of proteins:

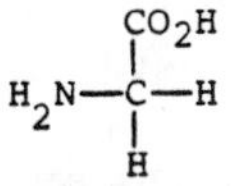

Glycine

Proline breaks the α-helix structure of proteins:

Proline

Alanine, being small, is usually found on the surface of proteins even though it is hydrophobic:

$$CH_3-C(-H)(-CO_2H)(-NH_2)$$

Alanine

The *basic amino acids* are lysine and arginine due to their extra amino ( – $NH_2$) groups. The *acidic amino acids* are aspartic acid and glutamic acid due to their extra carboxyl ( – $CO_2H$) groups. Histidine can act as a base or an acid depending upon the pH, and it is the best physiologic buffer of the AA's. All of the others are considered *neutral amino acids.*

Amino acids exist as *dipolar ions* due to the presence of both a basic part (the – $NH_2$) and an acidic part (the – $CO_2H$):

$$R-C(-\overset{\oplus}{N}H_3)(-H)-CO_2^{\ominus}$$

dipolar ion

The charge on the amino acid varies with the pH and the *isoelectric point*. The isoelectric point (pI) of an AA is the pH where the AA has no net charge:

$$R-C(-NH_2)(-H)-CO_2H$$

no net charge at isoelectric points

If the pH is above the isoelectric point or very basic, AA's have a net negative charge (anions):

$$R-C(-\overset{\oplus}{N}H_3)(-H)-CO_2^{\ominus} \xrightarrow[\text{(basic)}]{OH^{\ominus}} R-C(-NH_2)(-H)-CO_2^{\ominus}$$

anionic form

If the pH is below the isoelectric point or very acidic, AA's have a net positive charge (cations):

$$R-C(-\overset{\oplus}{N}H_3)(-H)-CO_2^{\ominus} \xrightarrow[\text{(acidic)}]{H^{\oplus}} R-C(-\overset{\oplus}{N}H_3)(-H)-CO_2H$$

cationic form

Proteins also have isoelectric points. Whether proteins are basic or acidic depends on the relative numbers of basic and acidic AA's present. If there is an excess of acidic AA's, the proteins are acidic and have an isoelectric point at a pH less than 7 (neutrality for water). So, at pH = 7, they have a net negative charge. If there is an excess of basic AA's, proteins are basic and have an isoelectric point at a pH greater than 7. At pH = 7, they have a net positive charge. Proteins undergo electrophoresis just like amino acids. In other words, if the pH of the medium is less than the pI of the protein, the protein must have a net positive charge. Or, if the pH of the medium is greater than the pI, the protein must have a net negative charge. Proteins are composed of AA's linearly linked by peptide bonds. A *peptide bond* is an amide bond (See Section 4.12.1.1) formed by the $\alpha$-amino group of an AA and the 1-carboxyl group of a second AA. Water is released when a peptide bond is formed and is added when it is hydrolyzed:

formation of peptide bond

peptide bond

hydrolysis of peptide bond

The structure of proteins is divided into primary (1°), secondary (2°), tertiary (3°) and quaternary (4°). The *1° structure* of a protein is the sequence of AA as determined by DNA (Section 2.4.1) and it determines the higher structures. *Secondary structure* is the orderly intermolecular or intramolecular hydrogen bonding of the protein chain assuming an $\alpha$-helix (e.g., in keratin) or $\beta$-pleated sheet (e.g., in silk), respectively. The *3° structure* is the further folding of the protein (many parts of it still remain $\alpha$-helical) onto itself. The molecule is stabilized by hydrogen bonding, van der Waals bonding, hydrophobic bonding, electrostatic bonding (see Section 3.4.1) and, especially, covalent bonding in the form of disulfide bonds (by cysteine). Globular proteins result and usually have an interior that is hydrophobic and an exterior that is hydrophilic; enzymes are examples. *Quaternary structures* is when two or more separate protein chains bind together by noncovalent bonds (e.g., hemoglobin).

## 4.13.2 Questions to Review Amino Acids and Proteins

(1) What characteristics of amino acids determine the primary structure of proteins?

(a) acid-base properties
(b) side chain composition
(c) hydrogen bonding properties
(d) sequence in proteins

(2) Which is an $\alpha$-amino acid?

(3) The peptide bond would be described chemically as which type of bond?

(a) ester
(b) amide
(c) ether
(d) anhydride

(4) When a peptide bond is hydrolyzed (split):

(a) water is released from the amino acid(s)
(b) water is added to the amino acid(s)
(c) oxidation of the amino acid occurs
(d) reduction of amino acid occurs

(5)   Primary structure of amino acids is:

(a) exemplified by $\alpha$-helical structure
(b) not found in quaternary proteins
(c) coded for by DNA
(d) all of the above

(6)   Secondary structure of proteins is associated with:

(a) sequence of amino acids
(b) not in globular proteins
(c) coded for by DNA
(d) $\alpha$-helix

(7)   Select the type(s) of bonding important in maintenance of tertiary structure of proteins:

(a) hydrophobic
(b) van der Waals
(c) covalent
(d) all are important

(8)   The highest level of protein structure found in monomeric globular proteins is:

(a) primary
(b) secondary
(c) tertiary
(d) quaternary

(9)   Which of the following would be considered a hydrophilic amino acid?

(a) 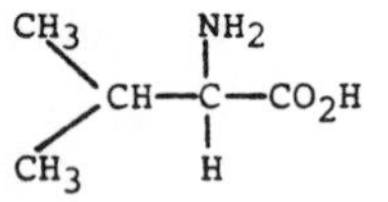 $(CH_3)_2CH-\underset{\underset{H}{|}}{\overset{\overset{NH_2}{|}}{C}}-CO_2H$

(b) [pyrrole ring]$-CH_2-\underset{\underset{NH_2}{|}}{CH}-CO_2H$

(c) [benzene ring with O]$-CH_2-\underset{\underset{H}{|}}{\overset{\overset{NH_2}{|}}{C}}-CO_2H$

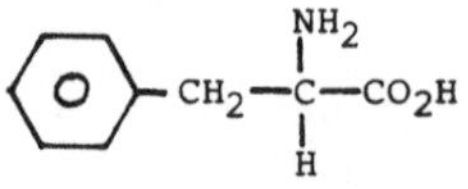

(d) none of the above

(10)   Select the basic amino acid:

(a) 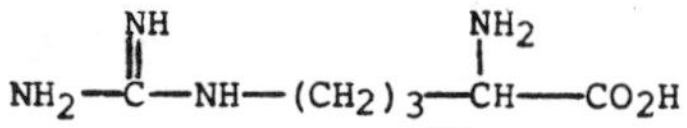 $NH_2-\overset{\overset{NH}{\|}}{C}-NH-(CH_2)_3-\underset{\underset{NH_2}{|}}{CH}-CO_2H$

(b) $HO_2C-CH_2-\underset{\underset{NH_2}{|}}{CH}-CO_2H$

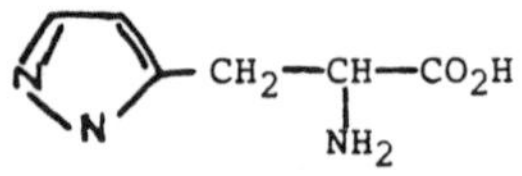

(c) $CH_3-S-CH_2-CH_2-\underset{\underset{NH_2}{|}}{CH}-CO_2H$

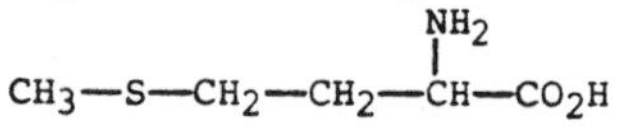

(d) none of the above

(11)   Select the acidic amino acid:

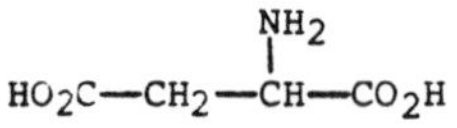

(a) 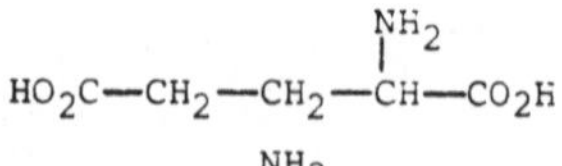 $HO_2C-CH_2-CH_2-\underset{\underset{NH_2}{|}}{CH}-CO_2H$

(b) 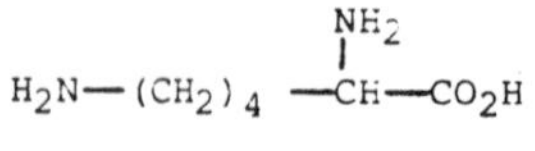 $H_2N-(CH_2)_4-\underset{\underset{NH_2}{|}}{CH}-CO_2H$

(c) 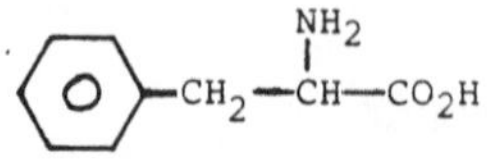 [benzene ring with O]$-CH_2-\underset{\underset{NH_2}{|}}{CH}-CO_2H$

(d) none of the above

(12)   Which amino acid in question #11 will most likely be found on the interior of globular proteins?

(a)
(b)
(c)
(d)

(13) Which of the following peptides probably has the highest pI?

(a) 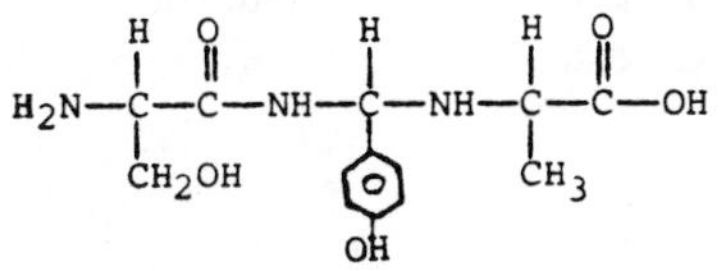 $H_2N$—C—C—NH—C—NH—C—C—OH
with side chains $CH_2OH$, phenyl ring with $OH$, $CH_3$

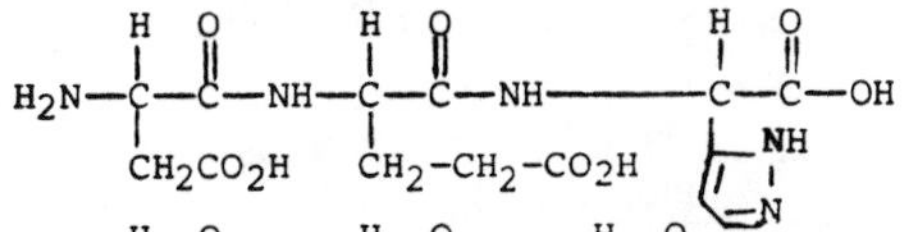

(b) $H_2N$—C—C—NH—C—C—NH——C—C—OH
with side chains $CH_2CO_2H$, $CH_2$—$CH_2$—$CO_2H$, imidazole ring ($NH$, $N$)

(c) $H_2N$—C—C—NH—C—C—NH—C—C—OH
with side chains $CH(CH_3)(CH_3)$, $HO$—$CH$—$CH_3$, $CH_2OH$

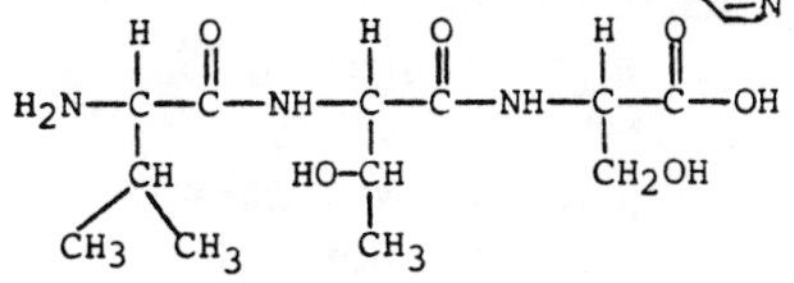

(d) 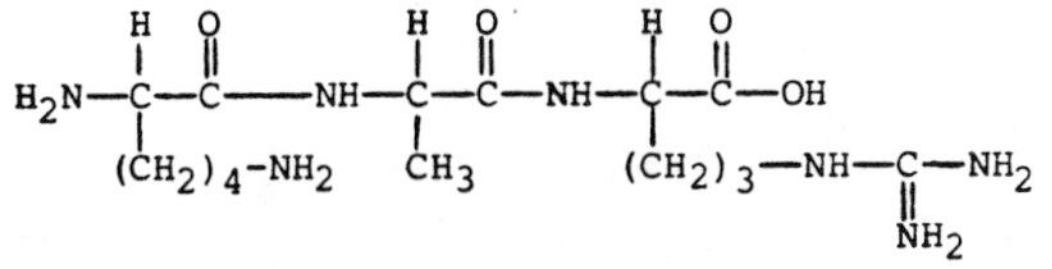 $H_2N$—C—C——NH—C—C—NH—C—C—OH
with side chains $(CH_2)_4$—$NH_2$, $CH_3$, $(CH_2)_3$—$NH$—C($NH_2$)=$NH_2$ (guanidino)

(14) Which of the peptides in #13 will probably migrate to the cathode at pH = 7.0?

(a)
(b)
(c)
(d)

(15) Which of the peptides in #13 will probably migrate to the anode at pH = 7.0?

(a)
(b)
(c)
(d)

## 4.13.3    Answers to Questions in Section 4.13.2

( 1) d   ( 2) d   ( 3) b   ( 4) b   ( 5) c   ( 6) d   ( 7) d   ( 8) c   ( 9) b   (10) a   (11) a
(12) c   (13) d   (14) d   (15) b

## 4.13.4    Discussion of Answers to Questions in Section 4.13.2

*Questions #1 to #8* Adequately discussed in text.

*Question #9-#11* Look at the R groups to determine the neutrality, basicity, acidity or hydrophilicity. Refer to Section if necessary.

*Question #12* (Answer: c) Hydrophobic AA's are found on the interior. The AA in option (c) with the phenyl group is hydrophobic.

*Question #13* (Answer: d) (a) and (c) have only polar or hydrophobic AA's, so its pI is around 7. (b) has two acidic AA's and one AA that may be basic or acidic; therefore, its pI is less than 7. (d) has two basic amino acids and, therefore, has a pI greater than 7. See Section for discussion.

*Question #14* (Answer: d) The cathode attracts the positive ion. Therefore, the peptide must be positively charged at pH = 7.0. This means pH = 7 must be acidic relative to the pI and that the pI must be greater than 7, which means it must contain basic AA's.

*Question #15* (Answer: b) The anode attracts the basic ion. Therefore, the peptide must be negatively charged at pH = 7.0. This means that pH = 7 must be alkaline relative to the pI, or that the pI must be less than 7. Therefore, there must be an excess of acidic AA's. See discussion in Section.

### 4.13.5    Vocabulary, Concepts, etc. Checklist for Amino Acids and Proteins

\_\_\_\_\_ classes of amino acids  
\_\_\_\_\_ protein structure  
\_\_\_\_\_ peptide linkage and hydrolysis  
\_\_\_\_\_ dipolar ions  
\_\_\_\_\_ isoelectric point, pI  
\_\_\_\_\_ basic amino acids  

\_\_\_\_\_ acidic amino acids  
\_\_\_\_\_ primary structure  
\_\_\_\_\_ secondary structure  
\_\_\_\_\_ tertiary structure  
\_\_\_\_\_ quaternary structure  
\_\_\_\_\_ classes of amino acids  

## 4.14    CARBOHYDRATES

### 4.14.1    Review of Carbohydrates

Carbohydrates have the general formula $C_n (H_2O)_m$ where n and m are whole numbers. *Monosaccharides* are the basic units of carbohydrates. They are classified by the number of carbons they contain, i.e., *hexoses* ($C_6$), *pentoses* ($C_5$), etc. Hexoses and pentoses exist in predominantly ring forms called *pyranoses* (six membered rings) or *furanoses* (five membered rings) in equilibrium with the open-chain forms. Ring forms are hemiacetals (see Section 4.7.1); open-chain forms are polyhydroxy aldehydes. In the ring forms, $\alpha$ or $\beta$-anomers are possible. The pyranoses exist in the stable chair conformation with most, if not all, of the hydroxyls in equatorial positions. When two monosaccharides differ by the configuration of one hydroxyl group, they are called *epimers*. If n is the number of asymmetric carbons, then $2^n$ is the number of optical *isomers* (based on open chain).

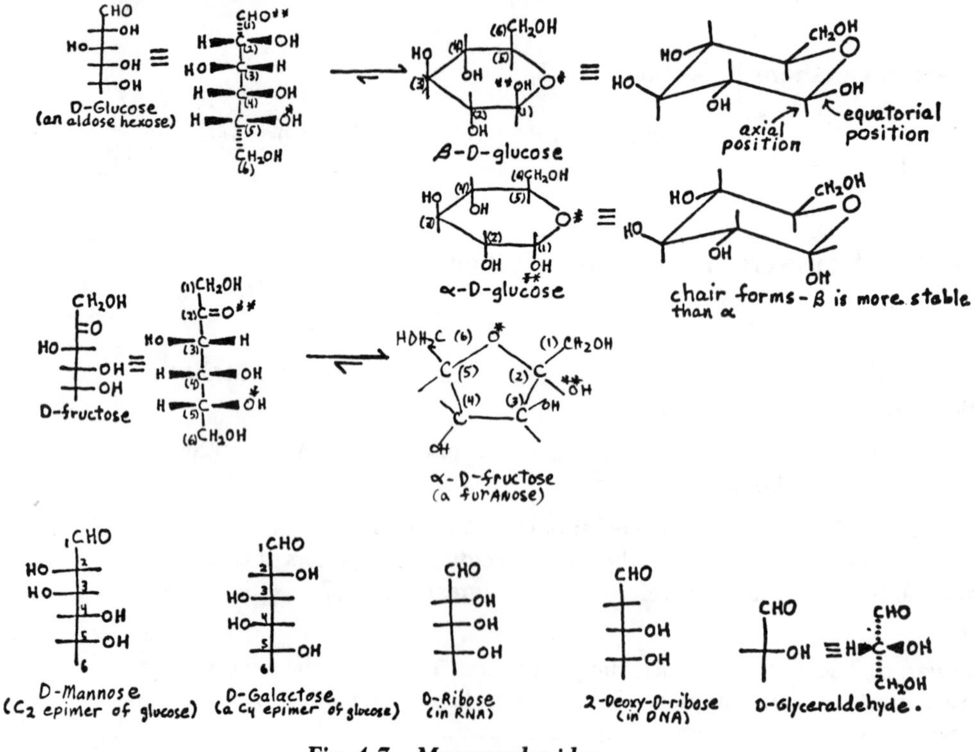

Fig. 4.7—Monosaccharides

Hexoses usually have n = 4 and pentoses usually have n = 3. Sugars are given a relative *configuration* on the basis of the orientation of the next to last carbon's hydroxyl group as compared to D-glyceraldehyde. Most naturally occuring sugars have the *D* configuration. A *ketose* is a carbohydrate with a ketone group; an *aldose* has an aldehyde group. Illustrations of the above points with the common monosaccharides are in Fig. 4.7.

Monosaccharides bond together to form *disaccharides* . The new bond is called a *glycosidic bond* and is between the hemi-acetal carbon and an hydroxyl group of the other sugar; water is released when the bond is formed. Hydrolysis (breaking) of the bond requires water. The glycosidic bond is an acetal grouping (see Section 4.7.1) (Fig. 4.8). *Sucrose* (common sugar) is made of glucose and fructose. *Lactose* (milk sugar) is made of galactose and glucose. *Maltose* ($\alpha$-1,4 bond) is made of two glucose units and is an hydrolysis product of starch or glycogen. *Cellobiose* ($\beta$-1,4 bond) is also made of two glucoses, and it is the breakdown product of the cellulose.

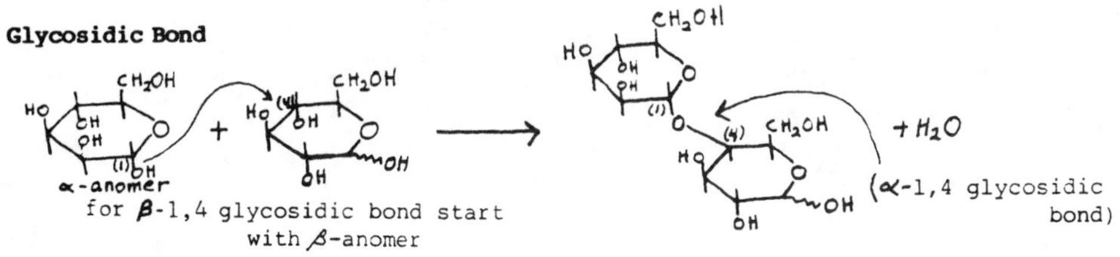

**Fig. 4.8—Glycosidic Bond**

*Polysaccharides* are many monosaccharides joined by glycosidic bonds; they may be branched also. *Starch* (plant energy storage), *glycogen* (animal short-term energy storage), and *cellulose* (plant structural component) are all made from glucose. Cellulose has $\beta$-1,4 bonds not found in the other two. Starch and glycogen both have $\alpha$-1,4 bonds but differ in the frequency and position of branch points ($\alpha$-1,6 bond).

Inulin is a polymer of fructose.

## 4.14.2    Questions to Review Carbohydrates

(1)    Which disaccharide has the *incorrect* monosaccharide components listed by it?

    (a) maltose—mannose and glucose
    (b) lactose—galactose and glucose
    (c) sucrose—fructose and glucose
    (d) cellobiose—two glucoses

(2)    Which of these is not a monosaccharide?

    (a) ribose
    (b) galactose
    (c) maltose
    (d) mannose

(3)    Which compound is the reference for the relative configuration of sugars and amino acids?

    (a) d-glucose
    (b) d-glyceraldehyde
    (c) l-glycine
    (d) d-alanine

(4) Both glycogen and cellulose are polymers of glucose. The main factor that makes them different is

(a) cellulose has more glucose units
(b) glycogen has more branch points
(c) glycogen has $\alpha$-1,4 bonds and cellulose has $\beta$-1,4 bonds between glucose units
(d) cellulose has more glucose units and more branch points

(5) For monosaccharides, the ring forms (pyranose or furanose) are:

(a) acetals
(b) hemiacetals
(c) carbonyls
(d) esters

Use the following structures for questions #6-#12.

I

II

III

IV

V

VI

VII

VIII

IX

X

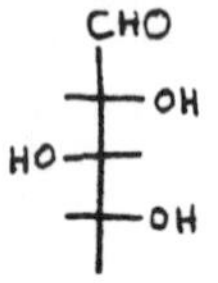

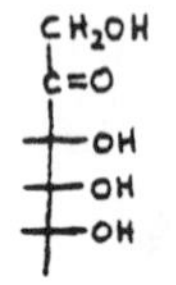

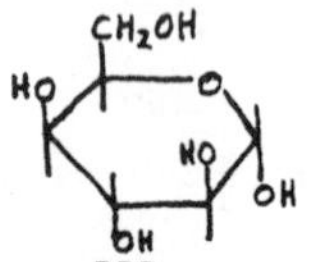

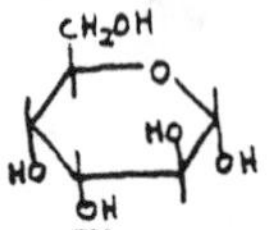

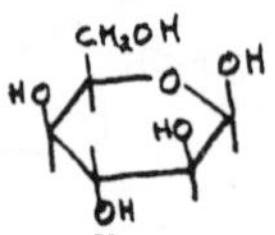

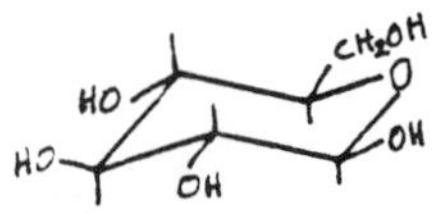

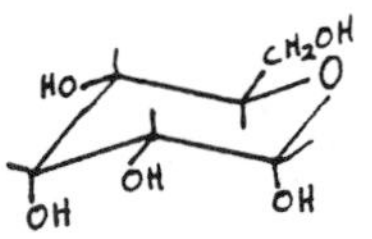

(6) Which structure is a furanose?

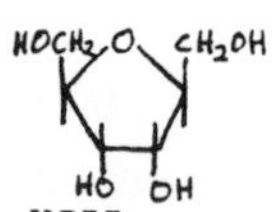

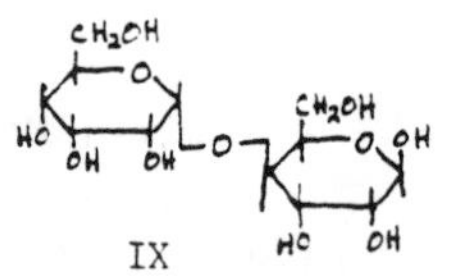

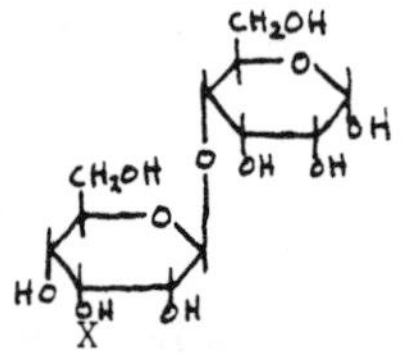

(a) III
(b) VI
(c) VIII
(d) IX

(7) Which structure is a ketose?

(a) I
(b) II
(c) III
(d) VI

(8) Which structure is the anomer of III?

(a) I
(b) IV
(c) V
(d) none of these

(9) Which structure is an epimer of IV?

(a) III
(b) V
(c) VI
(d) none of these

(10) Which conformation is more stable?

(a) VI
(b) VII
(c) both equal

(11)    Which compound is a pentose?

   (a) I
   (b) II
   (c) III
   (d) VIII

(12)    Which compound has an α-1,4 glycosidic bond?

   (a) IX
   (b) X
   (c) both
   (d) neither

## 4.14.3    Answers to Questions in Section 4.14.2

( 1) a   ( 2) c   ( 3) b   ( 4) c   ( 5) b   ( 6) c   ( 7) b   ( 8) c   ( 9) a   (10) a   (11) a
(12) a

## 4.14.4    Discussion of Answers to Questions in Section 4.14.2

*Questions #1 to #5* Adequately discussed in Section.

*Question #6* (Answer: c) A furanose is a ring form which contains five atoms.

*Question #7* (Answer: b) A ketose is a sugar which has a ketone functional grouping. (Section 4.7.1).

*Question #8* (Answer: c) Anomers are compounds in the ring that differ in configuration only at the former carbonyl carbon:

*Question #9* (Answer: a) Epimers are optical isomers that are different in configuration at a carbon other than the anomeric. III differs from IV at Carbon #4.

*Question #10* (Answer: a) The more stable conformation is where the maximum number of substituents, especially the larger substituents, are in equatorial positions.

*Question #11* (Answer: a) A pentose has a total of five carbons. See Section for symbolism.

*Question #12* (Answer: a) To have an α bond the compound must be an α-anomer:

### 4.14.5 Vocabulary, Concepts, etc. Checklist for Carbohydrates

_____ cyclic structures
_____ conformations of hexoses
_____ ketose
_____ aldose
_____ epimers
_____ anomers
_____ glycosidic bonds, hydrolysis
_____ monosaccharides
_____ hexoses
_____ pentoses
_____ pyranoses
_____ furanoses
_____ starch
_____ nomenclature and classification of carbohydrates
_____ glucose
_____ fructose
_____ galactose
_____ mannose
_____ maltose
_____ sucrose
_____ lactose
_____ glycogen
_____ cellulose

## 4.15 REFERENCES FOR REVIEW OF ORGANIC CHEMISTRY

Hendrickson, J.B., D.J. Cram, and G.S. Hammond. *Organic Chemistry.* McGraw-Hill Book Co.

Loudon, G.M. *Organic Chemistry.* Addison-Wesley Publishing Co., Inc.

Morrison, R.T., and R.N. Boyd. *Organic Chemistry.* Allyn & Bacon, Inc.

The above texts are excellent introductory texts. However, they are too detailed for the requirements of the MCAT. A selective review might be valuable.

Solomons, T.W. *Organic Chemistry.* John Wiley & Sons, Inc.

This book is an excellent reference to cover all the problem-solving aspects of organic chemistry. It is very similar to the MCAT topic outline and it contains clear illustrations and explanations.

*Chapter 5:*

# Review

# of

# Physics

## 5.1     TRANSLATIONAL MOTION

### 5.1.1     Review of Translational Motion

*Distance* depends upon the path taken, has an inconstant direction, and has magnitude only. *Speed* is the distance traveled divided by the change in time. Both speed and distance are scalar quantities—have magnitude but not direction. They have positive values only. *Displacement* is independent of the path taken (i.e., depends only on initial and final positions of the object) and has a constant direction and magnitude. *Velocity* is the displacement divided by the change in time. Both velocity and displacement are vector quantities (i.e., have direction and magnitude). *Acceleration* is the change in velocity divided by the change in time, and it is a vector also. (Fig. 5.1.)

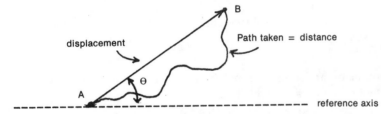

Note that displacement has a constant direction and magnitude and is independent of the path taken (there are many paths from A to B but the displacement is the same regardless of the path taken)

$$\text{speed} = \frac{\Delta \text{distance}}{\Delta \text{time}} = \frac{d_f - d_i}{t_f - t_i}$$

f = final
i = initial

$$\text{velocity} = \frac{\text{displacement}}{\Delta \text{time}}$$

$$\text{acceleration} = \frac{\Delta \text{velocity}}{\Delta \text{time}} = \frac{v_f - v_i}{t_f - t_i}$$

$\Delta$(delta) = change

*Fig. 5.1—Translational Motion Parameters*

The *units* of distance and displacement are length such as feet (ft), meters (m), miles and kilometers (km). The units of speed and velocity then become length divided by time such as feet/sec., miles/hour or meters/sec. Acceleration has the units of length/time/time (length/time$^2$) and examples are feet/sec$^2$, meters/sec$^2$ and miles/hour$^2$. Note the *sign* ( + or − ) of displacement, velocity or acceleration depends on the system under study and the specific values of the final (f) and initial (i) values. A displacement is negative if it is opposite to the direction designated as positive. The velocity is negative if the displacement is negative. The acceleration is negative if the velocity is decreasing. *Instantaneous* velocity or acceleration is for a given point in time. For velocity, it is the slope of the graph of distance vs. time at the given time. The *average* velocity or acceleration is for a period of time, and is conveniently taken as:

$$v = \frac{v_f + v_i}{2} \text{ if acceleration is constant,}$$

$$a = \frac{a_f + a_i}{2} \text{ if the force is constant.}$$

Note that these are different from the equations presented earlier.

*Force* is defined as the *action* of one particle on another, e.g., pushing a book with your hand.

Forces (Section 5.3.1) act upon objects to cause an acceleration. If a constant force is acting there is a constant (unchanging) acceleration. The motion produced in this case is called *uniform motion*. The acceleration (a) is causing a change in velocity (v) over time (t):

if a = 10 m/sec² and 5 secs elapse

then $v = at = \left(10\frac{m}{sec^2}\right)$ (5 secs) = 50 m/sec after 5 seconds.

The changing acceleration and velocity are both causing a change in displacement (d)—the directions of acceleration, velocity and displacement are all in the same direction:

$d_{vo} = v_o t$ displacement due to the initial velocity ($v_o$) at time = t;
$d_a$ = ½ at² displacement due to the acceleration at time = t
$d_o$ = initial displacement (if any) from a reference.

The total displacement (d) in a time (t) for uniform motion (equation for uniform linear motion) is:

$d = d_o + v_o t + ½ at^2$ (memorize)
or, final displacement (d) = initial displacement from a reference point ($d_o$) + change in displacement due to initial velocity ($v_o t$) + change in displacement due to acceleration (½at²).

*Translational motion* is the motion of an object through space. The above equations illustrate uniform translational motion along a straight line.

Displacements, velocity and accelerations are added (or subtracted) by methods of *vectors*.

It may be noted that speed, time and distance are *scalars*, whereas velocity, acceleration and displacement are *vectors*. In order to review vectors, study the section on vectors in Volume II *(Skills Development for the Medical College Admission Test)*. Make sure that you really understand how to break or resolve a vector into the sine and cosine components. On the actual MCAT, if a problem is asked about finding the resultant of 3 or 4 vectors, use the "quick graphical method" illustrated below:

*Quick graphical method:*

Let $v_1$ = 64 fps
$v_2$ = 83 fps
$v_3$ = 31 fps
$v_4$ = 47 fps

Scale: 50mm = 83fps

Example Problem

In order to find the resultant of the four vectors $v_1$, $v_2$, $v_3$, $v_4$, you can use the long method, which involves breaking down each vector into two components. Students get an average of 1 minute per problem to get an answer on the MCAT, hence the "quick graphical method" is recommended.

*Use of "quick graphical method"*

Select any vector to start with. For this example problem, select $v_3$ as the starting vector. Remember each vector has a *tip* (the arrowhead) and a *tail* (where it is attached to the particle). Start by drawing the vector $v_3$, making sure *your* measurements of *direction* and *length of vector* are fairly accurate. Now select *any other* vector such as $v_1$, and draw it so that the tail of $v_1$ coincides with the tip of $v_3$. Proceed to vector $v_2$ and draw it so that the tail of $v_2$ coincides with the tip of $v_1$. You are now left with vector $v_4$. Using the sequential procedure outlined above, draw $v_4$ attached to $v_2$ so that the tail of $v_4$ coincides with the tip of $v_2$. The vector diagram is now complete. To determine the answer as to the *direction* and *length of the resultant*, join the tip of $v_4$ to the tail of $v_3$.

$$AB = v_R = \text{Resultant velocity vector for the problem.}$$

This method is also called the "Tip-Tail method" and takes about one to two minutes. The question that might arise in your mind: "Can I use a protractor or ruler on the MCAT?" The answer is "NO." Use your answer sheet or the test booklet and your pencil to *measure* as you would with a ruler and a protractor. Your sense of direction and orientation will guide you. Draw the X-axis and Y-axis to improve your "angle sense" so that you have a better grip on finding the angles. PRACTICE THIS METHOD AT LEAST FIVE TIMES, before using it on the actual MCAT. Students who know this method have shown more confidence in solving such problems.

Approximate quick solution

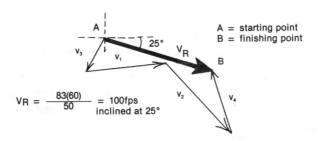

$$v_R = \frac{83(60)}{50} = 100\text{fps inclined at } 25°$$

*Free fall motion.* This is vertical motion (in reference to the earth), that is, upward or downward in a straight line. It is always uniformly accelerated motion with the acceleration equal to g. Values of g are:

$$32\text{ft/sec}^2 \text{ or } 980 \text{ cms/sec}^2 \text{ or } 9.8 \text{ m/sec}^2.$$

The equations for uniform linear motion (Section 5.1.1) are applicable when g is substituted for $a$:

$$d = d_0 + v_0 t + \tfrac{1}{2} gt^2$$
$$v = gt.$$

The reference point (origin) and positive and negative directions must be defined. As an example, in $g = 32$ ft/sec$^2$, what the g means is that for every second an object is falling under the influence of gravity (neglecting air resistance), the velocity is increasing by 32 ft/sec. For an object thrown straight up, its speed is decreasing by 32 ft/sec. for every second.

In the free fall of actual objects, the value of g is modified by buoyancy of air and resistance of air. What results is drag force and depends on the location on earth, weight, shape and size of the object, and the velocity of the object (as free fall velocity increases, the drag force increases). When the drag force reaches the force of gravity, the object reaches a final velocity called the terminal velocity and continues to fall at that velocity.

*Projectile motion* is conveniently thought of as having vertical (affected by g) and horizontal (independent of g) components. The vertical component is described by free fall motion (as above) and the horizontal component is described by uniform linear motion (Section 5.1.1) with a = 0. The projectile is generally fired at some angle (Θ) to the horizontal, and the motion is parabolic (see Fig. 5.2).

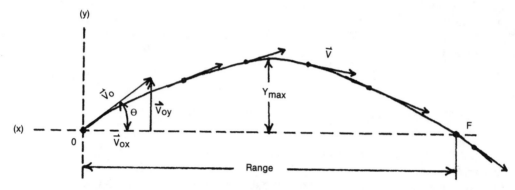

*Fig. 5.2—Projectile Motion*

*Vertical component (free fall)*

|  |  |
|---|---|
| initial speed | $v_{oy} = v_o \sin \Theta$ |
| distance at time = t | $y = v_{oy}t + \frac{1}{2} gt^2$ |
| speed at any time = t | $v_y = v_{oy} + gt$ |

(note that g is negative if it is opposite to the original displacement)

*Horizontal component (linear with constant speed)*

|  |  |
|---|---|
| initial speed | $v_{ox} = v_o \cos \Theta$ |
| distance at any time = t | $x = v_{ox}t$ |
| speed at any time = t | $v_x = v_{ox}$ (speed is constant) |

*Initial velocity vector (v̄) at any time = t*

| magnitude | $v^2 = (v_{ox})^2 + (v_{oy})^2$ (Pythagorean |
|---|---|
| direction (Θ) | $\tan\Theta = v_{oy}/v_{ox}$       Theorem) |

Points to note about the above are:
    (1) $v_{ox}$ is constant
    (2) $v_y$ is zero at $y_{max}$, then $v_y = 0 = v_{oy} + gt - v_{oy} = gt$
        (and can solve for t)
    (3) at O and F, the v's are equal but opposite in sign
    (4) the maximum range is attained when Θ = 45°

## 5.1.2    Questions to Review Translational Motion

(1)    Which of the following depends upon the path taken?

    (a) distance
    (b) displacement
    (c) both
    (d) neither

(2)　Which of the following is a vector?

(a) distance
(b) speed
(c) velocity
(d) all of these

(3)　The quantity below with the dimension of length/time² is:

(a) displacement
(b) velocity
(c) acceleration
(d) force

(4)　A constant acceleration is caused by a:

(a) constant force
(b) changing force
(c) constant displacement
(d) either (a) or (b)

(5)　An object was moving at 10m/sec; then a force was applied for 10 sec and the final velocity was 60m/sec. The acceleration was:

(a) 3 m/sec²
(b) 5 m/sec²
(c) 7 m/sec²
(d) none of the above

(6)　An object initially moving at 15m/sec is accelerated at the rate of 5m/sec² for 5 sec, the final velocity of the object is:

(a) 15 m/sec
(b) 25 m/sec
(c) 40 m/sec
(d) 100 m/sec

(7)　An object starts 5m from a reference point with an initial velocity of 10 m/sec and an acceleration of 5 m/sec². After 5 secs, the object is how far from the reference point?

(a) 75m
(b) 80m
(c) 117.5m
(d) 180.5m

Use the following speed-time graph for Questions #8 through #12. The motion is initially to the right and is in a straight line.

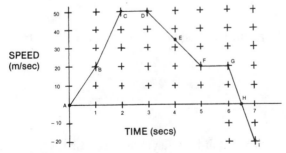

(8)　The slope of the graph at any point represents:

(a) acceleration
(b) displacement
(c) force
(d) kinetic energy

(9)    The instantaneous speed at point B is:

(a) 20 m/sec
(b) 25 m/sec
(c) 10 m/sec
(d) 35 m/sec

(10)   The instantaneous acceleration at point E is:

(a) 15 m/sec$^2$
(b) $-15$ m/sec$^2$
(c) 30 m/sec$^2$
(d) $-30$ m/sec$^2$

(11)   At point I, the object is:

(a) to the left of the origin
(b) moving to the right
(c) moving to the left
(d) not moving

(12)   The average speed from 0 to 2 secs is:

(a) 12.5 m/sec
(b) 20 m/sec
(c) 22.5 m/sec
(d) 25 m/sec

(13)   The analysis of projectile motion is greatly simplified by:

(a) using the formula for describing the motion as a parabola
(b) realizing that the time of ascent is one-half the time of descent
(c) neglecting the effect of gravity if the object is considered a point mass
(d) separating the motion into vertical (free fall) and horizontal (uniform linear motion) components

(14)   The maximum horizontal distance an object can attain is when the object is thrown at what angle to the horizontal?

(a) 15°
(b) 30°
(c) 45°
(d) 60°

(15)   An unbalanced force acting upon an object causes

(a) a change in the mass of the object
(b) an acceleration of the object
(c) the object to maintain a constant velocity
(d) none of the above

(16)   An object is thrown vertically upward at an initial velocity of 49 m/sec. It will rise to what height?

(a) 122.5 m
(b) 245 m
(c) 490 m
(d) the time must be given

(17)   An object dropped from the edge of a cliff will fall how far in 10 seconds?

(a) cannot be determined; need the mass of the object
(b) 98 m
(c) 980 m
(d) 490 m

Use the following information for Questions #18 and #19.

An object is thrown with an initial speed of 19.6 m/sec at an angle of 30° with the horizontal.

(18)   The maximum height the object reaches is:

(a) 2.45 m
(b) 4.9 m
(c) 9.8 m
(d) 98 m

(19)   The range (horizontal distance) of the object is:

(a) 19.6 m
(b) $19.6\sqrt{3}$ m
(c) 9.8 m
(d) $9.8\sqrt{3}$ m

## 5.1.3     Answers to Questions in Section 5.1.2

( 1) a   ( 2) c   ( 3) c   ( 4) a   ( 5) b   ( 6) c   ( 7) c   ( 8) a   ( 9) a   (10) b   (11) c
(12) c   (13) d   (14) c   (15) b   (16) a   (17) d   (18) b   (19) b

## 5.1.4     Discussion of Answers to Questions in Section 5.1.2

*Questions #1 to #4:* Adequately discussed in the Section.

*Question #5* (Answer: b) Use the formula for acceleration (a),

$$a = \Delta v / \Delta t = (v_f - v_i) / (t_f - t_i) = (60 - 10) / (10 - 0) = 50/10 = 5 \text{ m/sec}^2$$

*Question #6* (Answer: c) The final velocity ($v_f$) is:

$v_f$ = initial velocity + velocity change due to acceleration =
     15 m/sec + at = 15 + (5 m/sec²) (5 sec)  =  15 + 25  =  40 m/sec

*Question #7* (Answer: c) Use the formula for distance:

$$d = d_0 + v_0 t + \tfrac{1}{2} at^2 = 5 + (10)(5) + \tfrac{1}{2}(5)(5)^2$$
$$= 5 + 50 + (\tfrac{1}{2})(5)(25) = 55 + \tfrac{1}{2}(125)$$
$$= 55 + 62.5 = 117.5$$

*Question #8* (Answer: a) The slope of the curve of any graph is the ratio of the change in the y-axis ($\Delta y$) to the corresponding change in the x-axis ($\Delta x$). In this case,

$\Delta y$ = change in speed = $\Delta v$
$\Delta x$ = change in time = $\Delta t$

then:

slope = $\Delta y / \Delta x$ = $\Delta v / \Delta t$ = acceleration.

*Question #9* (Answer: a) The answer is 20 m/sec as read from the graph. Instantaneous speed is the speed at a given point in time.

*Question #10* (Answer: b) Since E is on the line DF, the instantaneous acceleration (i.e., the slope at a given point) at E is the same as the slope of line DF:

acceleration at E = (20 - 50) / (5 - 3) = -30/2 = -15 m/sec²

*Question #11* (Answer: c) Initially, a positive speed meant the object was moving to the right. A negative speed now means the object is moving to the left. The area between the curve and the time axis is the distance traveled. Since the area from A to H is much greater than the area from H to I, the object could not have moved back to the origin as (a) states. Also, only at points A and H is the object motionless.

*Question #12* (Answer: c) The average speed is,

$$\text{average speed} = \text{total distance/total time}.$$

The total distance is the area under the graph from A to C.

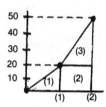

Total area = distance = Area #1 + Area #2 + Area #3
$$= (\tfrac{1}{2})(20)(1) + (20)(1) + (\tfrac{1}{2})(30)(1)$$
$$= 10 + 20 + 15 = 45m$$

Then: avg. speed = 45m/2 sec. = 22.5 m/sec. The formula $v = \dfrac{v_f + v_i}{2}$ cannot be used because the acceleration is not constant over this interval.

*Questions #13 to #15:* Adequately discussed in the Section.

*Question #16* (Answer: a) The object will rise for as long as it takes the downward acceleration (due to gravity-g) to overcome the initial upward velocity, i.e.:

$$v_o = gt$$

$$t = \frac{v_o}{g} = \frac{49 \text{ m/sec}}{9.8 \text{ m/sec}^2} = 5 \text{ secs.}$$

Then using the formula for uniform linear motion (Section 5.1.1):

$$d = d_o + v_ot + \tfrac{1}{2} gt^2 = 0 + 49(5) + \tfrac{1}{2}(-9.8)(5)^2 = 245 - 122.5$$
$$d = 122.5 \text{ m}.$$

Note that the g is negative because it opposes the original motion.

*Question #17* (Answer: d) Using the equations for linear motion (Section 5.1.1) and the fact that gravity is the accelerative force:

$$d = d_o + v_ot + \tfrac{1}{2} gt^2$$
$$= 0 + (0)(10) + (\tfrac{1}{2})(9.8)(10)^2 = (4.9)(100) = 490 \text{ m}.$$

This is an example of free fall motion.

*Question #18* (Answer: b) The maximum height would correspond to the height reached if the object was thrown vertically upward with the vertical component of the initial velocity ($v_o$)

$$v_y = v_o \sin 30° = (19.6)(\tfrac{1}{2}) = 9.8 \text{ m/sec}$$

$$v_x = v_o \cos 30° = (19.6)(\sqrt{3}/2) = 9.8\sqrt{3} \text{ m/sec}$$

Remember: $\sin \Theta = $ opposite/hypotenuse
$\cos \Theta = $ adjacent/hypotenuse

The distance can be calculated using the formula for linear motion (Section 5.1.1):

$$d = d_0 + v_0 t + \tfrac{1}{2} g t^2.$$

But the time is needed. This is found by reasoning that the object continues to rise until its upward motion is offset by the downward acceleration of gravity (g): $v_y = gt$

$$t = \frac{v_y}{g} = \frac{9.8 \text{ m/sec}}{9.8 \text{ m/sec}^2} = 1 \text{ sec.}$$

Note that 1 sec is the time required for half the trajectory. Using the above:

$$d = d_0 + v_0 t + \tfrac{1}{2} g t^2$$
$$d = 0 + (9.8)(1) + (\tfrac{1}{2})(-9.8)(1)^2 = 9.8 - 4.9 = 4.9\text{m}.$$

*Question #19* (Answer: b) From question #22, the time for half the trajectory was 1 sec, so the total time is two secs. To find the range, use the horizontal component of the initial velocity ($v_x$) as calculated in question #22. There is no force in the horizontal direction so the acceleration is zero in this direction. Then using the equation for linear motion applied in the horizontal direction (Section 5.1.1):

$$d = d_0 + v_0 t + \tfrac{1}{2} a t^2$$
$$d = 0 + (9.8\sqrt{3})(2) + (\tfrac{1}{2})(0)(2)^2$$
$$d = 19.6\sqrt{3} \text{ m.}$$

## 5.1.5    Vocabulary, Concepts, etc. Checklist for Translational Motion

_____ units and dimensions of distance, speed (velocity), acceleration
_____ equation for uniform linear motion
_____ speed
_____ distance
_____ displacement

_____ velocity
_____ acceleration
_____ translational motion
_____ projectile motion
_____ free fall motion
_____ Tip-Tail method

## 5.2    EQUILIBRIUM

### 5.2.1    Review of Equilibrium

When a force (Section 5.3.1) acts upon an object, the object will undergo translational motion or rotational motion. Translational motion is the motion of the object through space when the force is acting along an axis and/or the center of mass (that point whose motion can be described like a particle, Section 5.3.1). Rotational motion is the rotation of an object about an axis caused by a force not directed along that axis. The effective force causing rotation about an axis is the *torque (L)* (Fig. 5.3).

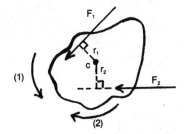

L = (force) (moment arm)
    moment arm is the perpendicular distance from the force to the axis
F = force
r = moment arm
c = center of mass or an axis
$L_1 = (F_1)(r_1)$ = counterclockwise (1) = positive
$L_2 = (F_2)(r_2)$ = clockwise (2) = negative

*Fig. 5.3—Torque (Rotational Moment)*

To determine the direction of rotation caused by the torque, imagine the direction the object would rotate if the force is pushing against its moment arm (at right angles). The net forces acting on an object is best determined by resolving them into the x and y components. The net torques acting on an object is obtained by summing the counterclockwise (+) and clockwise (-) torques. An object is at equilibrium when the net forces and torques acting on it are zero. Note that this means there is no acceleration but does not mean there is no velocity; it means either the object is motionless or moving with a constant velocity. The conditions of equilibrium are:

for translational equilibrium
$\Sigma F_x = 0$      ($\Sigma$ = sum over all)
$\Sigma F_y = 0$
for rotational equilibrium
$\Sigma L = 0$      (in a given geometric plane, must hold for three mutually perpendicular planes).

If the torques sum to zero about one point in an object, they will sum to zero about any point in the object. If the point chosen as reference includes the line of action of one of the forces, that force need not be included in calculating the torques.

*Newton's First Law* states that objects at rest or in motion tend to remain as such unless acted upon by an outside force. That is, objects have inertia (resistance to motion). For translational motion, the mass (m) is a measure of inertia. For rotational motion, a quantity derived from mass called the moment of inertia (I) is the measure of inertia. The $I = \Sigma mr^2$ in general, but its exact formulation depends on the structure of the object. See Section 5.6.1 for compressive and tensile forces.

*Momentum* (M) is a vector quantity. Its formulation for magnitude is:
$M = mv$
$m$ = mass
$v$ = velocity

For a discussion of vectors, refer to Volume II *(Skills Development for the Medical College Admission Test)*.


*Linear momentum* is a measure of the tendency of an object to maintain motion in a straight line. Notice that M is directly proportional to the mass of the object and its velocity (not acceleration). The larger the M, the greater the tendency of the object to remain moving along a straight line (in the same direction). The M is also a measure of the force needed to stop or change direction of the object. The *impulse* (I) is given by:
$I = F \Delta t = M = mv$
$F$ = force acting
$\Delta t$ = elapsed time which force is acting over

Impulse is a measure of the force required to impart or change momentum of an object. Impulse is also a vector.

Just like energy, *momentum is also conserved*. The total linear momentum of a system is constant when the resultant external force acting on the system is zero.

Remember, there are three conservation laws for ALL states of matter:

1. Law of Conservation of Mass
2. Law of Conservation of Momentum
3. Law of Conservation of Energy

Collisions are a form of interaction of matter during which momentum (remember, it is a vector) is conserved. During an elastic collision (objects do not stick), there is conservation of momentum and conservation of kinetic energy. During an inelastic collision (objects stick together), there is conservation of momentum but not of kinetic energy (the remainder of the energy is lost as heat or sound, so total energy is conserved).

Two special collisions will be mentioned. In the explosion of an object at rest, the total momentum of all the fragments must sum to zero (original momentum was zero). If one object collides elastically with a second identical object that is at rest, the first object comes to rest and the second moves off with the momentum of the first. Newton's Second Law and Third Law of Motion are discussed in the next section.

### 5.2.2 Questions to Review Equilibrium

(1) Rotational motion:

    (a) movement of an object along a curved line
    (b) movement of an object through space
    (c) motion of an object about a fixed point
    (d) motion of an object about an axis

(2) "An object at rest tends to remain at rest while objects in motion tend to remain in motion...;" this is Newton's First Law and it reflects the property of:

    (a) velocity
    (b) weight
    (c) potential energy
    (d) inertia

(3) If a force is acting on an object, but off an axis, what type of motion results?

    (a) rotational
    (b) translational

(4) The product of force times the moment arm is the:

    (a) energy
    (b) work
    (c) torque
    (d) force

(5) The net force (in newtons) on the following object (answers in nts) is:
$F_2 = 100$ nts

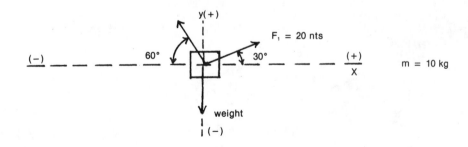

    (a) zero
    (b) $F_x = -32.7$; $F_y = -1.5$
    (c) $F_x = -15.4$; $F_y = +98.3$
    (d) $F_x = -80.0$; $F_y = -98.3$

(6)   What is the net force on the following object?

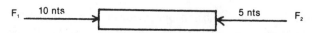

    (a) 15 nts
    (b) 5 nts to the right
    (c) 5 nts compressive force
    (d) none of these

(7)   What is the net torque acting about the axis through the center A (perpendicular to the paper) of the square with sides equal to 4m?

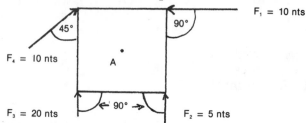

    (a) 38.2 nt – m counterclockwise
    (b) 76.4 nt – m clockwise
    (c) 38.2 nt – m clockwise
    (d) none of the above

(8)   The object below is in static and rotational equilibrium. What are the components of the force, $F_1$?

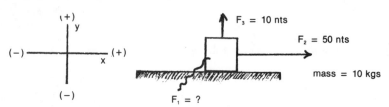

    (a) $F_x = -50$ nts; $F_y = -10$ nts
    (b) $F_x = -50$ nts; $F_y = +88$ nts
    (c) $F_x = +50$ nts; $F_y = -108$ nts
    (d) none of the above

(9)   The object below is in rotational equilibrium. What force, $F_1$, is required for this equilibrium (neglect the weight)?

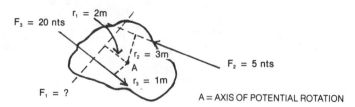

    (a) counterclockwise, 17.5 nts
    (b) clockwise, 5 nts
    (c) clockwise, 35 nts
    (d) none of the above

## 5.2.3    Answers to Questions in Section 5.2.2

(1) d    (2) d    (3) a    (4) c    (5) b    (6) b    (7) c    (8) b    (9) d

**5.2.4     Discussion of Answers to Questions in Section 5.2.2**

*Questions #1 to #4:* Adequately discussed in the text.

*Question #5* (Answer: b) The forces may be rediagrammed as:

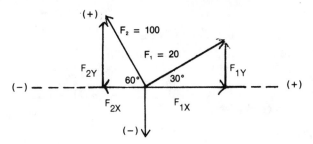

$$W_y = mg = (10)(9.8) = 98 \text{ nts}$$
(Weight has no x-component in this case.)

For a 30°-60° right triangle (see also Volume II: *Skills Development for the Medical College Admission Test*) use:

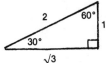

Then: for $F_1$: $F_{1y} = +(\frac{1}{2})(20) = +10$   $F_{1x} = +(\sqrt{3}/2)20 = +10\sqrt{3}$
for $F_2$: $F_{2y} = +(\sqrt{3}/2)(100) = +50\sqrt{3}$   $F_{2x} = -(\frac{1}{2})(100) = -50$

Then: $\Sigma F_x = F_{1x} + F_{2x} + W_x = 10\sqrt{3} - 50 + 0 = 17.3 - 50 = -32.7 \text{ nts}$
REMEMBER: $(\sqrt{3} \sim 1.73)$
$\Sigma F_y = F_{1y} + F_{2y} + W_y = +10 + 50\sqrt{3} - 98 = +50(1.73) - 88$
$= 86.5 - 88 = -1.5 \text{ nts.}$

The net force (F) would be:
$$F^2 = F_x{}^2 + F_y{}^2$$
$$F = \sqrt{F_x{}^2 + F_y{}^2} = \sqrt{(-32.7)^2 + (-1.5)^2} = 32.7 \text{ nts}$$

Try to calculate free-hand to get more practice.

*Question #6* (Answer: b) These are opposing forces acting along the same line of action. The net force is the algebraic sum (assume positive is to the right):

$$\text{net force} = +10 \text{ nts} - 5 \text{ nts} = +5 \text{ nts.}$$

*Question #7* (Answer: c) The forces, their moment arms (r) and directions of rotation (R) are:

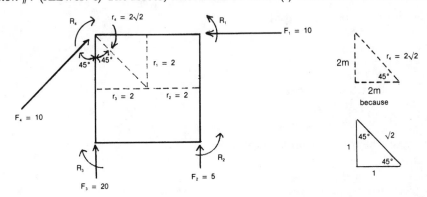

(Refer to Volume II: *Skills Development for the Medical College Admission Test*, the section on trigonometry.)

The torques are:

Counterclockwise ( + )
$$L_1 = F_1 \times r_1 = (10)(2) = +20 \text{ nt} \cdot \text{m}$$
$$L_2 = F_2 \times r_2 = (5)(2) = +10 \text{ nt} \cdot \text{m}$$

Clockwise ( − )
$$L_3 = F_3 \times r_3 = -(20)(2) = -40 \text{ nt} \cdot \text{m}$$
$$L_4 = F_4 \times r_4 = -(10)(2\sqrt{2}) = -20\sqrt{2} = -28.2 \text{ nt} \cdot \text{m}$$

The net torque (L) is:
$$L = L_1 + L_2 + L_3 + L_4 = +20 + 10 - 40 - 28.2 = +30 - 68.2$$
$$L = -38.2 \text{ nt} \cdot \text{m (which is clockwise)}.$$

*Question #8* (Answer: b) The force diagram is:

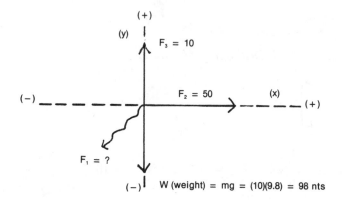

Components of forces:

| | |
|---|---|
| $F_1 : F_{1X} = ?$ | $F_{1y} = ?$ |
| $F_2 : F_{2X} = +50$ | $F_{2y} = 0$ |
| $F_3 : F_{3X} = 0$ | $F_{3y} = +10$ |
| $W : W_X = 0$ | $W_y = -98$ |

Net force (F):
$$\Sigma F_X = 0 = F_{1X} + F_{2X} + F_{3X} + W_X = F_{1X} + 50 + 0 + 0 = F_{1X} + 50$$
$$\text{then, } F_{1X} + 50 = 0$$
$$F_{1X} = -50 \text{ nts.}$$
$$\Sigma F_y = 0 = F_{1y} + F_{2y} + F_{3y} + W_y = F_{1y} + 0 + 10 - 98 = F_{1y} - 88$$
$$\text{then, } F_{1y} - 88 = 0$$
$$F_{1y} = 88 \text{ nts.}$$

Also, practice using quick graphical method as shown in Section 5.1.1.

*Question #9* (Answer: d) The directions of rotations are:
$F_2$ causes counterclockwise ( + ) motion
$F_3$ causes counterclockwise ( + ) motion

The individual torques are:
$$L_1 = F_1 \times r_1 = (F_1)(2) = 2F_1 \text{ (sign unknown)}$$
$$L_2 = +F_2 \times r_2 = +(5)(3) = +15 \text{ nt} \cdot \text{m}$$
$$L_3 = +F_3 \times r_3 = +(20)(1) = +20 \text{ nt} \cdot \text{m}.$$

Since rotational equilibrium exists the torques sum to zero:
$$\Sigma L = L_1 + L_2 + L_3 = 0$$
$$2F_1 + 15 + 20 = 0$$
$$2F_1 + 35 = 0$$
$$2F_1 = -35$$
$$F_1 = -17.5 \text{ nts and motion is clockwise}.$$

### 5.2.5    Vocabulary, Concepts, etc. Checklist for Equilibrium

_____ conditions for translational equilibrium    _____ torque
_____ conditions for rotational equilibrium    _____ Law of Conservation of Mass
_____ separation of forces into their components    _____ Law of Conservation of Momentum
_____ Newton's First Law    _____ Law of Conservation of Energy


## 5.3    FORCE, MOTION AND GRAVITATION

### 5.3.1    Review of Force, Motion and Gravitation

The *center of mass* (COM) of an extended body is that point whose motion can be described like a particle (e.g., as linear, circular, parabolic) even if the motion of the extended object cannot be so described. In collisions, the COM velocity (of the system) is not changed. The *center of gravity* (COG) is the COM but is conceptualized as that point where the sum of gravitational forces acting on an extended object can be represented by a summation force (acting at the COM). An object suspended from the COG is in rotational equilibrium (Section 5.2.1). The COG can be determined experimentally by suspending an object by a string at different points and noting that the direction of the string passes through the COG. The intersections of the projected lines in the different suspensions is the COG. The COG of a regular geometric object is the geometric center. The COG of an irregular object may be inside or outside the object. An object is in *stable equilibrium* if the COG is as low as possible, and any change in orientation will lead to an elevation of the COG. *Unstable equilibrium* is when the COG is high (relative to a surface supporting it, e.g.), and any change in orientation would lead to a lowering of the COG. *Neutral equilibrium* is an intermediate location of the COG and a change in orientation would not change the level of the COG. A force acting through the COG causes translational motion. A force acting off the COG causes rotational motion. *Mass* is a dimension that cannot be broken down into simpler units. This is to be contrasted with *weight* which is a force. Units of mass are slugs (weight in pounds divided by g = 32 ft/sec$^2$), kilograms, grams, etc. Units of weight are pounds (defined differently from the pounds of mass), dynes (gms·cm/sec$^2$) and newtons (kg·m/sec$^2$).

*Newton's Second Law* involved an unbalanced force acting upon an object and producing an acceleration in the direction of the force that is directly proportional to the force and inversely proportional to the mass of the body:

$$a = F/m$$
$$\text{or, } F = ma$$

For every action, there is an equal and opposite reaction. This is *Newton's Third Law.* If one object exerts a force, F, on a second object, the second object exerts a force, –F, on the first. These forces cannot neutralize each other because they act on different objects. Every force arises from three basic forces. These are gravitational (below), electromagnetic (Section 5.7), and nuclear (Section 5.13).

*Newton's Second Law of Motion* is considered to be the *most* important one for the MCAT student. Applications and uses of the *Second Law* include driving a nail into the wall, putting your foot on the accelerator of your car while driving, freely falling objects under the action of opposing forces such as friction, running compared to jogging, the movement of blood and drugs in your arteries and veins. Make sure that you draw a *"free-body"* diagram to solve problems which involve the second and third laws of motion.

As shown above, Force = mass × acceleration.
Momentum = mass × velocity.

Hence, $\dfrac{\text{Force}}{\text{Momentum}} = \dfrac{\text{acceleration}}{\text{velocity}}$

Also, $F = ma = \dfrac{m\,(v_f - v_i)}{(t_f - t_i)}$ (from earlier sections)

Therefore, $F\,(t_f - t_i) = m\,(v_f - v_i)$ = Impulse-Momentum Principle

Newton also formulated the *Law of Gravitation* as:

$$F = K_G(m_1 m_2/r^2)$$

This states that there is a gravitational force existing between any two bodies of masses $m_1$ and $m_2$. The force is proportional to the product of the masses:

$$F \propto m_1 m_2$$

and inversely proportional to the square of the distance between them:

$$F \propto 1/r^2$$

The $K_G$ is the universal constant of gravitation, and its value depnds upon the units being used. (Some books use 'G' instead of $K_G$.)

*Frictional forces* are illustrated in Fig. 5.4.

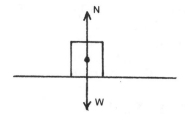

W = weight = mg = N (neglecting signs)

*Fig. 5.4—Frictional Forces*

$F = \mu N$, this is the maximal frictional force
$\mu$ = coefficient of friction
N = normal (perpendicular) force to the surface the object rests on.

*Friction* is the resistance offered to the motion of a body and is mostly caused by the roughness (ups and downs or indentations) between two rough bodies. Friction depends on the texture of the contact surface of two bodies.

Frictional forces are nonconservative (mechanical energy is not conserved) and are caused by molecular adhesions between tangential surfaces but are independent of the area of contact of the surfaces. Frictional forces always oppose the motion. Static friction is when the object is not moving, and it must be overcome for motion to begin. The coefficient of static friction, $\mu_s$, is given as:

$$\mu_s = \tan\Theta,$$

where $\Theta$ is the angle at which the object first begins to move on an inclined plane as the angle is increased from $0° \rightarrow \Theta°$:

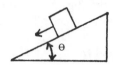

*Fig. 5.5—Inclined Plane*

there is also a coefficient of kinetic friction, $\mu_k$, which exists when surfaces are in motion. The $\mu_s > \mu_k$ always.

The analysis of *motion on an incline* is shown in Fig. 5.6.

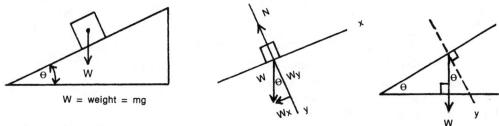

components of forces
  N = normal to surface
$W_y = W\cos\Theta$, $W_x = W\sin\Theta$

*Fig. 5.6—Motion on an Incline I (Neglecting Friction)*

The weight (W) due to gravity (g) may be sufficient to cause motion if friction is overcome. The reference axes usually chosen as shown such that one (the x) is along the surface of the incline. Additional forces on the object added to the basic set above is shown in Fig. 5.7.

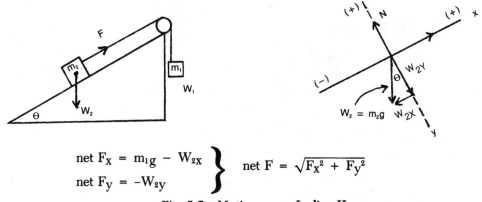

$$\left.\begin{array}{l} \text{net } F_x = m_1 g - W_{2x} \\ \text{net } F_y = -W_{2y} \end{array}\right\} \quad \text{net } F = \sqrt{F_x^2 + F_y^2}$$

*Fig. 5.7—Motion on an Incline II*

Note that N is the reactive force to $W_{2y}$, the axes are assigned ( + ) and ( − ) as one desires.


## 5.3.2    Questions to Review Force, Motion and Gravitation

(1)    One of Newton's Laws of Motion:

   (a) An unbalanced force acting upon an object produces an acceleration of that object.
   (b) Objects moving in circles at constant tangential velocity have no force acting upon them.
   (c) The square of the period of revolution is proportional to the cube of the radius of revolution.
   (d) Objects falling to earth describe a hyperbolic projectory.

(2)    In order for any object to undergo an acceleration, it must

   (a) lose energy
   (b) gain energy
   (c) be acted upon by balanced (net zero) forces
   (d) be acted upon by unbalanced forces

(3)     Newton's Second Law:

    (a) $E = \frac{1}{2} mv^2$
    (b) $F = -kx$
    (c) $U = mgh$
    (d) $F = ma$

(4)     Frictional forces exist between an object and the surface it is on, and they

    (a) are proportional to the normal force to the surface that the object rests on
    (b) are dependent on the area of contact between the surfaces
    (c) always augment the motion of the object
    (d) are conservative forces

(5)     For $\mu_s$ (coefficient of static friction) and $\mu_k$ (coefficient of kinetic friction)

    (a) $\mu_s > \mu_k$
    (b) $\mu_s = \mu_k$
    (c) $\mu_s < \mu_k$
    (d) any of the above

(6)     The motion of the center of mass is like a(n):

    (a) particle
    (b) extended object
    (c) both
    (d) neither

(7)     The force of gravity between two objects is

    (a) inversely proportional to the products of the masses
    (b) inversely proportional to the distance between them
    (c) directly proportional to the square of the radius
    (d) inversely proportional to the square of the distance between them

(8)     A force of 15 newtons acting upon a 5 kg object will produce an acceleration equal to:

    (a) $\frac{1}{3}$ m/sec²
    (b) $\frac{1}{75}$ m/sec²
    (c) 3 m/sec²
    (d) 75 m/sec²

(9)     An object has an acceleration of 2 m/sec² and a mass of 5 kg. The force necessary to impart this acceleration is:

    (a) 0.4 newtons
    (b) 2.5 newtons
    (c) 5 newtons
    (d) 10 newtons

(10)    If F = force, $\Delta U$ = potential energy change, $\Delta x$ = displacement over which $\Delta U$ occurs, then:

    (a) $F = \Delta U \Delta x$
    (b) $F = 1/\Delta U \Delta x$
    (c) $F = -\Delta x/\Delta U$
    (d) $F = -\Delta U/\Delta x$

(11)    An object first begins to slide down an inclined plane when the angle with the horizontal is 45°. The coefficient of static friction ($\mu_s$) of the object-surface is:

    (a) 0.5
    (b) 1.0
    (c) $\sqrt{2}/2$
    (d) need more information

Use the following speed-time graph for Questions #12 through #16.

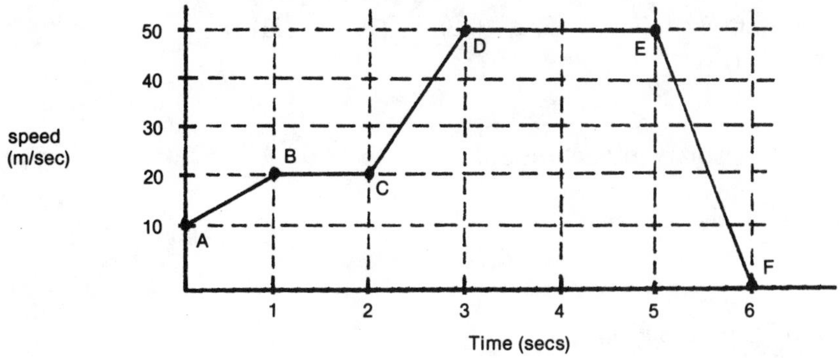

The above is a graph for a 2 kg object moving along a straight line to the right initially.

(12)    The area under the graph represents:

(a) distance
(b) acceleration
(c) force
(d) velocity

(13)    The greatest force is acting at:

(a) AB
(b) BC
(c) CD
(d) EF

(14)    No net force is acting along:

(a) AB
(b) BC
(c) CD
(d) EF

(15)    The distance traveled from A to B is:

(a) 5 m
(b) 10 m
(c) 15 m
(d) 20m

(16)    At point F, the object is:

(a) motionless
(b) moving backward
(c) moving forward
(d) at the origin

(17)    What value of Weight ($W_1$) is required such that the object (A) does not move down the incline (assume no friction)

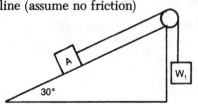

mass of A is 10 kg

(a) 5 newtons
(b) 10 newtons
(c) 49 newtons
(d) none of the above

**5.3.3**     **Answers to Questions in Section 5.3.2**

( 1) a   ( 2) d   ( 3) d   ( 4) a   ( 5) a   ( 6) a   ( 7) d   ( 8) c   ( 9) d   (10) d   (11) b
(12) a   (13) d   (14) b   (15) c   (16) a   (17) c

**5.3.4**     **Discussion of Answers to Questions in Section 5.3.2**

*Questions #1 to #7:* Adequately discussed in the Section.

*Question #8* (Answer: c)

$$F = ma$$
$$a = F/m = 15 \text{ newtons}/5 \text{ kgs} = 3(\text{nts/kg})$$
$$= 3[(\text{kg-m/sec}^2)/\text{kg}] = 3 \text{ m/sec}^2$$

*Question #9* (Answer: d)

$$F = ma = (5 \text{ kg})(2 \text{ m/sec}^2) = 10 \text{ kg-m/secs}^2 = 10 \text{ newtons}.$$

*Question #10* (Answer: d) If the relationship is not already known to you, it may be determined (in this case) by knowing unit interrelations (i.e., by doing dimensional analysis):

$$\text{energy} = \text{work} = Fd \text{ (Section 5.4.1)}$$

then to get force equal to some combination of energy and displacement:

Force $\propto$ energy/displacement, which is the *form* of answer (d).

Or, since Force = newtons and energy = joules = *newtons-meters* and d = meters, the only way to combine the units of energy and displacement to yield the units of force is:

$$\text{newtons (force)} \propto \frac{\text{newtons-meters (energy)}}{\text{meters (displacement)}} = \text{newtons}$$

or
$$\text{Force} \propto \frac{\text{energy}}{\text{displacement}}$$

Note that the best that can be said from this analysis is that force is proportional to energy over displacement. The exact form of answer (d) could not be arrived at in this manner.

*Question #11* (Answer: b) The $\mu_S$ is found by:

$$\mu_S = \tan \Theta$$
$$\mu_S = \tan 45°$$
$$\mu_S = 1/1 = 1$$

$$\tan \Theta = \text{opposite/adjacent}.$$

Refer to Volume II: *Skills Development for the Medical College Admission Test.*

*Question #12* (Answer: a) The area under any curve is proportional to the product of the axes:

y-axis is speed (v)
x-axis is time (t)
product = (v)(t) = distance.

*Question #13* (Answer: d) The greatest force is acting where the greatest acceleration (whether positive or negative) is also. This is because:

$$F = ma \text{ and } F \propto a.$$

The greatest acceleration is where the slope $\Delta v/\Delta t$ is the greatest in absolute value (neglecting signs). For each of the above line segments, the slope, and acceleration, is:

$$a = \Delta v/\Delta t = (v_f - v_i)/(t_f - t_i)$$

AB: $\quad a = (20-10)/(1-0) = 10/1 \quad = 10$
BC: $\quad a = (20-20)/(2-1) = \;\;0/1 \quad = \;\;0$
CD: $\quad a = (50-20)/(3-2) = 30/1 \quad = 30$
EF: $\quad a = \;\;(0-50)/(6-5) = -50/1 = -50.$

Hence, EF has the largest acceleration and the largest force.

*Question #14 (Answer: b) Again, since F* = ma *and F $\propto$ a, a zero acceleration gives a zero force. A zero acceleration occurs where the slope is zero.* See the discussion in Question #13 for the slopes of the segments. BC is the only one with a zero slope and, therefore, a zero acceleration and a zero force.

*Question #15* (Answer: c)

(I)  By geometry:

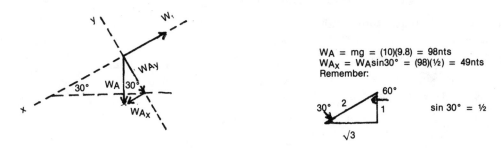

Area (1) $= (\frac{1}{2})(10)(1) = 5$m
Area (2) $= (10)(1) \;\;= \;\;10$ m
total $\;\;\;\; = 5 + 10 = 15$ m

(II) By formulas:

$d = d_0 = v_0 t + 1\, at^2$ $\qquad$ (Section 5.1.1)
$\quad d_0 = 0 \qquad v_0 = 10$ m/sec
$\quad\;\; a = \Delta v/\Delta t = (20 - 10)/(1 - 0) = 10/1 = 10$ m/sec$^2$
$\quad\;\; t = 1$ sec
$d = 0 + (10)(1) + (\frac{1}{2})(10)(1)^2 = 10 + 5 = 15$ m.

*Question #16* (Answer: a) The speed is zero at point F, so the object must not be moving. Also, note that at no point is the speed negative, so the object could not have returned to the origin.

*Question #17* (Answer: c) The schematic showing the forces is:

$W_A = mg = (10)(9.8) = 98$nts
$W_{Ax} = W_A \sin 30° = (98)(\frac{1}{2}) = 49$nts
Remember:

$\sin 30° = \frac{1}{2}$

In order for the object not to move, the $W_1$ should balance $W_{Ax}$. The $W_{Ay}$ has no effect on motion along x (the incline). Therefore, a $W_1$ of 49 nts is required. The mass would be:

$$m = W_1/g = 49/9.8 = 5 \text{ kgs}.$$

## 5.3.5 Vocabulary, Concepts, etc. Checklist for Force, Motion, Gravitation

_____ center of mass
_____ center of gravity
_____ Newton's Second Law
_____ motion on an incline
_____ Newton's Third Law

_____ Law of Gravitation
_____ friction
_____ mass
_____ weight

## 5.4     WORK AND ENERGY

### 5.4.1     Review of Work and Energy

Energy is a scalar (see Volume II: *Skills Development for the Medical College Admission Test*) and is generally conceptualized as the ability to do work. Note that objects exert forces upon other objects, and if a displacement results, work (see below) is performed which is not contained within the object. Energy, by contrast, is contained by the object (or system), and if work is performed, this energy either increases or decreases (for negative or positive work respectively).

$$\text{Work = Force times distance} = F \cdot d$$

Mechanical energy is divided into kinetic energy (K) and potential energy (U). *Kinetic energy* is the energy associated with the motion of objects. *Potential energy* is the energy that results by position or configuration (of a system); there is no motion. When motion begins, potential energy is converted into kinetic energy. The formulation of potential energy depends upon the system.

$U = mgh$ = gravitational potential energy
$m$ = mass
$h$ = height above earth's surface.
$k = \frac{1}{2}mv^2$ = kinetic energy
$v$ = speed of object

Additional features of potential energy are: (1) potential energy *cannot* be defined for frictional forces, and (2) the potential energy of a system is independent (in contrast to work) of the path to reach that system.

Potential energy can be of many types such as: magnetic, electric, chemical. Always remember potential energy as a *field* that exists around molecules.

The *Law of Conservation of Mechanical Energy* is:
Total Energy (TE) = kinetic energy (K) + potential energy (U) +
energy due to dissipative forces (e.g., friction).

In the absence of dissipative forces, this can be taken as:
TE = K + U

On the actual MCAT the questions normally reflect applications of energy conservation. Remember that potential and kinetic energies at *any* two points, along the path of movement of the particle, can be easily found by the following formula:

$$K_1 + U_1 = K_2 + U_2$$
(without considering friction)

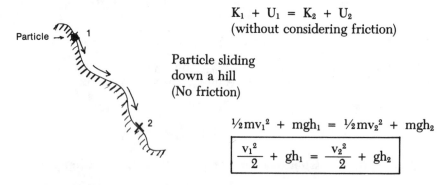

Particle sliding
down a hill
(No friction)

$$\frac{1}{2}mv_1^2 + mgh_1 = \frac{1}{2}mv_2^2 + mgh_2$$

$$\boxed{\frac{v_1^2}{2} + gh_1 = \frac{v_2^2}{2} + gh_2}$$

Potential and kinetic energy are scalar quantities.

*Work* (W) is a scalar also. Work results when a force (F) causes displacement (d):

$$W = Fd\cos\theta$$

Note that F cosΘ is the component of F along the displacement (d). When Θ = 0°, then cos 0° = 1, and W = Fd which is the result for forces in the same direction as the displacement. When Θ = 90°, then cos 90° = 0 and W = 0. That is, forces perpendicular to the displacement do no work. Remember, walking a dog illustrates the concept of work.

Another way of looking at work is as the change in mechanical energy of an object. Remember that the potential energy between two points (or positions) is the amount of work that would be required to move an object between those two points. The change in kinetic energy of an object is the work performed by the object assuming all the energy goes into work. To summarize:

$$W = E_f - E_i = \Delta E$$
$$E = K + U = \text{mechanical energy}$$
$$f = \text{final} \qquad i = \text{initial} \qquad \Delta = \text{change.}$$

This means work and energy have the same units:

$$W = (\text{force})(\text{distance}) = \text{newtons-meters} = \text{joules}$$
$$= \text{dynes-cms} = \text{ergs.}$$

Joules and ergs are units of work or energy.
Pressure (P) times volume (V) also yields work (W), W = (P)(V).
This is used to study heat engines.

*Power* (P) is a scalar and is the rate at which work is done:
$$P = \text{work}(W)/\text{time}(t) = W/t$$

The units of power are:
$$P = \text{work/time} = \text{joules/secs} \equiv \text{watts.}$$


## 5.4.2 Questions to Review Work and Energy

(1) When a system does work or work is done on a system

    (a) the force of the system changes
    (b) the momentum of the system changes
    (c) the torque of the system changes
    (d) the energy of the system changes

(2) All of the following statements are correct concerning potential energy (PE) except:

    (a) PE depends on the configuration rather than the motion of a system
    (b) PE may be converted to kinetic energy
    (c) PE cannot be defined for frictional forces
    (d) PE depends upon the path taken to reach a certain state

(3) The Law of Conservation of Energy takes into account all of the following except:

    (a) conversion of mass into energy
    (b) potential energy
    (c) kinetic energy
    (d) energy loss due to dissipative forces

(4) If W = work and t = time, then power (P) is:

    (a) P = W/t
    (b) P = t/W
    (c) P = Wt
    (d) P = 1/Wt

(5)     At what angle to the direction of the displacement would a force perform no work?

(a) 0°
(b) 45°
(c) 90°
(d) 180°

(6)     All are expressions of work except:

(a) changes in mechanical energy
(b) momentum times mass
(c) force times distance
(d) pressure times volume

(7)     A 5kg object is moving in a straight line at a velocity of 4 meters/sec. The kinetic energy (K) is:

(a) 40 joules
(b) 20 joules
(c) 10 joules
(d) 80 joules

(8)     An object weighing 10 kg is at a distance of 10 m above the earth's surface. The potential energy (U) of this object is:

(a) 980 joules
(b) 100 joules
(c) 9.8 joules
(d) 1000 joules

(9)     If a 5 kg object is 20 meters above the earth's surface and it falls to 10 meters above the surface, what is the change in potential energy (U)?

(a) gains 490 joules
(b) loses 490 joules
(c) loses 50 joules
(d) only the kinetic energy changes, the potential energy does not change

(10)    The shaded area under the graph might represent:

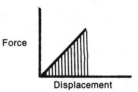

(a) momentum
(b) force field
(c) work
(d) pressure

(11)    A person does 20 joules of work in 10 seconds; the power (P) generated is:

(a) 2000 watts
(b) 200 watts
(c) 2 watts
(d) 0.5 watts

(12)    A force of 20 newtons is used to move a 10 kg object 20 meters in 10 seconds; the power (P) generated is:

(a) 40,000 watts
(b) 4,000 watts
(c) 400 watts
(d) 40 watts

(13)　A force of 10 newtons pushes a 5 kg object 20 meters. The work performed is:

(a) 200 joules
(b) 40 joules
(c) 10 joules
(d) 2.5 joules

(14)　How much work is performed in the diagram below?

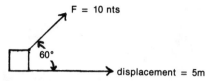

(a) 50 joules
(b) 50 cos 30° joules
(c) 25 joules
(d) 50 sin 60° joules

(15)　A 5 kg object moving at 4 m/sec strikes a second object. After the collision, the first object is moving at 2 m/sec. Assuming all the energy (E) was used to perform work (W) on the second object, the work performed is:

(a) 30 joules
(b) 60 joules
(c) 90 joules
(d) 120 joules

## 5.4.3　Answers to Questions in Section 5.4.2

( 1) d　( 2) d　( 3) a　( 4) a　( 5) c　( 6) b　( 7) a　( 8) a　( 9) b　(10) c　(11) c
(12) d　(13) a　(14) c　(15) a

## 5.4.4　Discussion of Answers to Questions in Section 5.4.2

*Questions #1 to #6:* Adequately discussed in the Section.

*Question #7* (Answer: a)
$$K = \tfrac{1}{2}mv^2 = (\tfrac{1}{2})(5)(4)^2 = (5/2)(16) = 40 \text{ joules.}$$

*Question #8* (Answer: a)
$$U = mgh = (10 \text{ kg})(9.8 \text{ m/sec}^2)(10\text{m}) = 980 \text{ joules.}$$

*Question #9* (Answer: b)
$$\Delta U = U_2 - U_1 = mgh_2 - mgh_1 = mg(h_2 - h_1)$$
$$= (5)(9.8)(10 - 20) = (5)(9.8)(-10) = -490 \text{ joules.}$$

The minus sign means U is lost.

*Question #10* (Answer: c) The area under the graph is given by the product of the axes. This is (force)(displacement), which is work (or energy).

*Question #11* (Answer: c)
$$P = \text{work/time} = 20 \text{ joules/10 secs} = 2 \text{ joules/sec} = 2 \text{ watts.}$$

*Question #12* (Answer: d)
$$P = \text{work/time} = 400 \text{ joules/10 secs} = 40 \text{ joules/sec} = 40 \text{ watts.}$$
$$\text{work} = (\text{force})(\text{distance}) = (20)(20) = 400 \text{ joules.}$$

*Question #13* (Answer: a)
$$W = Fd \cos\Theta$$
$$\Theta \text{ must be } 0° \text{ so } \cos\Theta = 1$$
$$W = Fd = (10)(20) = 200 \text{ joules.}$$

*Question #14* (Answer: c) Remember that:

$$\cos 60° = ½$$

Then: $W = Fd \cos\Theta = (10)(5) \cos 60° = 50(½) = 25$ joules.

*Question #15* (Answer: a)
$$\Delta E = W = E_f - E_i$$
$$E = ½mv^2$$
$$W = ½mv_f^2 - ½mv_i^2 = ½m(v_f^2 - v_i^2)$$
$$W = ½(5)(4^2 - 2^2) = (5/2)(16 - 4) = (5/2)(12) = 30 \text{ joules.}$$

## 5.4.5    Vocabulary, Concepts, etc. Checklist for Work and Energy

_____ work
_____ kinetic energy
_____ gravitational potential energy
_____ Law of Conservation of Energy

_____ power
_____ joules
_____ watts

## 5.5    THERMODYNAMICS

### 5.5.1    Review of Thermodynamics

*Heat* is a form of energy. Bodies *do not contain* heat; they either emit or absorb energy as heat. When a body absorbs or emits energy, all of the energy need not be in the form of heat. For example, a body emitting energy may emit some as heat and some as light energy. A body *does not contain thermal energy* (or internal energy) which is the *sum* of the potential and kinetic energies associated with the position or motion, respectively, of the molecules.

*Thermal equilibrium* results when the average kinetic energies per molecule of two bodies are equal. This is also when the heat flow between the bodies is zero, and when the temperatures of the two bodies are equal. *Temperature* is taken to be a measure of the average thermal energy of a body; it is also a measure of the amount of energy absorbed or emitted as heat by a body. Thus when temperature rises, the average kinetic energy per molecule rises, and the object absorbs more energy as heat, and vice versa.

$$\text{Temperature of molecules} = \text{Constant} \times mv^2 \text{ (average)}$$

*Measurement of temperature* is by thermometers. A *thermometer* has (1) a thermometric property (e.g., pressure, density, resistance) which varies directly as temperature; (2) a lower fixed point (e.g., freezing point (FP) of water); (3) a higher fixed point (e.g., boiling point (BP) of water); and (4) a scale calibrated between these two points and extrapolated beyond them. Relative temperature scales are the *Celsius* or *Centigrade* (FP of water = 0°C, BP of water = 100°C) and the *Fahrenheit* (FP of water = 32°F, BP of water = 212°F). Absolute scales (the zero point of the scale is the true absolute zero) are the *Rankine*

(°R) calibrated in °F units and the *Kelvin* (°K) calibrated in °C units. Interconversions of the scales are:

°C = 5/9 (°F-32)   or   °F = (9/5) °C + 32 and 5 units Celsius = 9 units Fahrenheit
°K = °C + 273          °R = °F + 460

The Celsius and Fahrenheit scales are equal at −40°.

Heat capacity is a measure of the amount of heat a body can gain (or lose) per change in temperature ($\Delta t$),

$$\text{heat capacity} = \text{heat gained/temperature change} = Q/\Delta t.$$

*Specific heat capacity* (C) is the heat capacity per unit mass of substance:

$$C = (Q/\Delta t)/m = Q/m\Delta t.$$

This can be rearranged to give the amount of heat exchanged (gained or lost) by a substance:

$$Q = (C)(m)(\Delta t).$$

The units of heat most commonly used are calories. A calorie is the amount of heat required to raise the temperature of 1 gram of water one degree Celsius.

A kilocalorie is 1000 calories. Since heat is a form of energy, its units must be equivalent to the unit of other energies (kinetic or potential) or work which is the Joule (or other similar units). *The interconversion of calories and joules is:*

| 4.184 joules = 1 kilocalorie |
| 4.2 joules ≈ 1 kilocalorie. |

(Memorize for the MCAT!)

The *specific heat of water is then:*

$$1 \ (\text{calorie/gm} - °C).$$

It is in the understanding of *phase transitions* that specific heat, heat of fusion and heat of vaporization have particular value. Below are the important features of phase transitions (See Sections 3.4.1 and 3.5.1):

| Phase Transition | Conditions | Heat Associated |
|---|---|---|
| (1) solid $\underset{\text{freeze}}{\overset{\text{melt}}{\rightleftharpoons}}$ liquid | Solid and liquid vapor pressure in equilibrium. Temperature called melting (or freezing) point (MP or FP). | heat of fusion ($H_f$) $H_f = Q/m$ at MP or $Q = m \ H_f$ $Q$ = heat transferred $m$ = mass |
| liquid $\underset{\text{condense}}{\overset{\text{evaporate (boil)}}{\rightleftharpoons}}$ gas | Gas and liquid vapor pressure in equilibrium. Temperature called the boiling point (BP). | Heat of evaporation ($H_V$) $H_V = Q/m$ at BP or $Q = H_V \ m$ |

Note that $H_V > H_f$ because usually more kinetic energy per molecule is required to separate liquid molecules to become gaseous than to separate solid molecules to become liquid. As a substance gains or loses energy as heat, it passes through the various phases. A scheme for substances gaining heat is:

| Phases & Temps | Solid Below (1) → MP | Solid at (2) MP → | Liquid at (3) MP → | Liquid at (4) BP → | Gas at (5) BP → | Gas above BP |
|---|---|---|---|---|---|---|
| Heat changes | (1) Heat is absorbed to raise the temperature as the specific heat of the solid:<br><br>$Q = C\,m\Delta t$<br>$C$ = of solid | (2) Heat is absorbed as heat of fusion to cause solid to melt to the liquid. Note that the temperature does not change:<br>$Q = H_f\,m$ | (3) Heat is absorbed as the specific heat of the liquid to raise its temperature:<br><br><br>$Q = C\,m\Delta t$<br>$C$ = of liquid | (4) Heat is absorbed as heat of vaporization to cause the liquid to be converted to gas. The temperature does not change.<br>$Q = H_v\,m$ | (5) Heat is absorbed as the specific heat of the gas to raise its temperature:<br><br><br>$Q = C\,m\Delta t$<br>$C$ = of gas | |

The reverse steps would hold if the substance was losing energy as heat. To summarize, heat is used to change the phase or the temperature of a substance. When two objects are in contact and at different temperatures, heat flows from the one with the higher temperature to the one with the lower temperature until the temperatures are equal. The above equations can be used to calculate heat flows and temperatures by using:

> Heat flow law:      heat loss = heat gain      (Memorize this equation and how to use it on the MCAT.)

As an illustration, study the following example and how it relates to the heat flow law.

> You are preparing a small pot of chicken soup in the kitchen. The pot is made of a special alloy with a specific heat of 0.10. The specific heat of chicken soup is 0.83. Suddenly you drop a large gold bracelet in the soup. The bracelet has a mass of 75 grams. There is about 1000 grams of chicken soup in the pot and the pot has a mass of 500 grams. The bracelet you were wearing had a temperature of 50°F. The specific heat of the bracelet is 0.032. The temperature of the pot and the soup inside it is 88°C. Find the final temperature of the bracelet.

Solution: Heat lost by hot substances = heat gained by cold substances.

The problem shows that chicken soup and the pot are *hot*, whereas the bracelet is *cold*. Convert the temperature of the bracelet to °C, using,

$$\frac{F - 32}{9} = \frac{C}{5}, \quad \frac{50 - 32}{9} = \frac{C}{5}$$

which gives temperature of bracelet to be 10°C.

> Heat lost by pot + heat lost by chicken soup =  Heat gained by gold bracelet.

Subscripts used are as follows:      s = chicken soup
b = gold bracelet
p = cooking pot

$$C_p\,(m_p)(t_p - t_f) + C_s\,(m_s)(t_s - t_f) = C_b\,(m_b)(t_f - t_b)$$
$t_f$ = Final temperature of bracelet and resulting mixture.
$0.1\,(500)(88 - t_f) + 0.83\,(1000)(88 - t_f) = 0.032\,(75)(t_f - 10)$

In order to solve this problem quickly on the MCAT, use guidelines given in Volume II: *Skills Development for the Medical College Admission Test* under "High Speed Mathematics Review," which shows how to multiply quickly.

Solving for $t_f$, one obtains 87.8°C. In other words, the bracelet's temperature is *almost* the same as the chicken soup, but it rose rapidly from 10°C to 87.8°C. On the MCAT you *could* have approximated the answer to this problem by looking at the relative *masses* of various objects. This illustrates the use of the heat flow equation.

When substances gain (or lose) heat they usually undergo *expansion (or contraction)*. Expansion (contraction) can be by linear dimensions, by area, or by volume. These are:

| Type | Final | Original | Change caused by heat |
|------|-------|----------|-----------------------|
| (1) Linear | L | $L_0$ | $\alpha \Delta t L_0$ |

$L = L_0 + \alpha \Delta t L_0 = L_0(1 + \alpha \Delta t)$
$\alpha$ = coefficient of linear thermal expansion, $\Delta t$ = change in temp

| | | | |
|------|-------|----------|-----------------------|
| (2) Area | A | $A_0$ | $\beta \Delta t A_0$ |

$A = A_0 + \beta \Delta A_0 = A_0(1 + \beta \Delta t)$
$\beta$ = coefficient of area thermal expansion = $2\alpha$

| | | | |
|------|-------|----------|-----------------------|
| (3) Volume | V | $V_0$ | $\gamma \Delta t V_0$ |

$V = V_0 + \gamma \Delta t V_0 = V_0(1 + \gamma \Delta t)$
$\gamma$ = coefficient of volume thermal expansion = $3\alpha$

*Heat flows between substances* by three mechanisms: conduction, convection and radiation. *Conduction* is a process in which heat energy is transferred by adjacent molecular collisions throughout a material medium—the medium does not move. The heat energy is carried off by the motion of the electrons. Good electrical conductors, therefore, are usually good heat conductors. The rate of heat transfer (H) by conduction is:

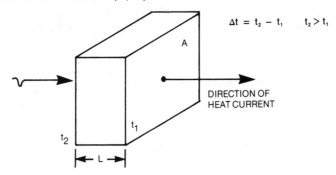

$\Delta t = t_2 - t_1 \qquad t_2 > t_1$

DIRECTION OF HEAT CURRENT

*Fig. 5.8—Heat Conduction*

$H = Q/T = kA(\Delta t/L)$
Q = heat exchanged
T = time elapsed
A = cross-sectional area
L = length over which transfer occurs
$\Delta t$ = temperature difference
k = thermal conductivity of the material.

Note that the rate (H) is directly proportional to A and $\Delta t$ and inversely proportional to L. The thermal conductivity, k is a property of the substance.

*Convection* is a process in which heat energy is transferred by the actual mass motion of a fluid (gas or liquid). Convection currents are set up which may be natural (caused by density differences, e.g., wind) or forced (as in a house ventilation system). The rate of energy transfer (H) is:

$H = Q/T = hA \Delta t$ (note the relations shown).

The convection coefficient h is not a property of the substance.

*Radiation* is a process in which heat energy is transferred by electromagnetic waves absorbed or emitted at the atomic level. All substances radiate heat regardless of the temperature. In general, as the absolute temperature (T) increases, the wavelength of the emitted heat decreases. The rate of emission (R) is:

$R = e \delta T^4$ (Stephan-Boltzmann Law)
T = absolute temperature
e = emissivity = the ability to absorb or emit thermal radiation
$\delta$ = Stephan's Constant.

The *key relation* is that the R is proportional to the fourth power of the absolute temperature. A body at the same temperature as its surroundings will radiate and absorb heat at the same rate. If not at the same temperature, the net rate of radiation is:

net rate of radiation = rate of energy emission − rate of energy absorption

$R = e\delta T_1^4 - e\delta T_2^4 = e\delta (T_1^4 - T_2^4)$
$T_1$ = temperature of body
$T_2$ = temperature of surroundings.

*Thermodynamics* is concerned with the energy states of molecules and chemical reactions. A system is the object under study. It is the reference point. When the system gains (e.g., energy), the (energy) change is positive. The environment is everything outside the system. Systems exchange energy by the processes of work or heat exchange. The systems do not contain work or heat. Work or heat exchange depends upon the path from the initial to the final state. This is in contrast to state functions which are independent of the path taken but depend upon the initial and final states only. The state functions to be discussed are pressure (P), volume (V), temperature (T), internal energy (E) and entropy (S). See section 3.8.1 for the discussion of other state functions, enthalpy (H) and free energy (G).

Energy is a property of a system and not a process (like heat or work). Specifically, the internal energy change ($\Delta E$), of a system depends on the work done and heat exchanged as follows:

$\Delta E = q - W$         *First Law of Thermodynamics*
q = + if heat is added to the system
q = − if heat is lost from the system
W = $+ p\Delta V$ if work is done by the system
    p = external pressure
  $\Delta V = V_f - V_i$ change in volume of the system
      Note: this gives the sign to the work.

The internal energy depends on the kinetic energies of the molecules, on the potential energies of forces between molecules, and the kinetic and potential energies of the electrons and nuclei. The First Law of Thermodynamics is a restatement of the Law of Conservation of Energy. The $\Delta E$ of a reaction is determined by running the reaction at constant volume and measuring the amount of heat exchanged:

$\Delta E = q - W = q - p\Delta V = q_V$
$\Delta V = 0$
$q_V$ = heat at constant volume.

A reversible process is one that occurs in such small increments that it can be reversed at any point. An irreversible process is one that cannot be easily reversed. As a concrete example, if you walked down a flight of stairs one step at a time, it would be fairly easy to reverse your direction at any step—this would be a reversible process. But if you jumped out of a window, equivalent to that flight of stairs, you could not reverse yourself—this would be an irreversible process. For reversible (rev) and irreversible (irrev) processes, the following are true:

$W_{rev} > W_{irrev}$
$q_{rev} > q_{irrev}$

These concepts lead into entropy (S) and the Second Law of Thermodynamics which is

$$\Delta S = (q_{rev}/T) \text{ for a reversible path}$$

Note: (1) $\Delta S$ is still independent of a particular reversible path,
(2) $\Delta S = \Delta S$ system + $\Delta S$ environment = 0,
(3) $\Delta S$ exists for an irreversible path but it is not equal to $(q_{rev}/T)$
(4) $\Delta S$ is increasing for an irreversible path.

Entropy is further discussed in Section 3.8.1.

## 5.5.2    Questions to Review Thermodynamics

(1)    Heat:

(a) is contained by an object
(b) is absorbed or emitted by an object
(c) both (a) and (b)
(d) neither (a) nor (b)

(2)    Temperature:

(a) is a measure of the average thermal energy of a body
(b) is a measure of the amount of heat a body absorbs or emits
(c) increases when the average kinetic energy per molecule increases
(d) all of the above

(3)    Thermal equilibrium occurs when:

(a) the average kinetic energy per molecule of two bodies is equal
(b) the heat flow between two bodies is zero
(c) the temperature between two bodies is equal
(d) all are correct

(4)    Heat capacity is:

(a) the amount of heat a body contains per degree of temperature
(b) the amount of heat a body can gain or lose per degree change in temperature
(c) represented as: temperature/heat
(d) both (a) and (c)

(5)    Specific heat capacity:

(a) the amount of heat contained by a substance
(b) the amount of heat contained per unit change of temperature by a substance
(c) the heat capacity per unit change in temperature
(d) the heat capacity per unit mass

(6)    If C = specific heat capacity, $\Delta t$ = change in temperature and m = mass, then the amount of heat (Q) exchanged is:

(a) $Q = C/m\Delta t$
(b) $Q = C\, m\Delta t$
(c) $Q = Cm/\Delta t$
(d) $Q = C\Delta t/m$

(7)    Heat of fusion refers to the phase change between:

(a) gas and solid
(b) liquid and gas
(c) liquid and solid
(d) all phases

(8)     When a solid is converted to a liquid:

   (a) heat is released
   (b) heat is required
   (c) temperature increases
   (d) both (a) and (c)

(9)     A net release of heat to the environment occurs during:

   (a) condensation
   (b) sublimation
   (c) evaporation
   (d) melting

(10)    Heat flows between substances by all the following processes except:

   (a) conjugation
   (b) conduction
   (c) convection
   (d) radiation

(11)    The process whereby heat is transferred by adjacent molecular collisions throughout a medium is:

   (a) convection
   (b) conduction
   (c) radiation
   (d) momentum

(12)    In heat transfer in a substance (e.g., a rod) by conduction, the rate of heat transfer is:

   (a) directly proportional to the length of heat transfer (end to end of the rod, e.g.)
   (b) indirectly proportional to the temperature difference
   (c) directly proportional to the cross-sectional area (e.g., of the rod)
   (d) independent of the nature of the substance

(13)    The process of transferring heat energy by the mass motion of a fluid is called:

   (a) bulk flow
   (b) radiation
   (c) conduction
   (d) convection

(14)    Heat loss or gain by the process of radiation:

   (a) occurs in all substances regardless of temperature
   (b) occurs only if the temperature is above the critical temperature of a substance
   (c) is independent of the nature of a substance
   (d) only (b) and (c)

(15)    As the absolute temperature increases, the wavelength of radiation emitted by a substance tends to:

   (a) increase
   (b) decrease
   (c) remain the same
   (d) totally unpredictable

(16)    The reference point in thermodynamics is called the:

   (a) surroundings
   (b) environment
   (c) state
   (d) system

(17)    Which of the following is independent of the path taken for its value?

(a) internal energy
(b) work
(c) heat
(d) none of these

(18)    A statement of the First Law of Thermodynamics is:

(a) $\Delta S = q_{rev}/T$
(b) $\Delta G = \Delta H - T\Delta S$
(c) $\Delta E = q - W$
(d) none of these

(19)    The internal energy ($\Delta E$) depends upon:

(a) kinetic energy of molecules
(b) potential energy of forces between molecules
(c) kinetic and potential energies of electrons and nuclei
(d) all of these

(20)    The Second Law of Thermodynamics involves a definition of:

(a) internal energy
(b) enthalpy
(c) entropy
(d) free energy

(21)    During the step of conversion of a liquid to a gas, the heat is

(a) used to overcome intermolecular forces between liquid molecules and convert
them to gaseous molecules
(b) used to raise the temperature of the gas
(c) used to raise the temperature of the liquid
(d) all of the above

(22)    The conversion of 10 grams of a solid to 10 grams of its liquid at the freezing point
(25°C) requires 100 cals of heat. The heat of fusion of this substance is:

(a) 0.40 cals/gm·°C
(b) 40 cals·gm/°C
(c) 10 cals/gm
(d) 250 cals·°C/gm

(23)    An object weighing 10 gms has a specific heat of 2 cals/gm/°C. To raise its
temperature from 10°C to 60°C would require how many calories?

(a) 10 cals
(b) 100 cals
(c) 1000 cals
(d) 5000 cals

(24)    A substance weighing 5 gms has its temperature raised from 25° to 75°C without a
phase change while absorbing 45 calories of heat. Its specific heat capacity is:

(a) 11,250 cals/gm·°C
(b) 450 cals/gm·°C
(c) 0.18 cals/gm·°C
(d) 4.50 cals/gm·°C

(25)    The amount of heat required to convert 10 gms of water (solid) at 0°C to water
(liquid) at 50°C (specific heat of solid water is 0.5 cals/gm·°C; specific heat of liquid
water is 1.0 cals/gm·°C; heat of fusion of water is 80 cals/gm) is:

(a) 1300 kilocalories
(b) 350 cals
(c) 1300 cals
(d) 1500 cals

(26) If a heating coil is supplying 50 cals/min to a tank containing water (ice) at 0°C, the amount of water (as a liquid) that can be formed in 10 min. (use specific heat and heat of fusion from question #25) is:

(a) 3.5 gms
(b) 6.25 gms
(c) 420 gms
(d) 500 gms

(27) A temperature of 50°C (Celsius) corresponds to what temperature Fahrenheit (F)?

(a) 122°F
(b) 90°F
(c) 82°F
(d) 27.8°F

(28) At what temperature are the Celsius (°C) and Fahrenheit (°F) scales equal?

(a) 100
(b) 37
(c) –40
(d) 0

(29) The coefficient of linear expansion ($\alpha$) of a substance is $2 \times 10^{-5}$°C$^{-1}$. The coefficient of volume expansion ($\gamma$) would be:

(a) $6 \times 10^{-5}$°C$^{-1}$
(b) $8 \times 10^{-5}$°C$^{-1}$
(c) $2 \times 10^{-15}$°C$^{-3}$
(d) need more information

(30) An object with a linear expansion coefficient ($\alpha$) of $2 \times 10^{-4}$°C$^{-1}$ has the volume of 10.000 liters. If the temperature increases 100°C, the new volume will be:

(a) 10.020 liters
(b) 10.008 liters
(c) 10.600 liters
(d) no change to three decimal places

(31) Heat is being conducted through a square-faced metal block 4 meters long with sides 2 meters in length. If another block of the same metal is constructed but with a square face of 4 meters on a side and 8 meters long, what is the rate of heat conduction through it, compared with the first block, for a given temperature difference? *Note:* the heat is passing through the square faces along the complete length.

(a) The second is four times the first.
(b) The second is twice the first.
(c) The second is one-half the first.
(d) The second is one-fourth the first.

(32) If the temperature of an object is changed from 20°C to 10°C, the rate of radiational heat loss is how much of the original?

(a) slightly more than 1.0
(b) slightly less than 1.0
(c) ½ as much
(d) ¹⁄₁₆ as much

## 5.5.3    Answers to Questions in Section 5.5.2

( 1) b  ( 2) d  ( 3) d  ( 4) b  ( 5) d  ( 6) b  ( 7) c  ( 8) b  ( 9) a  (10) a  (11) b
(12) c  (13) d  (14) a  (15) b  (16) d  (17) a  (18) c  (19) d  (20) c  (21) a  (22) c
(23) c  (24) c  (25) c  (26) b  (27) a  (28) c  (29) a  (30) c  (31) b  (32) b

## 5.5.4    Discussion of Answers to Questions in Section 5.5.2

*Questions #1 to #20:* Adequately discussed in the Section.

*Question #21* (Answer: a) During a phase conversion step, energy is used to break intermolecular bonds and is not used to increase the average kinetic energy of the molecules (raise the temperature).

*Question #22* (Answer: c)

heat of fusion = calories required for phase change/mass undergoing phase change
$$= 100 \text{ cals}/10 \text{ gms} = 10 \text{ cals/gm}$$

*Question #23* (Answer: c)

$Q = C \, m\Delta t = (2 \text{ cals/gm} \cdot °C)(10 \text{ gms})(60 - 10°C) = (2)(10)(50) \text{ cals}$
$Q = 1000 \text{ cals}$

*Question #24* (Answer: c)

$C = Q/m\Delta t = 45 \text{ cals}/(5 \text{ gms})(75 - 25°C) = 9/50 = 0.18 \text{ (cals/gm} \cdot °C)$

*Question #25* (Answer: c) The scheme is:

$$(1) \qquad\qquad (2)$$

water (solid) at 0°C→water (liquid) at 0°C→water (liquid) at 50°C
(1) heat of fusion ($H_f$) of water for phase change
    cals = ($H_f$)(mass) = (80 cals/gm)(10 gms) = 800 cals
(2) SH of water (liq) to raise temperature
    cals = (SH)(mass)(temp change) = C m$\Delta$t
    $= (1.0)(10)(50 - 0) = (10)(50) = 500 \text{ cals}$

Total:       (1) + (2) = 800 + 500 = 1300 cals.

*Question #26* (Answer: b) The total heat delivered in 10 mins. is:

cals = 50 cals/min)(10 mins) = 500 cals.

The scheme for water changes is:
$$(1)$$
water (solid) at 0°C→water (liquid) at 0°C
(1) heat of fusion ($H_f$) of water for phase change
    $H_f$ = heat change/mass = Q/m
    m = Q/$H_f$ = 500 cals/(80 cals/gm) = 6.25 gms.

*Question #27* (Answer: a) Use ratio and proportion and known facts about temperature scales:

| °C | | °F |
|----|----|----|
| | BP | |
| 100 | ┬ | 212 |
| | │ | |
| 50 | ┼ | ?°F |
| | │ | |
| 0 | ┴ | 32 |
| | FP | |

$(50 - 0)/(100 - 0) = (F - 32)/(212 - 32) = (F - 32)/180$
$(50)(180)/100 = F - 32$
$90 = F - 32$
$122 = F$

BP = boiling point
FP = freezing point

(The key to understanding this is noting that the distances on the scales are equal even though the calibrations differ.)

*Question #28* (Answer: c) This is similar to Question #27:

```
°C   BP   °F
100 ──┬── 212
      │
?°C ──┼── ?°F
      │
0  ──┴── 32
     FP
```

$$C - 0/100 - 0 = F - 32/212 - 32$$
$$C/100 = F - 32/180$$
$$\text{now } C = F \text{ for problem}$$
$$F/100 = F - 32/180$$
$$180F/100 = F - 32$$
$$9F/5 = F - 32$$
$$9F = 5F - 160$$
$$4F = -160$$
$$F = -40° = C$$

*Question #29* (Answer: a) The following relationship holds:

$$\gamma = 3\alpha = (3)(2 \times 10^{-5} °C^{-1}) = 6 \times 10^{-5} °C^{-1}.$$

*Question #30* (Answer: c) The coefficient of volume expansion ($\beta$) is:

$$\gamma = 3\alpha = (3)(2 \times 10^{-4} °C^{-1}) = 6 \times 10^{-4} °C^{-1}.$$

The formula for volume expansion is:

$$V = V_0 (1 + \gamma \Delta t)$$
$$= (10.000)[1 + (6 \times 10^{-4})(100)] = 10.00 [1 + (6 \times 10^{-4})(10^2)]$$
$$= (10.000)(1 + 6 \times 10^{-2} = (10.000)(1 + 0.06)$$
$$= (10.000)(1.06) = 10.600 \text{ liters.}$$

*Question #31* (Answer: b) The formula for heat rate in conduction is:

$$H = k(A/L)\Delta t \qquad \text{(see in section)},$$

or could remember that,

$$H \propto A \quad \text{and } H \propto 1/L \text{ or,}$$
$$H \propto A/L.$$

Then k and $\Delta t$ are constants. And,

$$A_1 = (2)(2) = 4 \text{ m}^2 \qquad \text{(area of a square)}$$
$$L_1 = 4 \text{ m}$$
$$A_2 = (4)(4) = 16 \text{ m}^2$$
$$L_2 = 8 \text{ m}$$

Putting these in either of the formulas above

$$\frac{H_2}{H_1} = \frac{k\dfrac{A_2}{L_2}\Delta t}{k\dfrac{A_1}{L_1}\Delta t} = \frac{\dfrac{A_2}{L_2}}{\dfrac{A_1}{L_1}} = \frac{A_2}{L_2} \cdot \frac{L_1}{A_1} = \frac{(16)}{(8)} \cdot \frac{(4)}{(4)} = 2$$
$$H_2 = 2H_1$$

*Question #32* (Answer: b) Using the Stephan-Boltzman Law:

$$R = e\delta T^4$$
$$1 = \text{original} \qquad 2 = \text{final}$$
$$T_1 = 20° + 273° = 293°, \quad T_2 = 10° + 273° = 283°$$
$$\frac{R_2}{R_1} = \frac{e\delta T_2^4}{e\delta T_1^4} = \frac{T_2^4}{T_1^4} = (283/293)^4 = 0.89$$
$$R_2 = 0.89R_1$$

### 5.5.5　Vocabulary, Concepts, etc. Checklist for Thermodynamics

_____ First Law of Thermodynamics
_____ Second Law of Thermodynamics
_____ equivalence of Joules and calories
_____ Celsius (Centigrade)
_____ Fahrenheit
_____ Rankine
_____ Kelvin
_____ interconversions of temperature scales
_____ coefficients of thermal expansion

_____ conduction
_____ convection
_____ radiation (of heat)
_____ specific heat
_____ heat capacity
_____ heat of fusion
_____ heat of vaporization
_____ internal energy
_____ entropy


## 5.6　SOLIDS AND FLUIDS

### 5.6.1　Review of Solids and Fluids

| Solids | Liquids | Gases |
| --- | --- | --- |
| 1. Solids are rigid. | Liquids are fluid. | Gases are extremely fluid. |
| 2. Solids have a definite shape. | Liquids have no definite shape, but have a well-defined surface. | Gases are shapeless; they occupy the entire container. |
| 3. Solids have a definite volume. | Liquids have a definite volume. | Gases have no definite volume. |
| 4. Solids have a higher density because their molecules are closely packed together. | Liquids are lighter than solids because molecules are farther apart. | Gases are extremely light because their molecules are far apart. |
| 5. Solids are extremely cohesive. | Liquids, except for mercury, are less cohesive. | Gases have almost no cohesion at all. There is almost no interaction between their molecules. |
| 6. Solids diffuse at an extremely slow rate, e.g., lead and gold diffuse into each other when left for six months or more. | Liquids exhibit various types of diffusion such as convective, turbulent and molecular, e.g., preparing coffee or tea in boiling water. | Gases diffuse at high speeds, e.g., air freshener in a room. |
| 7. Well-known theories and laws have been established to study solid behavior. | As of today, there is a large gap in the study of liquid behavior. No good model exists to represent a liquid. | Well-known theories have been established to study behavior of gases. |
| 8. Solids are almost incompressible. | Liquids are slightly compressible (do not confuse the slipping of liquid molecules under pressure with compression). | Gases are highly compressible, which gives them the property of resiliency. |

When a force acts on a solid, the solid is deformed. If the solid returns to its original shape, it is called _elastic_. The effect of a force depends on the area over which it acts. Stress is defined as the ratio of the force to the area over which it acts. Strain is defined as the relative change in dimensions or shape of the object caused by the stress. This is embodied in the definition of the modulus of elasticity (ME) as:

$$ME = stress/strain.$$

An important reminder for the MCAT student is to understand elastic solids. As an example, steel is more elastic than rubber. Rubber is more stretchable, but not more elastic, than steel. Do not confuse the words "elastic" and "stretchable."

Some different types of stresses are *tensile stress* (equal and opposite forces directed away from each other), *compressive stress* (equal and opposite forces directed toward each other), and *shearing stress* (equal and opposite forces which do not have the same line of action). There are two commonly useful moduli of elasticity:

(1) Young's Modulus (Y) for compressive or tensile stress:

$$Y = \text{longitudinal stress/longitudinal strain} = (F/A)/(\Delta l/l)$$
$$= Fl/A\Delta l$$

The A is the area normal (perpendicular) to the force

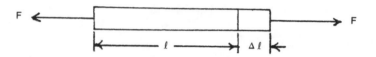

*Fig. 5.9(a)—Tensile Stress*

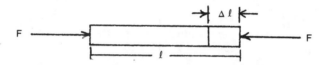

*Fig. 5.9(b)—Comprehensive Stress*

(2) Shear modulus (S) or the modulus of rigidity is:

$$S = \text{shearing stress/shearing strain} = (F/A)/\phi = (F/A)/\tan\phi =$$
$$(F/A)/(d/l) = Fl/dA. \text{ See Fig. 5.9(c).}$$

The A is the area tangential to the force. $\phi = \tan\phi$ for small angles.

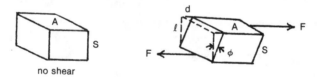

*Fig. 5.9(c)—Shear Stress*

### 5.6.1.1 DENSITY AND ITS PHYSICAL MEANING

What is meant by "heavy as lead" and "light as a feather?" Clearly, a grain of lead is light, while a mountain of feathers has considerable weight. Use of such comparisons are based not on a body's mass, but on the density of the material from which it is made.

The mass of a unit volume of a body is called its *density*. A grain of lead and a massive block of lead have the same density. Density is an *intensive* property.

In denoting density, usually shown is the number of grams (g) a cubic centimeter (cm)³ of the body weighs—the symbol g/cm³ is placed after this number. In order to determine the density, the number of grams is divided by the number of cubic centimeters (the fractional line in the symbol is a reminder).

Certain metals are among the heaviest materials—osmium, whose density is equal to 22.5 g/cm³, iridium (22.4), platinum (21.5), tungsten and gold (19.3). The density of iron is 7.88, that of copper is 8.93. Lighter substances include air with density .0013 g/cm³.

It should be stipulated that this discussion assumes continuous bodies. If there are pores in a solid, it will be lighter. Porous bodies—cork, sponge, steel wool—are frequently used in technology. The density of sponge may be less than 0.5, although the solid matter from which it is made has a higher density. As all other bodies whose density is less than one, sponge floats superbly on water unless soaked.

The lightest liquid is liquid hydrogen; it can only be obtained at extremely low temperatures. One cubic centimeter of liquid hydrogen has a mass of 0.07 g. Organic liquids—alcohol, benzene, kerosene—do not differ significantly from water in density. Mercury is very heavy—it has a density of 13.6 g/cm³.

Gases occupy whatever volumes contain them. Even though emptied into vessels of different volumes, gas-bags with the same mass of gas will always fill the volumes uniformly.

The density of gases is defined under so-called normal conditions as temperature of 0°C and pressure of one atmosphere. The density of air under normal conditions is equal to 0.00129 g/cm³; chloride is 0.00322 g/cm³. Gaseous hydrogen, like the liquid, is the lightest gas with density of 0.00009 g/cm³.

Density represents the packing of material in a certain volume.

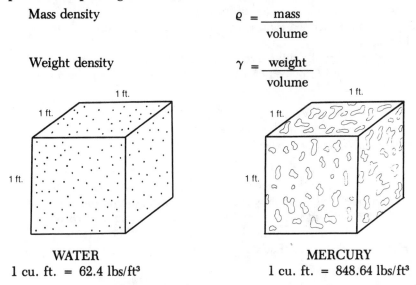

Mass density     $\varrho = \dfrac{\text{mass}}{\text{volume}}$

Weight density     $\gamma = \dfrac{\text{weight}}{\text{volume}}$

WATER
1 cu. ft. = 62.4 lbs/ft³

MERCURY
1 cu. ft. = 848.64 lbs/ft³

*Fig. 5.10—Illustration of the Concept of Density*

As an example, an average human being weighing 150 lbs. with 90% water is like a container of water about the same weight:
150 × 0.90 = 135 lbs. The weight density of water = 62.4 lbs./ft³.
Using, weight density = weight/volume:

$$62.4 = \frac{135}{\text{volume}}$$

This results in the average volume of the human body at 2.16 ft³. The above example shows the fundamental use of the density equation.

Generally, solids are more dense than liquids, which are more dense than gases. The *specific gravity* (SG) is defined as:

$$SG = \left(\frac{\text{density of a substance}}{\text{density of water}}\right) \text{ at a given temperature.}$$

The density of water is about 1 gm/ml over most common temperatures. So in most instances the specific gravity of a substance is the same as its density. Note that the units of density are mass/volume, whereas SG has no units.

Density is one of the key properties of fluids (liquids or gases) and the other is pressure. Pressure (P) is defined as force (F) per unit area (A):

$$P = F/A.$$

The F is the normal (perpendicular) force. Fluids can only exert P at an enclosed surface or body. Otherwise, fluids will flow under a shearing stress instead of being deformed elastically as solids would (see above). Pressure is also formulated as potential energy per unit volume as follows:

$$P = F/A = mg/A = (mg/A)(h/h) = mgh/V = \varrho gh$$

$$\varrho = \text{density} \qquad h = \text{depth below surface.}$$

Characteristics of force and pressure of fluids are:

(1) Forces exerted by fluids are always perpendicular to the container.
(2) The fluid pressure (hydrostatic) is directly proportional to the depth of the fluid and to its density:

$$P \propto \varrho h.$$

(3) At any particular depth, the fluid pressure is the same in all directions.
(4) Fluid pressure is independent of the shape or area of its container.
(5) An external pressure applied to an enclosed fluid is transmitted uniformly throughout the volume of the liquid (*Pascal's Law*).
(6) An object which is completely or partially submerged in a fluid experiences an upward force equal to the weight of the fluid displaced (Archimedes' Principle). This *buoyant force* ($F_B$) is:

$$F = V\varrho g = mg$$
$$\text{buoyant force} = \text{weight of displaced fluid.}$$

An object that floats must displace its own weight (not volume) in fluid.

Looking at Fig. 5.11 below, assume the body is totally immersed in the liquid. Now suppose the fluid inside the surface to be removed and replaced by a solid body having exactly the same shape. The pressure at every point will be exactly the same as before, so that the force exerted on the body by the surrounding fluid will be unaltered. That is, the fluid exerts on the body an upward force, $F_y$, which is equal to the weight, mg, of the fluid originally occupying the boundary surface and whose line of action passes through the original center of gravity.

The submerged body, in general, will not be in equilibrium. Its weight may be greater or less than $F_y$, and if it is not homogeneous, its center of gravity may not be on the line of $F_y$.

The weight of a dirigible floating in air, or of a submarine floating at some depth below the surface of the water, is just equal to the weight of a volume of air, or water, that is equal to the volume of the dirigible or submarine. That is, the average density of the dirigible equals that of the air, and the average density of the submarine equals the density of the water.

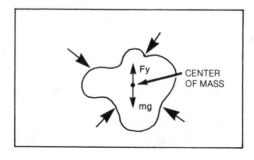

*Fig. 5.11—Buoyancy*

If $p_1$ and $p_2$ are the pressures at elevations $y_1$ and $y_2$ above some reference level and when p and g are constant,

$$p_2 - p_1 = -pg\,(y_2 - y_1).$$

Apply this equation to a liquid in an open vessel, as in Fig. 5.12 below. Take point 1 at any level and let p represent that pressure at this point. Take point 2 at the top where the pressure is atmospheric pressure, $p_a$. Then:

$$p_a - p = pg\,(y_2 - y_1),$$
$$p = p_a + pgh.$$

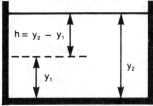

Fig. 5.12—*Hydrostatic Pressure*

Note that the shape of the containing vessel does not affect the pressure, and that the pressure is the same at all points at the same depth.

*Concept of Mass Flux*

Mass flux can be defined as the rate of change of mass of a fluid. It represents mass flow per unit time. It is an extremely important parameter to measure flow of blood from the heart, flow of substances into the kidneys, and also the flow of air into the lungs. Remember, mass flux is proportional to the rate of flow R mentioned below.

*Fluids in motion* are described by two equations, the continuity equation and Bernoulli's Equation. Fluids are assumed to have streamline flow which means that the motion of every particle in the fluid follows the same path as the particle that preceded it. Turbulent flow occurs when one path is not followed, molecules collide, energy is dissipated and frictional drag is increased. Rate of flow (R) is:

$$R = \text{volume past a point/time} = Avt/t = Av$$
$$\text{volume} = (\text{cross-sectional area})(\text{length}) = (A)(vt) = Avt$$
$$\text{length} = \text{distance} = (\text{velocity})(\text{time}) = vt$$

The equation can also be written as (the continuity equation):

$$A_1v_1 = A_2v_2 = \text{constant (see Fig. 5.13)}$$

where subscripts 1 and 2 refer to different points in the line of flow. Note that the velocity of the fluid is faster where the cross-sectional area is smaller and vice versa. Also, where the velocity is faster, the pressure (P) exerted is smaller and vice versa.

*Bernoulli's Equation* is an application of the Law of Conservation of Energy and is:

$$P + \varrho gh + \tfrac{1}{2}\varrho v^2 = \text{constant}$$
$$\text{pressure energy} + \text{potential energy} + \text{kinetic energy} = \text{constant}$$

This can be equivalently written as:

$$P_1 + \varrho gh_1 + \tfrac{1}{2}\varrho v_1^2 = P_2 + \varrho gh_2 + \tfrac{1}{2}\varrho v_2^2. \text{ (See Fig. 5.13)}$$

where the subscripts 1 and 2 refer to different points in the flow. All symbols are as defined previously.

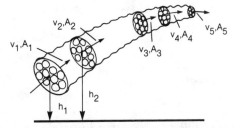

Fig. 5.13—*Concept of Mass Flux/Bernoulli's Equation*

Another important property of fluids is viscosity. Viscosity is analogous to friction between moving solids. It may, therefore, be viewed as the resistance to flow of layers of fluid (as in streamline or laminar flow) past each other. This also means that viscosity, as friction, results in dissipation of mechanical energy. As one layer flows over another, its motion is transmitted to the second layer and causes this layer to be set in motion. Since a mass (m) of the second layer is set in motion (v) and some of the energy of the first layer is lost, there is a transfer to momentum (mv) between the layers. The greater the transfer of this momentum from one layer to another, the more energy ($\alpha v^2$) that is lost and the slower the layers move. The viscosity coefficient ($\eta$) is a measure of the efficiency of transfer of this momentum. Therefore, the higher the viscosity coefficient, the greater the transfer of momentum and loss of mechanical energy and, thus loss of velocity. The reverse situation holds of low viscosity coefficients. Then a high viscosity (coefficient) substance flows slowly (e.g., molasses), and a low viscosity (coefficient) substance flows relatively fast (e.g., water or, especially, helium). Note that the transfer of momentum to adjacent layers is, in essence, the exertion of a force upon these layers to set them in motion (Newton's 1st Law—5.2.1). Whether flow is streamline (laminar) or turbulent (loss of layers flowing past each other and their replacement with eddies and whirlpool, etc., with the resultant dissipation of much mechanical energy) depends on a combination of factors already discussed. A convenient measure is Reynolds Number (R):

$$R = vd\varrho/\eta$$

v = velocity of flow; d = diameter of tube; $\varrho$ = density of fluid; $\eta$ = viscosity coefficient. In general, if R<2000 the flow is streamline; if R>2000 the flow is turbulent. Note that as v↑, d↑, $\varrho$↑ or $\eta$↓, the flow becomes more turbulent.

*Flow of Blood in Small Arterioles, Venuoles*

The Hagen-Poiseuille law for laminar viscous flow of blood through small size tubes can be calculated by:

$$\text{Flow rate} = Q = \frac{\pi R^2 p_d}{8\eta L} = v\pi R^2$$

Q = Flow rate = $m^3$/sec
R = Radius of flow tube or blood vessel (m)
$p_d$ = Pressure difference causing flow (m/sec²)
$\eta$ = Viscosity of blood ($\frac{nt \cdot s}{m^2}$)
L = Length of tube or blood vessel (m)
v = Average velocity of blood flow (m/s)

Use proportional reasoning to remember that flow rate is directly proportional to (Radius)², pressure difference is inversely proportional to (Radius)².

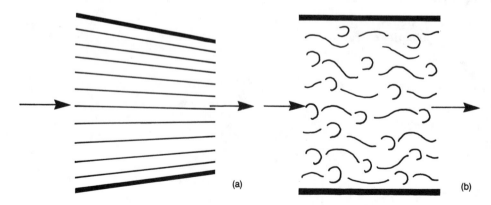

*Fig. 5.14—Illustrations of Laminar Flow (a) and Turbulent Flow (b)*

*Surface Tension*

Molecules of a liquid exert attractive forces toward each other (*cohesive forces*), and exert attractive forces toward surfaces they touch (*adhesive forces*). If a liquid is in a gravity-free space without a surface, it will form a sphere (smallest area relative to volume). If the liquid is lining an object, the liquid surface will contract (due to cohesive forces) to the lowest possible surface area. The forces between the molecules on this surface will create a membrane-like effect. Due to the contraction, a potential energy (PE) will be present in the surface. This PE is directly proportional to the surface area (A). An exact relation is formed as follows:

$$PE = \gamma A$$
$$\gamma = \text{surface tension} = PE/A = \text{joules}/m^2$$

An alternative formulation for surface tension ($\gamma$) is:

$$\gamma = F/l$$
$$F = \text{force of contraction (of surface)}$$
$$l = \text{length along surface.}$$

Because of the contraction, small objects which would ordinarily sink in the liquid may "float" on the surface membrane.

The liquid will rise or fall on a wall or in a capillary tube if the adhesive forces are greater than cohesive or cohesive are greater than adhesive forces, respectively:

cohesive > adhesive          adhesive > cohesive

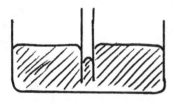    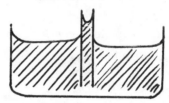

The distance the liquid rises or falls in the tube is directly proportional to the $\gamma$ and inversely proportional to the liquid density and radius of the tube.

### 5.6.2    Questions to Review Solids and Fluids

(1)    Stress, as used in physics, is defined as:

(a) the maximum weight an object can support
(b) the force per unit length
(c) the ratio of the force to the area over which it acts
(d) the relative change in dimensions of an object caused by a force

(2)    When an object is deformed by forces acting on an object along the same line of action but in the opposite directions, the stress resulting is called:

(a) tensile stress
(b) traction stress
(c) compressive stress
(d) shearing stress

(3)    If D = density, m = mass and V = volume occupied by that mass, then density is:

(a) $D = (m)(V)$
(b) $D = 1/(m)(V)$
(c) $D = m/V$
(d) $D = V/m$

(4)    Pressure is defined as:

(a) force per unit volume
(b) force per unit area
(c) mass per unit volume
(d) work times volume

(5)    Pressure may be formulated as:

(a) force per unit volume
(b) work times volume
(c) potential energy per unit volume
(d) weight per unit volume

(6)    All are characteristics of forces and pressures exerted by fluids except:

(a) forces are always perpendicular to the container walls
(b) pressure is directly proportional to the product of depth and fluid density
(c) pressure depends on the shape and size of the container
(d) buoyant force of submerged object equals the weight of the displaced fluid

(7)    Pascal's Law (of fluids):

(a) an external pressure applied to an enclosed fluid is transmitted uniformly through
    the volume of the fluid
(b) at any depth, the fluid pressure is the same in all directions
(c) fluid pressure is dependent on the shape or area of its container
(d) an object completely or partly submerged in a fluid experiences an upward force
    equal to the weight of the fluid displaced

(8)    Bernoulli's Equation is an application of:

(a) the 2nd Law of Thermodynamics
(b) the Law of Conservation of Momentum
(c) the Law of Conservation of Mass
(d) the Law of Conservation of Energy

(9)    All are true of viscosity except:

(a) it is analogous to friction
(b) there is no dissipation of mechanical energy
(c) there is transfer of momentum between adjacent layers
(d) as viscosity increases, rate of flow decreases

(10)   A certain metal has a mass (m) = 36 gm and occupies a volume (V) = 4 mls. The
       density (d) of it is:

(a) 144 gm-mls
(b) 9 gms/ml
(c) ⅑ mls/gm
(d) $\frac{1}{444}$ gms$^{-1}$ mls$^{-1}$

(11)   A substance has a density (d) of 7 gms/ml. If 42 gms are required, what volume (V) of
       the substance is this?

(a) ⅙ mls
(b) 6 mls
(c) 294 mls
(d) need more information

(12)   A fluid has a density (d) of 5 gms/ml and fills a container up to a height (h) of 10 cm's.
       The pressure (P) on the floor of the container is:

(a) 49,000 dynes/cm$^2$
(b) 50 nts/m$^2$
(c) 50 V dynes/cm$^2$ where V = volume in ml/s
(d) need more information

(13)    If an object is moved from 4 meters to 8 meters beneath the surface of a large tank of water, the pressure on it will:

(a) remain the same
(b) quadruple
(c) halve
(d) double

(14)    At a depth of 10 meters in a large container of water, 3 sheets of glass are placed parallel to the surface. Sheet A is 3m × 5m, sheet B is 4 × 4 and sheet C is 2 × 9. Which sheet has the greatest fluid pressure on its surface?

(a) A
(b) B
(c) C
(d) all are equal

(15)    The buoyant force ($F_B$) on an object that has a mass of 10 gms, a volume of 10 mls and displaces 2 mls of a liquid with a density of 5 gms/ml is:

(a) 10 dynes
(b) 9800 dynes
(c) 1000 dynes
(d) 40 dynes

(16)    In order for an object to float in a fluid, it must

(a) be made of a substance more dense than the fluid
(b) be made of a substance less dense than the fluid
(c) displace its own weight in the fluid
(d) displace its own volume in the fluid

(17)    The key feature of an object that sinks when placed in a fluid is that

(a) it displaced its weight in the fluid
(b) it displaced less than its weight in the volume it displaced
(c) it displaced its weight before it displaced its volume
(d) both (a) and (b)

(18)    A pipe has a section A of diameter = 10 meters and a section B of 5 meters. A given quantity of fluid flowing through it would

(a) move at the same speed at A and B
(b) move faster at A
(c) move faster at B
(d) would need volume of fluid to evaluate

(19)    Fluid is flowing as shown in the pipe below. At what point is the pressure exerted by the fluid the highest (pipe is filled with fluid at all points)?

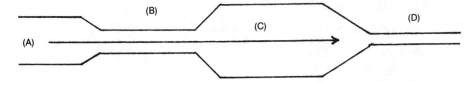

(a) A
(b) B
(c) C
(d) D

(20) At which point is the pressure exerted by the fluid the *least* in the constant diameter pipe below?

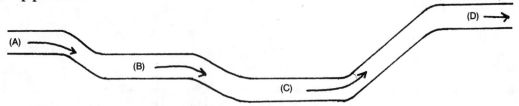

(a) A
(b) B
(c) C
(d) D

(21) The relative diameters of the blood vessels of the body and the relative flows are:

arteries > arterioles > capillaries.

In which of the above is turbulent flow most likely?

(a) artery
(b) arteriole
(c) capillary
(d) all equal

## 5.6.3    Answers to Questions in Section 5.6.2

( 1) c  ( 2) a  ( 3) c  ( 4) b  ( 5) c  ( 6) c  ( 7) a  ( 8) d  ( 9) b  (10) b  (11) b
(12) a  (13) d  (14) d  (15) b  (16) c  (17) b  (18) c  (19) c  (20) d  (21) a

## 5.6.4    Discussion of Answers to Questions in Section 5.6.2

*Questions #1 to #9:* Adequately discussed in the text.

*Question #10* (Answer: b)

$$d = m/V = 36 \text{ gms}/4 \text{ mls} = 9 \text{ gms/ml}$$

*Question #11* (Answer: b)

$$d = m/V$$
$$V = m/d = 42 \text{ gms}/7 \text{ gms per ml} = 6 \text{ mls}$$

*Question #12* (Answer: a)

$$F = F/A = \varrho gh$$
$$P = (5 \text{ gms/cm}^3)[(980)(\text{cms/sec}^2)](10 \text{ cms}) = 49{,}000 \text{ (gm-cm/sec}^2)/\text{cm}^2$$
$$P = 49{,}000 \text{ dynes/cm}^2$$
$$\text{dyne} = (\text{gm} - \text{cm})/\text{sec}^2.$$

*Question #13* (Answer: d) The pressure (P) exerted by the fluid is:

$$P = \varrho gh \text{ or } P \propto h$$
$$h = \text{depth under surface.}$$

So, P is directly proportional to h and if h doubles (8/4 = 2) Then P doubles. *OR*

$$P_1 = \varrho gh_1 = \text{original depth}$$
$$P_2 = \varrho gh_2 = \text{final depth}$$
$$P_2/P_1 = \varrho gh_2/\varrho gh_1 = h_2/h_1 = 8m/4m = 2$$
$$P_2 = 2P_1.$$

*Question #14* (Answer: d) Fluid pressure (P) is independent of the area or shape of its container or objects. The $P \propto \varrho h$ where $\varrho$ = density and h = depth. So at any particular depth the pressure is equal in all directions.

*Question #15* (Answer: b) From Archimedes' Principle:

$$F = V\varrho g$$

V = volume displaced = 2 mls
$\varrho$ = density of fluid = 5 gms/ml
g = 980 cms/sec$^2$

$$F = (2)(5)(980) = 9800 \text{ dynes.}$$

*Question #16* (Answer: c) If (b) were true, large ships would never float by virtue of their shape which makes the density of the whole object (not the steel material) less than that of water.

*Question #17* (Answer: b) According to Archimedes' Principle an object must displace its weight to float. The maximum volume of fluid that an object can displace is its (the object's) own volume. If a weight of fluid displaced in that maximum volume is not greater than the weight of the object, then it will sink.

*Question #18* (Answer: c) The continuity equation is:

$$A_1 v_1 = A_2 v_2.$$

Note that the larger the cross section, the smaller the fluid velocity and vice versa.

*Question #19* (Answer: c) The velocity (v) is slowest where the cross-sectional area (A) is greatest from the continuity equation ($A_1 v_1 = A_2 v_2$). At faster velocities, the pressure is lower, and at slower velocities the pressure (P) is higher from Bernoulli's Equation:

$$P + \varrho g h + \tfrac{1}{2}\varrho v^2 = \text{constant}$$

$\varrho g h$ does not change if h = constant
then $\tfrac{1}{2}\varrho v^2$ increases as v increases, and P must decrease because the whole expression is constant.

As the fluid moves faster, pressure energy (P) is converted to kinetic energy ($\tfrac{1}{2}\varrho v^2$) and the pressure drops.

*Question #20* (Answer: d) Since the diameter is constant, the velocity of fluid flow is constant by the continuity equation ($A_1 v_1 = a_2 v_2$). From Bernoulli's Equation:

$$P + \varrho g h + \tfrac{1}{2}\varrho v^2 = \text{constant}$$

$\tfrac{1}{2}\varrho v^2$ does not change
$\varrho$ = density     v = velocity

$\varrho g h$ changes because h (height above some arbitrary reference point) is changing, the larger h means the larger this term; the larger $\varrho g h$ means the smaller the P term becomes; then, the higher the pipe (due to h), the smaller the pressure (P).

*Question #21* (Answer: a) Turbulence is best estimated using Reynolds number (R) or by remembering the relations from R. The viscosity and density of the fluid (i.e., the blood) is constant. Since diameter (d) and velocity (v) are greatest in the arteries and

$$\text{turbulence} \propto (v)(d)$$

they have the highest turbulence. The velocity is greater in the arteries because the total cross-sectional area of the arteries is less than the total cross-sectional area of the capillaries.

### 5.6.5　Vocabulary, Concepts, etc. Checklist for Solids and Fluids

_____ density
_____ elastic properties
_____ specific gravity
_____ buoyancy
_____ hydrostatic pressure

_____ Pascal's Law
_____ viscosity
_____ Bernoulli's Equation
_____ tensile forces
_____ compressive forces

## 5.7　ELECTROSTATICS

### 5.7.1　Review of Electrostatics

The elementary charges are called positive $(+)$ or negative $(-)$. Each has a charge of $1.6 \times 10^{-19}$ coulombs but differ in sign. The electron is the negative charge carrier, and the proton is the positive charge carrier. Substances with an excess of electrons have a net negative charge. Substances with a deficiency of electrons have a net positive charge. One way of charging substances is by rubbing them (i.e., by contact). For example, glass rubbed on fur becomes positive and rubber rubbed on fur becomes negative. Objects can also be charged by induction which occurs when one charged object brought near another causes a charge redistribution in the latter to give net charge regions. *Conductors* transmit charge readily. *Insulators* resist the flow of charge.

Charges exert *forces* upon each other. Like charges repel each other and unlike charges attract. For two charges the force is given by *Coulomb's Law:*

$$F = k(q_1 q_2 / r^2) = (\tfrac{1}{4} \pi E_O)(q_1 q_2 / r^2)$$

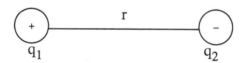

*Fig. 5.15—Illustration of Coulomb's Law*

$q$ = charges　　$k$ = constant = $9.0 \times 10^9$ nt-m²/coul²
$E_O$ = permittivity of air to the forces = $8.85 \times 10^{-12}$ coul²/nt-m²
$r$ = distance between the charges.

A charge generates an *electric field (E)* in the space around it. Fields (force fields) are vectors (have direction and magnitude). A field is generated by an object and is that region of space around an object that will exert a force on a second object when it is brought into the field. The field exists independently of the second object and is not altered by its presence. The force exerted on the second object depends upon that object and the field. The electric field $(E)$ is:

$$E = F/q = kQ/r^2 \qquad (\text{i.e., } F = kQq/r^2)$$

E and F are vectors
$Q$ = charge generating the field
$q$ = charge place in it.

Charges exert forces upon each other through fields. The direction of a field is the direction a positive charge would move if placed in it. *Electric field lines* are imaginary lines which are in the same direction as E at that point. The direction is away from positive charges and toward negative charges.

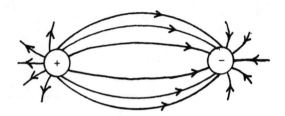

*Fig. 5.16—Electric Field Lines*

The *potential energy (PE)* of a charged object in a field would equal the work done on that object to bring it from infinity to a distance (r) from the charge setting up the electric field or,

$$PE = work = Fr = (qE)r = kQq/r$$
$$Q = \text{charge setting up field}$$
$$q = \text{charge brought in to a distance r.}$$

When a $+q$ moves against E, its PE increases. When a $-q$ moves against E, its PE decreases. Realize that if you brought two positive charges together, work would have to be done to the system (and PE would increase), and vice versa for a $+q$ and a $-q$.

The *electric potential (V)* is a scalar, and it is defined at each distance (r) from a charge (Q) generating an electric field. It represents the negative of the work per unit charge in bringing a $+q$ from infinity to r:

$$V = PE/q = kQ/r = \text{volts} = \text{joules/coulomb}$$
$$V = Ed \text{ for a parallel plate capacitor (Section 5.8.1).}$$

Lines (and surfaces) of equal V are perpendicular to electric field lines. Work can only be done when moving between surfaces of Vs and is, therefore, independent of the path taken. No work is done when a charge (q) is moved along an equal potential (equipotential) surface (or line), because the component of force is zero along it. Potential (V) is defined in terms of positive charges such that V is positive when due to a $+Q$ and negative when due to a $-Q$. Potential (V) is added algebraically at a point (because it is a scalar).

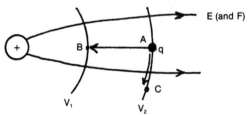

*Fig. 5.17—Electrical Potential*

(1) $V_1$, $V_2$ are two potential surfaces perpendicular to E and F;
    the values of $V_1$ or $V_2$ cannot be measured, only the
    difference between them can be measured.
(2) $V_2 - V_1$ (or $V_1 - V_2$) is the potential difference (PD, see below);
(3) charge (q) moved from A to B has work (W) done on it
    $$W = q (V_1 - V_2) = q (PD) \text{ see below;}$$
(4) charge (q) moved from A to C has no work done because this is along an
    equipotential surface and the component of force (F) is perpendicular to it;
(5) the lines of F are along the lines of E.

The *potential difference (PD)* is the difference in V between two points, or it is the work per unit positive charge done by electric forces moving a small test charge from the point of higher potential to the point of lower potential (Fig. 5.18):

$$PD = V_A - V_B = \text{volts} = \text{work/charge or joules/coulomb}$$
$$Work = q (V_A - V_B) = q (PD).$$

An *electric dipole* consists of two charges separated by some finite distance (d). Usually the charges are equal and opposite. The laws of forces, fields etc., above, apply to dipoles. A dipole is characterized by its *dipole moment (D.M.)* which is the product of the charge (q) and d. Dipoles tend to line up with the electric field. Motion of dipoles against an electric field requires energy as discussed above.

Dipole with equal and opposite charges        Alignment of dipole with E

E = electric field
F = forces exerted by E on the dipole

$$\text{dipole moment} = \text{(distance)(charge)} = qd.$$

**Fig. 5.18—Dipoles**

### 5.7.2  Questions to Review Electrostatics

(1)  Concerning fields, which is *incorrect*?

(a) They exist in space and are generated by objects (e.g., mass).
(b) Gravitational and electrical fields are examples.
(c) They are scalars.
(d) They exist independently of other objects.

(2)  Coulomb's Law of electrical forces (q = charge, r = distance between charges, k = constant, F = force) is:

(a) $F = k(q_1q_2/r^2)$
(b) $F = k(q/r^2)$
(c) $F = k(q_1q_2/r)$
(d) $F = k(q_2/r)$

(3)  If $F = \text{force} = kq_1q_0/r^2$ and $q_0 = $ an electric charge, then $F/q_0$ is:

(a) the electric field generated by $q_1$
(b) the force acting on $q_0$
(c) the electric potential set up by $q_0$
(d) the work done by the force on $q_1$

(4)  Electric field lines are:

(a) directed away from negative charges
(b) directed away from positive charges
(c) directed toward positive charges
(d) any of the above may be correct

(5)  The electric potential:

(a) represents the negative of the work per unit charge in bringing a positive charge from infinity to a distance (r) from an object generating an electric field
(b) is a vector
(c) has the units of henries
(d) all of the above

(6)    Formulations for electric potential (V) include all except: (q = charge, r = distance, E = electric field, F = force)

(a) $V = (\frac{1}{4}\pi E_O)(q/r)$
(b) $V$ = potential energy/charge
(c) $V = Er$
(d) $V = Fq$

(7)    A volt is a:

(a) newton/coulomb
(b) joule/coulomb
(c) coulomb/newton
(d) coulomb/joule

(8)    Electrical work is:

(a) dependent on the path taken by a charge between equipotential surfaces
(b) zero when a charge is moved along an equipotential (electric potential) line
(c) zero when a charge moves between surfaces of different electric potential
(d) both (a) and (c)

(9)    The potential difference as used in electricity is

(a) the difference in potential energy between two points
(b) the difference in electric potential between two points
(c) the difference in work between two points
(d) both (a) and (c)

(10)   Which of the following is a correct formulation of electrical work (W) done on moving a charge (q) in an electric field (E)? (V = electric potential, PD = potential difference, F = electrical force, r = distance between charges)

(a) $W = q(PD)$
(b) $W = Fq$
(c) $W = Vr$
(d) $W = Eq$

(11)   All are true about electric dipoles except:

(a) they consist of two charges separated by finite distance
(b) the dipole moment is a product of the charge and the distance between them
(c) the motion of dipoles against an electric field requires no energy
(d) the positive end of the dipole points in the direction of the electric field

(12)   If the distance between two electrical charges is doubled, the force between them is:

(a) decreased by $\frac{1}{4}$
(b) decreased by $\frac{1}{2}$
(c) doubled
(d) quadrupled

(13)   The charge (q) on each of two objects is doubled and they are moved twice as far apart (r); the force between them is:

(a) increased by a factor of 8
(b) increased by a factor of 4
(c) increased by a factor of 2
(d) unchanged

(14)   As two electrical charges move further apart, the force between them:

(a) increases proportionally to the inverse square of their separation
(b) increases proportionally to their separation
(c) decreases proportionally to the inverse square of their separation
(d) decreases proportionally to their separation

(15) If charge #1 ($q_1$) is doubled in size and charge #2 ($Q_2$) is tripled in size and the distance (r) between them is not changed, the force (F) between them is:

(a) decreased by a factor of 36
(b) increased by a factor of 36
(c) increased by a factor of 6
(d) unchanged

(16) What is the force between charge #1 ($q_1$) and charge #2 ($q_2$) in the diagram below?

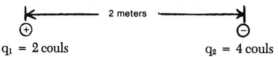

$q_1 = 2$ couls               $q_2 = 4$ couls

(a) repulsive, 2 nts
(b) attractive, 2 nts
(c) repulsive, 2k nts
(d) attractive, 2k nts

(17) The net force on charge C ($q_C$) is:

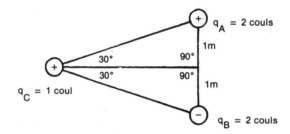

(a) zero
(b) horizontally and to the right, ½k nts
(c) horizontally and to the left, ½k nts
(d) vertical and down, ½k nts

(18) The electric field (E) generated by a charge

(a) is constant at all distances from the charge
(b) decreases directly as distance from the charge increases
(c) decreases proportional to the inverse square of the distance from the charge
(d) decreases proportional to the inverse distance from the charge

(19) All of the following are correct formulations for the potential energy (PE) of a charged object (q) in an electric field except:
(F = force on charge, V = electric potential, E = electric field, r = distance of charge from object setting up the electric field)

(a) PE = Vq
(b) PE = Fr
(c) PE = Eq
(d) PE = qEr

(20) A positive charge is moved against (in the opposite direction of) an electric field. The potential energy of this object:

(a) remains the same
(b) decreases
(c) increases
(d) cannot be evaluated

(21) A negative charge is moved against (in the opposite direction of) an electric field. The potential energy of this negative charge:

(a) stays the same
(b) increases
(c) decreases
(d) cannot be evaluated from the information given

(22) What is the electrical potential (V) at point A?

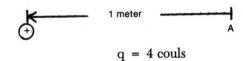

$$q = 4 \text{ couls}$$

(a) $+4$ volts
(b) $-4$ volts
(c) $+4k$ volts
(d) $-4k$ volts

(23) Determine the electric potential at point A.

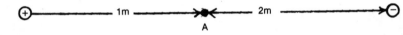

$q_1 = +4$ couls                              $q_2 = -16$ couls

(a) $-28$ volts
(b) $+28$ volts
(c) $+4k$ volts
(d) $-4k$ volts

(24) What is the work done in moving a charge $q_1$ from A to B?

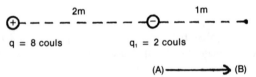

(a) $-10\pi$ joules
(b) $+10\pi$ joules
(c) $+(8/3)k$ joules
(d) $-(8k/3)$ joules

### 5.7.3 Answers to Questions in Section 5.7.2

( 1) c  ( 2) a  ( 3) a  ( 4) b  ( 5) a  ( 6) d  ( 7) b  ( 8) b  ( 9) b  (10) a  (11) c
(12) a  (13) d  (14) c  (15) c  (16) d  (17) d  (18) c  (19) c  (20) c  (21) c  (22) c
(23) d  (24) c

### 5.7.4 Discussion of Answers to Questions in Section 5.7.2

*Questions #1 to #11* Adequately discussed in the Section.

*Question #12* (Answer: a) From Coulomb's Law:

$$\frac{F_f}{F_o} = \frac{k\dfrac{q_1 q_2}{r_f^2}}{k\dfrac{q_1 q_2}{r_o^2}} = \frac{\dfrac{1}{r_f^2}}{\dfrac{1}{r_o^2}} = \frac{\dfrac{1}{r_f^2}}{\dfrac{r_o^2}{1}} = \frac{r_o^2}{r_f^2} = \frac{r_o^2}{(2r_o)^2} = \frac{r_o^2}{4r_o^2} = \frac{1}{4}$$

$$(r_f = 2r_o)$$

$$\frac{F_f}{F_o} = \frac{1}{4}$$

$$F_f = \tfrac{1}{4}F_o \qquad f = \text{final} \qquad o = \text{original}$$

Or reason from Coulomb's Law that force is proportional to the inverse square of distance $(1/r^2)$; this is $(\tfrac{1}{2})^2 = \tfrac{1}{4}$ for this case.

*Question #13* (Answer: d) From Coulomb's Law:

$$f = \text{final} \qquad\qquad o = \text{original}$$

$$q_{1f} = 2q_{10} \qquad q_{2f} = 2q_{20} \qquad r_f = 2r_o$$

$$\frac{F_f}{F_o} = \frac{k\dfrac{q_{1f}q_{2f}}{r_f^2}}{k\dfrac{q_{10}q_{20}}{r_o^2}} = \frac{q_{1f}q_{2f}}{r_f^2}\cdot\frac{r_o^2}{q_{10}q_{20}} = \frac{2q_{10}2q_{20}}{(2r_o)^2}\cdot\frac{r_o^2}{q_{10}q_{20}} = \frac{2\cdot2\cdot q_{10}\cdot q_{20}\cdot r_o^2}{4\cdot r_o^2\cdot q_{10}\cdot q_{20}} = \frac{4}{4} = 1$$

$$\frac{F_f}{F_o} = 1$$

$$F_f = F_o$$

Or, by reasoning from Coulomb's Law that since force is directly proportional to the product of the charges, the doubling of each charge would increase the force by a factor of $(2)(2) = 4$. Since force is proportional to the inverse square of the separation, the increase in separation decreases the force by $(\tfrac{1}{2})^2 = \tfrac{1}{4}$. Multiplying these factors together to get the net change as $(4)(\tfrac{1}{4}) = 1$ or no change.

*Question #14* (Answer: c) From Coulomb's Law:

$$F \propto 1/r^2$$

*Question #15* (Answer: c) From Coulomb's Law:

$$f = \text{final} \qquad\qquad o = \text{original}$$

$$q_{1f} = 2q_{10} \qquad\qquad q_{2f} = 3q_{20}$$

$$\frac{F_f}{F_f} = \frac{k\dfrac{q_{1f}q_{2f}}{r^2}}{k\dfrac{q_{10}q_{20}}{r^2}} = \frac{q_{1f}q_{2f}}{q_{10}q_{20}} = \frac{(2q_{10})(3q_{20})}{(q_{10})(q_{20})} = \frac{2\cdot3}{1} = 6$$

$$F_f = 6F_o$$

Or, by reasoning from Coulomb's Law that since force is directly proportional to the product of the charges, since this product is increased $(2)(3) = 6$ times so the force must be also.

*Question #16* (Answer: d) From Coulomb's Law:

$$F = k(q_1 q_2/r^2) = k(+2)(-4)/(2)^2 = -2\,k \text{ nts}$$

Since the sign is negative, the force is attractive.

*Question #17* (Answer: d) This problem may be solved by the symmetry of the system, Coulomb's Law and geometry. The forces (vectors) and their components exerted by $q_A(F_A)$ and $q_B$ ($F_B$) on qc are:

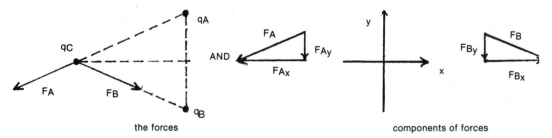

the forces                                            components of forces

The x-components ($F_{A_x}$ and $F_{B_x}$) cancel (because they are equal and opposite by the symmetry of the system) and the y-components sum to a vertically downward force. So, by elimination the answer is (d). OR, first by applying Coulomb's Law:

$$F_A = k(q_A q_C/r^2) = k[(+2)(+1)/(2)^2] = k/2$$
$$F_B = k(q_B q_C/r^2) = k[(-2)(+1)/(2)^2] = -k/2$$
the r = 2 m (meters) is derived by:

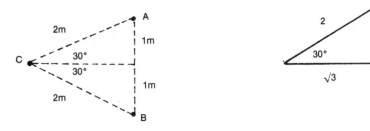

the side opposite the 30° angle is ½ the hypotenuse (which must then be 2 m)

The x-components still cancel and the y-components are:

$$F_{Ay} = +(½)F_A = -½(k/2) = -k/4$$
$$F_{By} = (½)F_B = ½(-k/2) = -k/4$$
$$F_y = F_{Ay} + F_{By} = -k/4 - k/4 = -k/2 \text{ nts}$$
the minus sign means the $F_y$ is directed down the y-axis.

*Question #18* (Answer: c) The formula for the electric field (E) is:

$$E = F/q_0 = kq/r^2; \text{ hence, } E \propto 1/r^2.$$

*Question #19* (Answer: c) Eq = force generated by E on q.

*Question #20* (Answer: c) The directions of the lines of an electric field is the direction a positive charge would move if placed in it. To move a positive charge in the opposite direction requires energy, and this energy is stored as the potential energy which increases. The potential energy of the system may be used to move any charge along the direction of the field lines.

*Question #21* (Answer: c) The direction of the field lines of an electric field is the direction a positive charge would move if placed in it. So, a negative charge would normally move in the opposite direction or against the field. When a charge moves in the expected direction in an electric field, the potential energy of the charge system decreases. This is like the potential energy of a rock decreasing as it fell toward the earth, because this is its expected direction to move in the gravitational field.

*Question #22* (Answer: c) The formula for V is:

$$V = kq/r = k(+4/1) = +4k \text{ volts.}$$

*Question #23* (Answer: d) Since the electric potential (V) is a scalar, the V contribution by each charge is determined separately and added algebraically to get the net potential at point A:

$$\text{For } q_1: V_1 = k(q_1/r_1) = k(+4/1) = +4k \text{ volts}$$
$$\text{For } q_2: V_2 = k(q_2/r_2) = k(-16/2) = -8k \text{ volts}$$
$$\text{Total: } V_A = V_1 + V_2 = +4k - 8k = -4k \text{ volts}.$$

*Question #24* (Answer: c) The work done in this instance can be calculated by using the following formulations:

$$W = q_1 (V_B - V_A) = q_1 (PD)$$
$$V_B = k(q/r_A) = k(+8/3) = (+8/3) k \text{ volts}$$
$$V_A = k(q/r_A) = k(+8/2) = +4 k \text{ volts}$$

for both the q is generating the potential

PD (Potential difference) $= V_B - V_A = (8/3)k - 4k = (8-12/3)k = -4k/3 \text{ volts}$

$$W = q_1 (PD) = (-2)(-4k/3) = (+8/3) k \text{ joules}.$$

The positive sign means that work must be put into (done to) the system.

## 5.7.5    Vocabulary, Concepts, etc. Checklist for Electrostatics

_____ charges

_____ conductors

_____ insulators

_____ Coulomb's Law

_____ electrical forces

_____ electric field

_____ volts

_____ dipole moment

_____ potentials

_____ potential differences

_____ electrical dipoles

## 5.8    DC CIRCUITS

### 5.8.1    Review of DC Circuits

*DC (direct current)* electricity is generated to AC (Section 5.9.1) with one important exception. The AC electricity is converted to DC by substituting a split ring commutator for the slip rings. This causes the connections to the brush to reverse twice per revolution to coincide with the current change in the armature. The current that is carried away is all in one direction.

The main elements in a DC circuit are the emf source (V) and the resistors (R). The current (I) results from their interaction. These three quantities are interrelated in *Ohm's* Law as:

$$V = IR.$$

V, I, R are the total of each in the circuit. Capacitors may also be used in DC circuits.

Circuit elements may be in series, in parallel, or in combinations of both. Two components are in *series* when they have only one point in common; that is, the current traveling from one of them back to the emf source *must* pass through the other. In a complete series circuit, or for individual series loops of a larger mixed circuit, the current (I) is the same over each component and the total voltage ($V_t$ is the sum of all the emf sources) is the sum of voltages across each resistor (including the internal resistances of emf sources--see below). Two components are in *parallel* when they are connected to two common points in the circuit; that is, the current traveling from one such element back to the source of emf (assume current started at source of emf) need not pass through the second component because there is an alternate path. In a parallel circuit, the total current is the sum of currents for each path (i.e., each path has a different current), and the voltage is equal for all paths and thus equals $V_t$. Circuits can be simplified into subunits that are either series or parallel, and the above rules are applied to them.

*Electromotive force* (V) maintains a constant potential difference and thereby maintains a continuous current. The emf source replaces energy lost by the moving electrons. Sources of emf are batteries (conversions of chemical energy to electrical energy) and generators (conversion of mechanical energy to electrical energy). A source of emf is symbolized in a circuit as in Fig. 5.19.

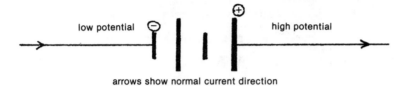

arrows show normal current direction

*Fig. 5.19—Electromotive Force*

The source of emf does work on each charge to raise it from a lower potential to a higher potential. Then as the charge flows around the circuit (naturally from higher to lower potential) it loses energy which is replaced by the emf source again, etc. Therefore work (energy) must be supplied at the rate energy is lost by the current flowing through the circuit,

energy supplied = energy lost.

Energy is lost whenever a charge (as current) passes through a resistor.

The *units of emf (E)* are volts (Section 5.7.1). The actual voltage delivered to a circuit is not equal to the V value of the source.

This is reduced by an Ir which represents the voltage loss by the *internal resistance (r)* of the source itself. The net voltage is called the terminal voltage ($V_t$) and is:

$V_t = V - Ir = IR_t$
$IR_t$ = totals for the whole circuit
$V$ = maximal voltage output of emf source.

The $V_t$ is the voltage delivered to the circuit by that emf source.

Normally, a charge gains energy as it flows through a source of emf. But when two sources of emf are connected in opposition (positive pole to positive pole), the charge flows from the higher emf source to the lower emf source. In this instance, it loses energy when passing through the smaller emf because it passes in the opposite direction to normal. If there is more than one source of emf in a circuit, the *total emf* is a sum of these by taking into account the differences in polarity (i.e., reversed emf's are negative):

$V_t$ (total) = $\Sigma V_{ti}$, i = 1, 2, . . . .

A voltmeter is used to measure voltages (potential differences) in circuits and is *symbolized* as:

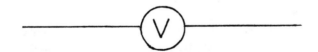

*Resistance* (R) is the opposition to the flow of electrons in a substance. *Resistivity* ($\varrho$) is an inherent property of a substance and is directly related to resistance. Resistivity varies directly as resistance and cross-sectional area, and indirectly as length.

Resistance has a fixed value for a given material and depends on the size, shape and temperature but not on the emf or current. Note these relations ($R \propto 1/A$):

R increases as 1 increases
R increases as A decreases
R increases as temperature increases.

Resistance increases with temperature because the thermal motion of atoms (molecules) increases and results in more collisions with electrons which impede their flow. The units of resistance are ohms symbolized by $\Omega$ (omega). From Ohm's Law, an ohm = volt/ampere.

When a $+I$ (current) flows across a resistor, there is a voltage decrease and an energy loss:

$$\text{energy loss} = Vq = VIt = \text{joules}$$
$$\text{power loss (P)} = VIt/t = VI = \text{watts} = \text{volt-amperes} = \text{joules/sec.}$$

The energy loss may be used to perform work. These relations hold for power (P),

$$P = VI = (IR)(I) = I^2R = V(V/R) = V^2/R.$$

Resistance in a circuit is *symbolized* by,

A variable resistance (as with a rheostat) is symbolized by:

*Resistance in a series* circuit is:

$$R = R_1 + R_2 + R_3 + \ldots$$

*Resistance in a parallel* circuit is,

$$1/R = 1/R_1 + 1/R_2 + 1/R_3 + \ldots \text{The R's are the total resistances.}$$

*Current* (I) is the amount of charge (Q) that flows past a point in a given amount of time (t),

$$I = Q/t = \text{amperes} = \text{coulombs/sec.}$$

Current is caused by the movement of electrons. The velocity (not current) of electrons is slowed by impurities in the conductor and by the thermal motion of atoms. A transient current is set up when a capacitor discharges (below). A continuous current is set up when a source of emf is present to replace the energy lost by moving electrons (see above). The direction of current is taken as the direction a positive charge moves, by convention. It is represented on a circuit diagram by arrows. Ammeters are used to measure the flow of current and are symbolized as:

*Capacitance* (C) is an inherent property of a conductor and is formulated as:

$$C = \text{charge/electric potential} = Q/V = \text{farad} = \text{coulomb/volt.}$$

This means that C is the number of coulombs that must be transferred to a conductor to raise its potential by one volt. The amount of charge that can be stored is determined by the size, shape and surroundings of the conductor. A smaller conductor usually has a smaller capacitance. A greater degree of curvature (or more pointed) usually means a greater capacity to store charge. The higher the dielectric strength (i.e., the electric field strength at which a substance ceases to be an insulator and becomes a conductor) of the medium, the greater the capacitance of the conductor.

A *capacitor* is two or more conductors with opposite but equal charges placed near each other. A common example is the parallel plate capacitor. The formulas of importance for capacitors are:

(1) $C = Q/V$

      V = potential difference between the plates

(2) $V = Ed$

    $E$ = electric field strength

    $d$ = distance between the plates

(3) C is directly proportional to the area of the plates

    C is inversely proportional to the distance between the plates;

        i.e.: $C_0 = E_0\, A/d$ for air and vacuum (as the medium) between the plates.

(4) $K = C/C_0 = $ *dielectric constant*

    $K = V_0/V = E_0/E$ also

    $C = KC_0$.

The *dielectric substances* set up an opposing electric field to that of the capacitor which decreases the net electric field and allows the capacitance of the capacitor to increase ($C = Q/Ed$). The molecules of the dielectric are dipoles which line up in the electric field.

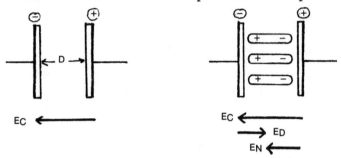

Fig. 5.20—*Capacitor without Dielectric*    Fig. 5.21—*Capacitor with Dielectric*

    $E$ = electric field

    $D$ = dielectric

    $C$ = capacitor

    $N$ = net

The C's are the total capacitances. (See also 5.9.1)

The *energy associated with each charged capacitor* is:

$$V_{avg} = \tfrac{1}{2}V$$
$$\text{Potential Energy (PE)} = W = (\tfrac{1}{2}V)(Q) = \tfrac{1}{2}QV = \tfrac{1}{2}(CV)(V) = \tfrac{1}{2}CV^2$$
$$= \tfrac{1}{2}\,Q(Q/C) = \tfrac{1}{2}Q^2/C.$$

The *symbol for a capacitor* is:

In a *DC circuit, the capacitor* charges up until the charge ($Q_{max}$) equals $V_t\, C$ and then the current stops. If the $V_t$ is then removed, the capacitor will discharge. In an *AC circuit*, there is an alternating surge of charge onto and off the capacitor, and a current exists there even though there is no transfer of charge between the plates. The behavior of a capacitor in a circuit is derived from calculus. Some of the key results are as follows:

(1) When a C is combined in series with an R:

    $V_t = IR + Q/C$

(2) $RC$ = time constant    $\tau$ = (ohms)(farads) = seconds

    (a) The capacitor takes about $5\tau$ to become fully charged ($Q_{max} = CV_t$).

    (b) In one $\tau$, the capacitor is 63% charged and has 37% of its final current ($V_t/R$) delivered to it (these numbers arise from the solution and the base of the natural logs which is e = 2.7183, $\therefore$ $1/e = 0.37$, $1 - 1/e = 0.63$)

    (c) The capacitor will be nearly fully discharged after $5\tau$.

    (d) The capacitor will have discharged down to 37% of $Q_{max}$ after one $\tau$.

### 5.8.2    Questions to Review DC Circuits

(1)    In a DC circuit:

     (a) if series, the currents are different for each component (e.g., resistors, capacitors)
     (b) if series, the voltages are the same for each component
     (c) if parallel, the currents are equal for all paths (of the circuit)
     (d) if parallel, the voltages are equal for all paths

(2)    The following graph represents which type of current(s)?

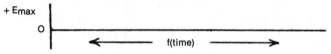

     (a) AC only
     (b) DC only
     (c) AC or DC
     (d) neither AC nor DC

(3)    Ohm's Law is:

     (V = potential difference, I = current, R = resistance, C = capacitance, Q = charge, L = inductance, t = time):

     (a) $C = Q/V$
     (b) $L = -\Delta V/(\Delta I/\Delta t)$
     (c) $V = IR$
     (d) $V = QLt$

(4)    The actual voltage output of an electromotive source

     (a) may be equal to, less than, or greater than the expected voltage of the source
     (b) is always equal to the expected voltage
     (c) is always more than the expected voltage
     (d) is always less than the expected voltage

(5)    All are correct concerning electromotive force (emf) sources except:

     (a) the units of emf are microfarads
     (b) maintains constant potential differences in a circuit
     (c) replaces energy lost by the moving electrons in a circuit
     (d) sources include both batteries and generators

(6)    A source of emf (electromotive force):

     (a) generates positive and negative charges
     (b) decreases the resistance an electron faces in moving through a circuit
     (c) does work on each charge to raise it from a lower potential (electrical) to a higher potential
     (d) changes the sign of the charge during each transit of the circuit

(7)    Normally, a charge gains energy as it moves through a source of emf, but it can lose energy if

     (a) the emf source has an internal resistance
     (b) the emf source has a reversed polarity
     (c) the emf source is a generator
     (d) the emf source is of low voltage

(8)    Resistance, as used in electricity, is

     (a) the opposition to flow of electrons in a substance
     (b) the opposition to the generation of emf
     (c) the location of storage of energy of electrons
     (d) has the units of farads

(9)    Resistance, as used in electricity, is:

    (a) inversely proportional to the density of the conductor
    (b) inversely proportional to the resistivity of the conductor
    (c) directly proportional to the cross-sectional area of the conductor
    (d) directly proportional to the length of the conductor

(10)   Resistance (electrical) has a fixed value for a given material and depends on all except:

    (a) size of a conductor
    (b) current in a conductor
    (c) shape of a conductor
    (d) temperature

(11)   The resistance of a substance can be expected to increase for all the following situations except:

    (a) increasing cross-sectional area
    (b) increasing length
    (c) increasing temperature
    (d) increasing resistivity of materials

(12)   The unit of power is the:

    (a) joule
    (b) volt
    (c) ampere
    (d) watt

(13)   Current is:

    (a) time/charge
    (b) charge/time
    (c) (charge)(time)
    (d) none of these

(14)   An ampere is:

    (a) coulombs/secs
    (b) (coulombs)(secs)
    (c) (volts)(ohms)
    (d) ohms/volts

(15)   Current is:

    (a) caused by the movement of positive charge
    (b) increased by the thermal motion of atoms
    (c) decreased by impurities in the conductor
    (d) all of the above.

(16)   To set up a continuous current, as opposed to a transient current, in a circuit, one may use a(n):

    (a) source of emf
    (b) capacitor
    (c) capacitor and resistor
    (d) capacitor and inductor

(17)   Capacitance is:

    (a) charge/potential
    (b) (charge)(potential)
    (c) (resistance)(current)
    (d) charge/resistance

(18) The farad is a unit of capacitance and is equal to:

(a) coulombs/volts
(b) (volts)(coulombs)
(c) amperes/ohms
(d) (amperes)(ohms)

(19) All of the following are associated with increased capacitance of a conductor except

(a) increased inducibility
(b) increased size
(c) increased curvature
(d) increased dielectric strength of the medium

(20) In a parallel plate capacitor,

(a) both plates are the same charge
(b) capacitance is directly proportional to the distance between the plates
(c) capacitance is independent of the medium between the plates
(d) capacitance is directly proportional to the area of the plates

(21) A capacitor will charge up to a certain point and then will cause the current to stop in a(n):

(a) DC circuit
(b) AC circuit
(c) both DC and AC
(d) neither DC nor AC

(22) In an AC circuit with a capacitor in series with a resistor, the voltage of the battery (neglecting internal resistance) is:

(a) (capacitor voltage)(resistor voltage)
(b) voltage across the capacitor minus voltage across the resistor
(c) voltage across the resistor minus voltage across the capacitor
(d) voltage across the resistor plus voltage across the capacitor

(23) If total resistance is 9 ohms and total voltage is 3 volts the current is:

(a) $\frac{1}{27}$ ampere
(b) $\frac{1}{3}$ ampere
(c) 3 amperes
(d) 27 amperes

(24) A current of 2 amperes and a resistance of 8 ohms requires what voltage (in a circuit):

(a) $\frac{1}{16}$ volt
(b) $\frac{1}{4}$ volt
(c) 4 volts
(d) 16 volts

(25) If it requires 20 volts to cause a current of 5 amperes in a wire, the resistance of the wire is:

(a) $\frac{1}{100}$ ohm
(b) $\frac{1}{4}$ ohm
(c) 4 ohms
(d) 100 ohms

(26) Assuming internal resistances of circuit elements is negligible, a charge would lose the most energy when it passes through a(n):

(a) capacitor
(b) inductor
(c) resistor
(d) battery

(27)  A battery has a voltage of 6V marked on it and an internal resistance of 0.5 ohm. If it is placed in the circuit below, what is the actual voltage it is producing in that circuit?

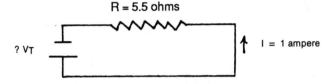

(a) 10 volts
(b) 8.5 volts
(c) 5.5 volts
(d) 5 volts

(28)  Calculate the internal resistance of the 20-volt battery in the following circuit:

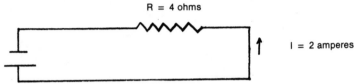

(a) 16 ohms
(b) 10 ohms
(c) 6 ohms
(d) 2 ohms

(29)  Determine the total emf (electromotive force) in the following circuit:

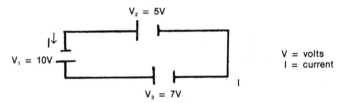

(a) 2 volts
(b) 8 volts
(c) 12 volts
(d) 22 volts

(30)  All are formulations of power (P) in a circuit with an emf (V) source and a resistor (R) with a current (I), except:

(a) P = VI
(b) P = IR/V
(c) P = I²R
(d) P = V²/R

(31)  A circuit has a current of 2 amperes and a resistance of 4 ohms. The maximal power that can be delivered is:

(a) 16 watts
(b) 8 watts
(c) 2 watts
(d) ½ watt

(32)  If the cross-sectional area of a conductor is quadrupled (× 4), the resistance:

(a) increases by a factor of 16
(b) increases by a factor of 4
(c) decreases by a factor of ¼
(d) decreases by a factor of ¹⁄₁₆

(33)    If the length of a conductor is doubled, the resistance:

(a) is not affected
(b) decreases by a factor of ½
(c) decreases by a factor of ¼
(d) increases by a factor of 2

(34)    In a circuit with a voltage of 10 volts and a resistance of 10 ohms and a current passing for 10 secs, the maximum possible number of Joules of heat produced is:

(a) 100 joules
(b) 1000 joules
(c) 1 joule
(d) 10 joules

(35)    Determine the current (I) in the following circuit:

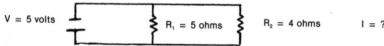

(a) 5/9 amperes
(b) 1.8 amperes
(c) 2.25 amperes
(d) 45 amperes

(36)    The voltage (V) of the following battery is (neglect internal resistance of battery):

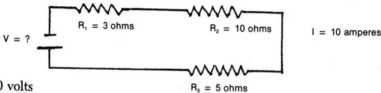

(a) 180 volts
(b) 18 volts
(c) 1.8 volts
(d) 0.55 volts

(37)    A current of 8 amperes will deliver what charge in 4 seconds?

(a) 2 statcoulombs
(b) 2 coulombs
(c) 32 statcoulombs
(d) 32 coulombs

(38)    If 10 coulombs pass a point in 2 seconds, the current is:

(a) 0.20 amps
(b) 5 amps
(c) 20 amps
(d) 200 amps

(39)    A conductor discharges (i.e., cannot hold any more charge) when 40 coulombs is placed on it at a voltage of 10 volts. What is its capacitance?

(a) 4000 farads
(b) 400 farads
(c) 0.25 farads
(d) 4 farads

(40)    The capacitance of a parallel plate capacitor in air is 20 farads. This capacitor is placed in a medium with a dielectric constant equal to 5. What is the capacitance now?

(a) 20 farads
(b) 4 farads
(c) 400 farads
(d) 100 farads

(41) In air, a parallel plate capacitor has a capacitance of 4 farads. In medium A, the capacitance is 32 farads. What is the dielectric constant of medium A?

(a) ⅛
(b) 8
(c) 128
(d) need the dielectric constant of air

(42) The units of resistance times capacitance is:

(a) voltage
(b) amperes
(c) henries
(d) seconds

(43) Convert the following circuit into a simple single equivalent resistance

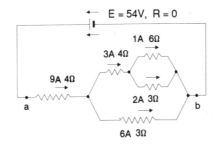

## 5.8.3    Answers to Questions in Section 5.8.2

( 1) d  ( 2) b  ( 3) c  ( 4) d  ( 5) a  ( 6) c  ( 7) b  ( 8) a  ( 9) d  (10) b  (11) a
(12) d  (13) b  (14) a  (15) c  (16) a  (17) a  (18) a  (19) a  (20) d  (21) a  (22) d
(23) b  (24) d  (25) c  (26) c  (27) c  (28) c  (29) b  (30) b  (31) a  (32) c  (33) d
(34) a  (35) c  (36) a  (37) d  (38) b  (39) d  (40) d  (41) b  (42) d
(43) See discussion of answer to question #43.

## 5.8.4    Discussion of Answers to Questions in Section 5.8.2

*Questions #1 to #22:* Adequately discussed in the Section.

*Question #23* (Answer: b) From Ohm's Law:

$$V = IR$$
$$I = V/R = 3 \text{ volts}/9 \text{ ohms} = \text{⅓ amp.}$$

*Question #24* (Answer: d) Solve using Ohm's Law:

$$V = IR = (2 \text{ amps})(8 \text{ ohms}) = 16 \text{ volts.}$$

*Question #25* (Answer: c) Use Ohm's Law:

$$V = IR$$
$$R = V/I = \frac{20 \text{ volts}}{5 \text{ amps}} = 4 \text{ ohms}$$

*Question #26* (Answer: c) Energy is lost when a charge passes through a resistance.

*Question #27* (Answer: c) The terminal voltage ($V_t$) of an emf source is determined by taking into account the internal resistance:

$r$  = 0.5 ohms         $V_t = V - Ir = I R_t$
$R_t$ = 5.5 ohms      $V - I r = 6 - 1 (.5) = 5.5$ volts
$V$  = 6 volts           $I R_t = 1 (5.5) = 5.5$ volts
$I$  = 1 amp             $V_t = 5.5$ volts

*Question #28* (Answer: c) See Section for an explanation of the formula:

$$V = 20 \text{ volts} \qquad r = ? \qquad\qquad V_t = V - I\,r = I\,R_t$$
$$R_t = 4 \text{ ohms} \qquad\qquad\qquad 20 - 2\,r = 2\,(4)$$
$$I = 2 \text{ amps} \qquad\qquad\qquad 20 - 2\,r = 8$$
$$r = 6 \text{ ohms}$$

*Question #29* (Answer: b) The total emf's around the loop of the circuit is:

$$V_{total} = \Sigma V = V_1 + V_2 - V_3 = 10 + 5 - 7 = 8$$

$V_3$ is negative because the current is moving through it in the reverse direction.

The internal resistances of the batteries have been neglected.

*Question #30* (Answer: b) Try to remember how to convert it to the others using Ohm's Law, although this is not explicitly required for the test.

*Question #31* (Answer: a) The appropriate formula is:

$$P = I^2\,R = (2)^2(4) = 16 \text{ watts}$$

The units are arrived at as follows:

$$P = (\text{amperes})^2(\text{ohms}) = (\text{amps})^2(\text{volts/amps}) = (\text{amps})(\text{volts})$$
$$= (\text{coulomb/sec})\text{volts} = \text{volt-coulomb/sec} = \text{joules/sec} = \text{watts}$$

Remember: joule = volt · coulomb.

*Question #32* (Answer: c) Resistance $(R) \propto 1/\text{Area}(A)$. Then if A increases by a factor of 4, the R decreases by ¼.

*OR:*
$$R_2/R_1 = (\varrho l/A_2)/(\varrho l/A_1) = (1/A_2)/(1/A_1) = (1/A_2)(A_1/1) = A_1/A_2$$
$$= A_1/(4A_1) = ¼ \qquad\qquad (A_2 = 4A_1)$$
$$\therefore R_2 = ¼\,R_1.$$

*Question #33* (Answer: d) Resistance $(R) \propto \text{length}\ (l)$. So, if length doubles, the R is doubled.

*OR:*
$$R_2/R_1 = (\varrho l_2/A)/(\varrho l_1/A) = l_2/l_1 = 2l_1/l_1 = 2$$
$$\therefore R_2 = 2R_1. \qquad\qquad (l_2 = 2l_1)$$

*Question #34* (Answer: a) $P = V^2/R$ (see Section)

$$P = (10)^2/10 = 10 \text{ watts}$$
$$(\text{Power})(\text{time}) = \text{joules} = (10)(10) = 100 \text{ joules}.$$

*Question #35* (Answer: c) $R_1$ and $R_2$ are in parallel. Then:

$$1/R_T = 1/R_1 + 1/R_2 = ⅕ + ¼ = ⁴/_{20} + ⁵/_{20} = ⁹/_{20}$$
$$\therefore R_T = ^{20}/_9 \text{ ohms.}$$

Then using Ohm's Law: $V = IR$
$$I = V/R = 5 \text{ volts}/(^{20}/_9 \text{ ohms}) = 5(^9/_{20}) = ^9/_4 = 2.25 \text{ amps.}$$

*Question #36* (Answer: a) This is a series circuit because the current (I) *must* pass through each resistor (R) before returning to the voltage source (V). The total resistance $(R_T)$:
$$R_T = R_1 + R_2 + R_3 = 3 + 10 + 5 = 18 \text{ ohms.}$$

Calculate V using Ohm's Law: $V = IR = (10 \text{ amps})(18 \text{ ohms})$
$$= 180 \text{ volts.}$$

*Question #37* (Answer: d)

$$I = q/t$$
$$q = (I)(t) = (8 \text{ amps})(4 \text{ seconds}) = 32 \text{ coulombs.}$$

*Question #38* (Answer: b)

$$I = q/t = 10 \text{ couls}/2 \text{ secs} = 5 \text{ amps}$$

*Question #39* (Answer: d) $C = q/V = 40 \text{ coulombs}/10 \text{ volts} = 4 \text{ farads}$

*Question #40* (Answer: d) $C = K C_O$      $C_O = $ capacitance of air
$$C = (5)(20) = 100 \text{ farads}.$$

*Question #41* (Answer: b) $C = K C_O$
$$K = C/C_O = {}^{32}\!/_4 = 8.$$

*Question #42* (Answer: d)

resistance (R) = ohms = volts/amperes = volts/(coulombs/sec)
$$= \text{(volt-sec)/couls}$$

capacitance (C) = farads = couls/volt

Then: (R)(C) = (volt-sec/coul)(coul/volt) = secs.

*Question #43*

Use principles of parallel/series resistors

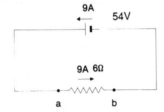

## 5.8.5     Vocabulary, Concepts, etc. Checklist for DC Circuits

_____ current
_____ battery
_____ internal resistance
_____ Ohm's Law
_____ resistors
_____ resistivity
_____ resistance
_____ capacitors
_____ capacitance

_____ DC electricity
_____ series circuits
_____ parallel circuits
_____ emf
_____ volts
_____ farad
_____ ohm
_____ dielectric constant
_____ dielectrics

## 5.9     AC CIRCUITS

### 5.9.1     Review of AC Circuits

*AC (alternating current)* electricity constitutes 99% of that used in the U.S. It is made by converting mechanical energy to electrical energy. An armature, which is a loop of wire, is rotated in a magnetic field using mechanical energy. A current is induced (see inductance below) in the wire of the armature. This current changes direction because the direction of the velocity of the loop and the magnetic field changes. Slip rings are fused to each end of the wire loop and rotate with it. Since the direction of the current alternates, the slip rings alternate in conducting the current away from the loop (hence AC). Graphite brushes are on the slip rings and these brush against conducting materials which carry away from the generator. AC looks like a sine wave (Fig. 5.22).

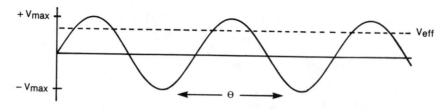

*Fig. 5.22—AC Electricity*

Note that the maximum voltages (V) are not the same as $V_{eff}$ (effective voltage, or root-mean square voltage). Similarly, the maximum current is not the effective (root-mean square) current delivered ($I_{eff}$). These relations are,

$$V_{eff} = 0.707 \, V_{max}$$
$$I_{eff} = 0.707 \, I_{max}.$$

One effective volt of AC will develop one effective ampere of current through a resistance of one ohm. The frequency of alternation of the cycle is also important in determining the V and I values. A typical frequency is 60 cycles/second.

The combined effect of a resistance and a reactance is known as apparent resistance or "*impedance*". The letter Z is generally used to indicate impedance. Thus, in an AC circuit, we can write Ohm's Law as:

$$I \text{ (amperes)} = \frac{V \text{(volts)}}{Z \text{(Ohms)}}$$

Impedance can be represented vectorially as the hypotenuse of the right triangle whose two sides are the ohmic resistance and the reactance, thus:

$$Z = \sqrt{R^2 + X_L^2}$$
$$I = \frac{V}{Z} = \sqrt{R^2 + (2\pi f L)^2}$$

Impedance Z

Reactance $X_L$

$\phi$ Phase angle

Resistance R

*Fig. 5.23—Vector Triangle Relating Resistance, Reactance, and Impedance*

The angle $\phi$ between R and Z is called the phase angle and is equal to the lag of the current behind the voltage, in electrical degrees.

*Concept of Capacitance*

The capacitance C of the capacitor is defined as the ratio of the charge Q on either conductor to the potential difference $V_{ab}$ between the conductors.

$$C = \frac{Q}{V_{ab}}$$

The net charge on the capacitor as a whole is zero and "the charge on a capacitor" is understood to mean the charge on either conductor, without regard to sign. From the definition, note that capacitance is expressed in coulombs per volt. Since one volt is equivalent to one joule per coulomb, one coulomb per volt is equivalent to one coul²/joule. A capacitance of one coulomb per volt is called one farad (for Faraday). That is, the capacitance of a capacitor is one farad if one coulomb is transferred from one conductor to the other, per volt of potential difference between the conductors.

Capacitors find many applications in electrical circuits. A capacitor is used to eliminate sparking when a circuit containing inductance is suddenly opened. The ignition system of the automobile engine contains a capacitor for this purpose. Capacitors are used in radio circuits for tuning, and for "smoothing" the rectified current delivered by the power supply. The efficiency of alternating current power transmissions can often be increased by the use of large capacitors.

*Dielectric Coefficient*

Most capacitors utilize a solid, nonconducting material or dielectric between their plates. A common type is the paper and foil capacitor, in which strips of metal foil form the plates and a sheet of paper impregnated with wax is dielectric. By rolling up such a capacitor, a capacitance of several microfarads can be obtained in a relatively small volume. The "Leyden jar," constructed by cementing metal foil over a portion of the inside and outside surfaces of a glass jar, is essentially a parallel-plate capacitor, with the glass forming the dielectric.

Electrolytic capacitors utilize as their dielectric an extremely thin layer of nonconducting oxide between a metal plate and a conducting solution. Because of the small thickness of the dielectric, electrolytic capacitors of relatively small dimensions may have a capacitance of the order of 50 $\mu f$.

### 5.9.2 Questions to Review AC Circuits

(1)  In an AC circuit, the effective value of the current is

   (a) equal to the maximum value of the AC current
   (b) greater than the maximum value of the DC current
   (c) less than the maximum value of AC current
   (d) greater than the maximum value of DC current

(2)  When a coil whose resistance is $15\Omega$ is connected to a 120-V, 60 Hz source, it draws 2.5A. Find (i) the impedance and (ii) the inductance of the coil.

   (a) $17.5\Omega$, $12.5\Omega$
   (b) $8\Omega$, $48\Omega$
   (c) $48\Omega$, $45.6\Omega$
   (d) $24\Omega$, $22.8\Omega$

### 5.9.3 Answers to Questions in Section 5.9.2

(1) c    (2) c

### 5.9.4 Discussion of Answers to Questions in Section 5.9.2

*Question #1* Adequately discussed in the Section.

*Question #2* Solution:

(a) First solve for the impedance of the circuit.

$$Z = \frac{V}{I}$$
$$= \frac{120 \text{ V}}{2.5 \text{ A}}$$
$$= 48\Omega.$$

(b)
$$Z^2 = R^2 + X_L^2$$
$$X_L = \sqrt{Z^2 - R^2}$$
$$= \sqrt{(48\Omega)^2 - (15\Omega)^2}$$
$$= 45.6\Omega$$

But since $X_L = 2\pi fL$, or $L = X_L/2\pi f$,

$$L = \frac{45.6\Omega}{6.28 \times 60 \text{ cycles/sec}} = 0.1210\text{H}$$

_____ AC circuits                        _____ impedance
_____ AC electricity                   _____ capacitance
_____ root mean-square current/voltage      _____ dielectric

## 5.10      GENERAL WAVE CHARACTERISTICS

### 5.10.1      Review of General Wave Characteristics

A _wave_ is a disturbance in a medium such that each particle in the medium vibrates about an equilibrium point in a simple harmonic motion (below). If the direction of vibration is perpendicular to the direction of propagation of the wave, the wave is called a _transverse wave_ (e.g., light). If the direction of vibration is in the same direction as propagation of the wave, the wave is called a _longitudinal wave_ (e.g., sound). Longitudinal waves are characterized by condensations (regions of crowding of particles) and rarefactions (regions where particles are far apart) along the wave in the medium See Fig. 5.24(b).

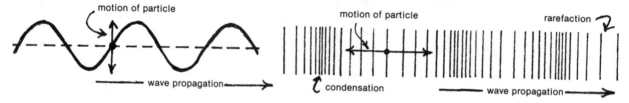

Fig. 5.24(a)—Transverse Wave           Fig. 5.24(b)—Longitudinal Wave

The _wavelength_ ($\lambda$) is the distance from crest to crest (or valley to valley) of a transverse wave. It may also be defined as the distance between two particles with the same displacement and direction of displacement. In a longitudinal wave, the wavelength can be taken as the distance from one rarefaction (or condensation) to another. The _amplitude_ (A) is the maximum displacement of a particle in one direction from its equilibrium point. _Frequency_ (f) is the number of wavelengths (cycles) that pass a point per unit time. _Period_ (T) is the time required for one wavelength to pass a point. _Speed_ (v) of a wave refers to its propagation through the medium. Speed increases as the inertia of the medium decreases (e.g., as density decreases). _Phase_ ($\phi$) is the difference in displacement and direction of a particle due to two different waves. Two waves are in phase if each particle has the same displacement and direction of motion ($\phi = 0$)(Fig. 5.25):

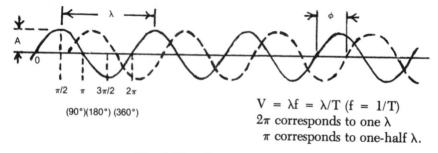

$\pi/2$   $\pi$   $3\pi/2$   $2\pi$
(90°)(180°) (360°)

$V = \lambda f = \lambda/T \ (f = 1/T)$
$2\pi$ corresponds to one $\lambda$
$\pi$ corresponds to one-half $\lambda$.

Fig. 5.25—Characteristics of Waves

The _superposition principle_ states that the effect of two or more waves on the displacement of a particle are independent. This means the displacement of a particle by simultaneous waves in a medium are algebraically additive. _Interference_ is the summation of the displacements of different waves in a medium. _Constructive interference_ is when the waves add to a larger resultant wave than either original. This occurs maximally when the phase difference ($\phi$) is a whole wavelength ($\lambda$) which corresponds to multiples of $360°$ ($2\pi$). So, this occurs at $\phi = 0, 2\pi, 4\pi$, etc. Since $\phi = 2\pi\Delta L/\lambda$, where $\Delta L$ equals the difference in path to a point of two waves (of equal wavelength), these waves interfere constructively when $\Delta L = 0, \lambda, 2\lambda, 3\lambda$, etc. *Destructive interference* is when the waves add to a smaller resultant wave than either original wave. This occurs maximally when $\phi = \pi, 3\pi, 5\pi$, etc., which are multiples of one-half wavelengths ($180° = \pi$ corresponds to $\frac{1}{2}\lambda$). This occurs when $\Delta L = \lambda/2, 3\lambda/2, 5\lambda/2$, etc.

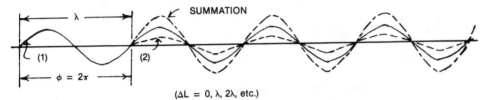

Waves (1) and (2) begin at the points shown, have the same $\lambda$ but different A's.
The summation wave is maximal since $\Delta L = \lambda$ in this example.

**Fig. 5.26—*Maximal Constructive Interference***

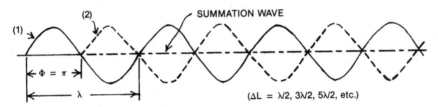

Waves (1) and (2) begin as shown, have the same $\lambda$ and the same A's.
The summation wave is the horizontal line (or the minimum) since $\Delta L = \lambda/2$ in this example.

**Fig. 5.27—*Maximal Destructive Interference***

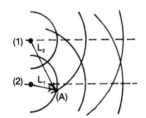

$L_1$, $L_2$ are distances from origins of waves to point A
$\Delta L = |L_2 - L_1|$ (absolute value).

**Fig. 5.28—*Schematic for* $\Delta L$**

*Standing waves* result when waves are reflected off a stationary object back into the oncoming waves of the medium, and superimposition (see above) results. *Nodes* are points where there is no particle displacement, which are similar to points of maximal destructive interference (above). Nodes occur at fixed end points (points that cannot vibrate). *Antinodes* are points that undergo maximal displacements and are similar to points of maximal constructive interference. Antinodes occur at open or free end points.

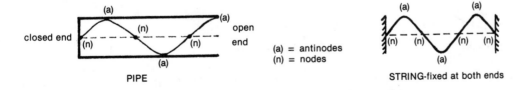

**Fig. 5.29—*Standing Waves***

The particles that are undergoing displacement when a wave passes through a medium undergo motion called simple harmonic motion (SHM) and are acted upon by a force described by Hooke's Law. SHM is caused by an inconstant force (called a restoring force) and as a result has an inconstant acceleration. The force is proportional to the displacement (distance from the equilibrium point) but opposite in direction,

$$F = -kx \qquad \textit{Hooke's Law}$$
$$k = \text{constant} \qquad x = \text{displacement from equilibrium}$$

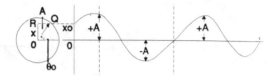

Fig. 5.30(a)—Simple Harmonic Motion

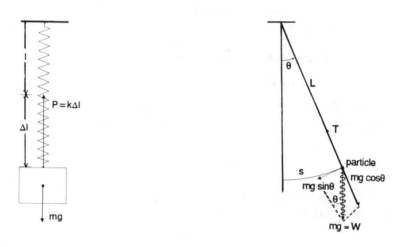

Fig. 5.30(b)—Simple Harmonic Motion      Fig. 5.30(c)—Simple Harmonic Motion

Features of SHM and Hooke's Law are:

(1) Force and acceleration are always in the same direction.
(2) Force and acceleration are always in the opposite direction of the displacement.
(3) Force and acceleration have their maximal values at $+A$ and $-A$; they are zero at the equilibrium point.
(4) Velocity direction has no constant relation to displacement or acceleration.
(5) Velocity is maximum at equilibrium and zero at A and $-A$.

The *electromagnetic spectrum* has the sequence below from long wavelength ($\lambda$) and low frequency (f) to short wavelength and high frequency. Many regions overlap,

*Long* $\lambda$                                                     *Short* $\lambda$
radiowaves / microwaves / infrared / visible / ultraviolet / X-rays / gamma rays
*Low f*                                                        *High f*

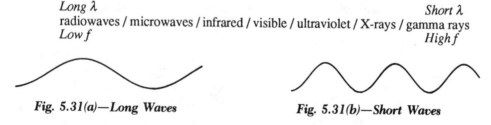

Fig. 5.31(a)—Long Waves          Fig. 5.31(b)—Short Waves

The visible light is broken down into colors remembered by the mnemonic, ROY G. BIV:

Red, Orange, Yellow, Green, Blue, Indigo, Violet

*Planck* developed the relation between energy (E) and the frequency (v) of electromagnetic radiation,

$$E = hv$$
$$h = \text{Planck's Constant}$$

Since, $v \propto 1/\lambda$, then, $E \propto 1/\lambda$. That is, high frequencies but short wavelengths correspond to high energy and vice versa. See Section 5.11.1 for resonance and beats.

## 5.10.2    Questions to Review General Wave Characteristics

(1)    If the direction of vibration of particles of a medium is in the direction of propagation of a wave, the wave is called:

(a) longitudinal
(b) transverse
(c) both
(d) neither

(2)    Condensations and rarefactions would be found in

(a) light waves
(b) electromagnetic radiation
(c) transverse waves
(d) longitudinal waves

(3)    "The effect of two or more waves on the displacement of a particle are independent" is a statement of:

(a) Interference Principle
(b) Huygens' Principle
(c) Correspondence Principle
(d) Superposition Principle

(4)    At the node of a wave:

(a) the displacement is maximal
(b) there is no displacement
(c) there may be an open or a free point
(d) both (a) and (c)

(5)    Select the *incorrect* relationship between the energy (E) of a wave and the parameters given:
(f = frequency, $\lambda$ = wavelength, A = amplitude)

(a) $E \propto f$
(b) $E \propto A^2$
(c) $E \propto 1/\lambda$
(d) all are correct

(6)    The restoring force that causes an object to undergo simple harmonic motion is

(a) a constant force
(b) inversely proportional to the displacement (from equilibrium) and in the same direction
(c) directly proportional to the displacement but opposite in direction
(d) both (a) and (b)

(7)    All of the following are true about simple harmonic motion *except*:

(a) force and acceleration have their maximum values at the equilibrium point
(b) force and acceleration are always in the same direction
(c) velocity direction has no constant relation to displacement or acceleration
(d) velocity is maximal at the equilibrium point

(8)    Which of the following colors of visible light has the shortest wavelength?

(a) green
(b) blue
(c) yellow
(d) red

(9)    Which of the following colors of visible light has the longest wavelength?

(a) yellow
(b) orange
(c) blue
(d) green

(10)    If f = frequency and $\lambda$ = wavelength of light, then the speed of light (c) is:

(a) c = 1/f
(b) c = $\lambda$/f
(c) c = f/$\lambda$
(d) c = f$\lambda$

(11)    The relation, E = h$\upsilon$, was put forth by

(a) Planck
(b) Einstein
(c) Newton
(d) Maxwell

(12)    Constructive interference occurs when:

(a) phase differences are 0, $2\pi$, $4\pi$, etc.
(b) path differences are 0, $\lambda$, $2\lambda$, $3\lambda$, etc.
(c) neither
(d) both

(13)    If the frequency of a wave is 10,000 hertz and it is travelling at 5000 m/sec, then its wavelength is:

(a) 5 m
(b) 2m
(c) 0.5 m
(d) 0.2 m

(14)    The speed of light (c) is $3.0 \times 10^{10}$ cm/sec. If the wavelength ($\lambda$) of red-light is approximately 400 nm (nm = $10^{-9}$m), then the frequency (f) of red-light is:

(a) $7.5 \times 10^{12}$/sec
(b) $7.5 \times 10^{14}$/sec
(c) $1.2 \times 10^{4}$/sec
(d) $1.2 \times 10^{6}$/sec

(15)    Electromagnetic radiation (e.g., light) with frequency (f) of 50,000 hertz (hertz = 1 cycle/sec) would have a wavelength ($\lambda$) of:

(a) 1/50,000 cms
(b) $6.0 \times 10^{-5}$ cms
(c) $6.0 \times 10^{5}$ cms
(d) cannot be determined

(16)    In a vibrating column of air

(a) open ends can only have nodes
(b) nodes can occur at open or closed ends
(c) open ends can only have antinodes
(d) antinodes may occur at closed ends

*Use the following data for Questions #17 through #22*

The particle of mass = 2 kg below is moving about the fixed point 0 as shown. Given are some values of the force on the particle at different values of displacement (X) from 0. The maximal displacement from 0 in any one direction is ± A and A = 5 m.

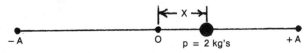

| X (meters)  | + 3   | + 1   | − 2   | − 4   |
|-------------|-------|-------|-------|-------|
| F (newtons) | − 0.6 | − 0.2 | + 0.4 | + 0.8 |

(17) This type of motion is called:

(a) uniform linear motion
(b) simple harmonic motion
(c) projectile motion
(d) free fall motion

(18) The force is described by:

(a) Faraday's Law
(b) Newton's First Law
(c) Hooke's Law
(d) none of the above

(19) If the above motion and force follow Hooke's Law, the value of k (neglect the units) is:

(a) 0.1
(b) 0.2
(c) 0.5
(d) 1.0

(20) The value of F at A = − 5m is:

(a) 0.2 nts
(b) 0.5 nts
(c) 1.0 nts
(d) 5 nts

(21) The force has a value of zero at x = ?

(a) 0 m
(b) +5 m
(c) −5 m
(d) ±2m

(22) At x = − 2 m, the acceleration (a) is (in m/sec²):

(a) 4.0
(b) 2.0
(c) 1.0
(d) 0.2

(23) A standing wave is established in a string fixed at both ends between two points 1m apart. Which of the following is not a possible wavelength of waves for this system?

(a) 4 m
(b) 2 m
(c) 1.0 m
(d) 0.5 m

(24) A standing wave is established in a pipe which is open at one end and is 2m long. All of the following are possible wavelengths of waves for this system except:

(a) 8 m
(b) 6 m
(c) 2⅔ m
(d) all are possible

(25) The wavelength of ultraviolet waves is $10^3$ angstroms. Find the energy of the ultraviolet waves, given Planck's constant = $6.626 \times 10^{-34}$ joule-sec. (1 angstrom = 1Å = $10^{-10}$m)

(a) $6.626 \times 10^{-31}$J
(b) $6.626 \times 10^{-41}$J
(c) $2 \times 10^{18}$J
(d) $2 \times 10^{-18}$J

## 5.10.3 Answers to Questions in Section 5.10.2

( 1) a  ( 2) d  ( 3) d  ( 4) b  ( 5) d  ( 6) c  ( 7) a  ( 8) b  ( 9) b  (10) d  (11) a
(12) d  (13) c  (14) b  (15) c  (16) c  (17) b  (18) c  (19) b  (20) c  (21) a  (22) d
(23) a  (24) b  (25) d

## 5.10.4 Discussion of Answers to Questions in Section 5.10.2

*Questions #1 to #11, #16* Adequately discussed in the text.

*Question #12* (Answer: d) It takes one whole cycle (2 $\pi$ = 360°) for a sine wave to completely repeat itself. So, for two waves to add constructively at every point, their phase must differ by multiples of $2\pi$, i.e.,

$2n\pi$ where n = 0, 1, 2, 3, etc.

The phase difference ($\phi$) for any given path difference to a given point is $\phi = 2\pi(\Delta L/\lambda)$ for a given wave with wavelength = $\lambda$. This is reasoned from the graph below:

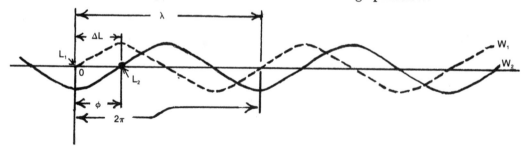

W$_1$ and W$_2$ are two waves out of phase.
L$_1$, L$_2$ are distances from O (origin).
the phase difference is $\phi$
the path difference is $\Delta L$
the following ratio holds because the corresponding distances are equal in the diagram above:
part/whole = $\phi/2\pi$ = $\Delta L/\lambda$
then: $\phi = 2\pi(\Delta L/\lambda)$

For constructive interference:
$$\phi = 2n\pi = 2\pi(\Delta L/\lambda)$$
$$n = \Delta L/\lambda$$
$$\Delta L = n\lambda \text{ where n = 0, 1, 2, 3 etc.}$$

*Question #13* (Answer: c)

$$v = \lambda f$$
$$\lambda = v/f = 5,000/10,000 = 0.5 \text{ m}$$

*Question #14* (Answer: b)

$$c = f\lambda$$
$$f = c/\lambda = (3.00 \times 10^{10} \text{cm/sec})/4 \times 10^{-5}\text{cm} = 0.75 \times 10^{15}/\text{sec} = 7.5 \times 10^{14}/\text{sec}$$
$$(\lambda = 400 \times 10^{-9} = 4.0 \times 10^{-7}\text{m} = 4 \times 10^{-5}\text{cm})$$

*Question #15* (Answer: c)

$$c = f\lambda = 3.00 \times 10^{10}\text{cm/sec}$$
$$f = 50,000/\text{sec} = 5 \times 10^4/\text{sec}$$
$$\lambda = c/f = 3.00 \times 10^{10}/5.0 \times 10^4 = 0.60 \times 10^6\text{cms}$$
$$\lambda = 6.0 \times 10^5 \text{ cms.}$$

*Question #17* (Answer: b) The particle is oscillating about a fixed point (0) which is called simple harmonic motion.

*Question #18* (Answer: c) The force is a restoring force and the motion is SHM. This is described in Hooke's Law as $F = -kx$.

*Question #19* (Answer: b) The motion follows Hooke's Law: $F = -kx$.
So, to find the k, any set of F and x may be substituted in the equation:

$$k = -(F/x) = -(-0.6 \text{ nts}/+3\text{m}) = +0.2 \text{ nt/m}$$
$$k = -(F/x) = -(-0.2 \text{ nts}/+1\text{m}) = +0.2 \text{ nt/m, etc.}$$

*Question #20* (Answer: c) Use the data from #19:

$$F = -kx$$
$$F = -(0.2)(-5) = +1.0 \text{ nts}$$

Note at $\pm A$, F has its maximal value.

*Question #21* (Answer: a)

$$F = -kx = 0$$
$$-kx = 0$$
$$x = 0 \text{ because k is not equal to zero.}$$

*Question #22* (Answer: d)

Can use:      $F = +0.4$ nts from chart at $x = -2$,

OR:        $F = -kx$ from Hooke's Law

$F = ma$ from Newton's 2nd Law (Section 5.3.1)

$$ma = -kx$$
$$a = -kx/m = -(0.2)(-2)/2 = +0.2\text{m/sec}^2.$$

*Question #23* (Answer: a) If the string is fixed at both ends, then only nodes can occur at these points. Then the smallest part of a wave that can exist between these points is $\frac{1}{2}\lambda$ which then equals 1 m:

Then the $\lambda$ of the above situation is 2 m as shown. This is the maximal allowed $\lambda$ for this set-up. Other $\lambda$s are possible as follows:

the next node after $\frac{1}{2}\lambda$ is $\frac{1}{2}\lambda$ away and the next node after that is another $\frac{1}{2}\lambda$ away. These then are $n(\frac{1}{2}\lambda)$ where $n = 0, 1, 2, 3$ etc., are the possible $\frac{1}{2}\lambda$'s that can fit into the distance ($l = 1$m) then: $n(\frac{1}{2}\lambda) = 1m = l$

$n\lambda/2 = l$

$\lambda = 2l/n =$ allowable $\lambda$'s

Then, the 1.0m and 0.5m are allowable $\lambda$'s:

$n = 2 l/\lambda = (2)(1)/0.5 = 4$ for $\lambda = 0.5m$

$n = 2 l/\lambda = (2)(1)/1 = 2$ for $\lambda = 1.0m$

Also, the $\lambda = 4m$ is not allowable because it does not give a value of n that is a whole number:

$n = 2l/\lambda = (2)(1)/4 = 0.5$ which is not acceptable.

Note that the allowable frequencies (f) are:

$f = v/\lambda = v/(2l/\lambda) = nv/2l$

$v =$ velocity of wave proportion.

*Question #24* (Answer: b) At the closed end of the pipe there must be a node and at the open end there must be an antinode. The shortest fraction of a wave that has a node and antinode in sequence is $\frac{1}{4}\lambda$ which must equal the 2m:

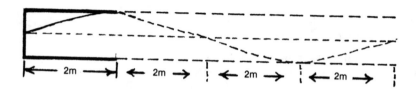

$\frac{1}{4}\lambda = 2m$

$\lambda = 8m$ as the longest possible allowable $\lambda$. The next antinode occurs $\frac{1}{2}\lambda$ beyond $\frac{1}{4}\lambda$ and then the next is $\frac{1}{2}\lambda$ beyond that, etc. (Only worry about next antinode because these go at the open end of the pipe.) The sequence of possible fractions of $\lambda$'s for this system is:

$\frac{1}{4}\lambda$

$\frac{1}{4}\lambda + \frac{1}{2}\lambda = \frac{3}{4}\lambda$

$\frac{3}{4}\lambda + \frac{1}{2}\lambda = \frac{5}{4}\lambda$

$\frac{5}{4}\lambda + \frac{1}{2}\lambda = \frac{7}{4}\lambda$ etc.

or to generalize this: $n\lambda/4$ where $n = 1, 3, 5, 7, 9$ etc.

(note that only the odd numbers are possible.)

Then each of these fractional $\lambda$s must fit into the 2m = *l*:

$n\lambda/4 = 2m = l$

$n\lambda/4 = l$

$\lambda = 4l/n \qquad n = 1, 3, 5, 7$ etc.

Then any $\lambda$ is possible as long as it gives $n = 1, 3, 5, 7$, etc., when substituted in the above equation:

$n = 4l/n$

for $\lambda = 8m$: $n = (4)(2)/8 = 1 \qquad \therefore$ possible

for $\lambda = 6m$: $n = (4)(2)/6 = \frac{4}{3} \qquad \therefore$ not possible

for $\lambda = \frac{8}{3} m$: $n = (4)(2)/(\frac{8}{3}) = 8(3/8) = 3 \qquad \therefore$ possible

Note that the frequencies (f) in this case are

$f = v/\lambda = v/(4l/n) = vn/4l \qquad n = 1, 3, 5$

$v =$ velocity of wave propagation.

*Question #25* (Answer: d)

$$E = h\nu, \ v = \nu\lambda$$
$$v = 2.998 \times 10^8 \text{ m/sec}$$
$$1J = 1 \text{ Newton-meter}$$
$$\lambda = 10^3\text{Å} = 10^3 10^{-10} = 10^{-7}\text{m}$$
$$\nu = \frac{v}{\lambda} = \frac{2.998 \times 10^8}{10^{-7}} = 2.998 \times 10^{15} \text{ Hz}$$
$$E = \text{Planck's Constant} \times \nu = h\nu$$
$$= 6.626 \cdot 10^{-34} \times 2.998 \cdot 10^{15}$$
$$= 1.99 \times 10^{-18} \text{ joules}$$

## 5.10.5    Vocabulary, Concepts, etc. Checklist for General Wave Characteristics

\_\_\_\_\_ simple harmonic motion
\_\_\_\_\_ constructive interference
\_\_\_\_\_ destructive interference
\_\_\_\_\_ frequency
\_\_\_\_\_ velocity
\_\_\_\_\_ amplitude
\_\_\_\_\_ transverse waves
\_\_\_\_\_ longitudinal waves
\_\_\_\_\_ superposition of waves
\_\_\_\_\_ electromagnetic radiation
\_\_\_\_\_ energy of waves
\_\_\_\_\_ gamma rays
\_\_\_\_\_ phase

\_\_\_\_\_ period
\_\_\_\_\_ Hooke's Law
\_\_\_\_\_ wavelength
\_\_\_\_\_ standing waves
\_\_\_\_\_ nodes
\_\_\_\_\_ antinodes
\_\_\_\_\_ radiowaves
\_\_\_\_\_ microwaves
\_\_\_\_\_ infrared
\_\_\_\_\_ visible
\_\_\_\_\_ ultraviolet
\_\_\_\_\_ x-rays
\_\_\_\_\_ $E = h\nu$

## 5.11    SOUND

### 5.11.1    Review of Sound

*Sound* is a longitudinal (Section 5.10.1) mechanical wave which travels through an elastic medium. Sound is thus produced by vibrating matter. There is no sound in a vacuum (because there is no matter). Compressions (condensations) are regions where particles (of matter) are close together and are high pressure regions. Rarefactions are regions where particles are sparse and are low pressure regions of sound waves.

The *speed* (v) of sound is proportional to the square root of the elastic restoring force and inversely proportional to the square root of the inertia of the particles (e.g., density, $\varrho$, is a measure of inertia),

$$v \propto \sqrt{F}$$
$$v \propto 1/\sqrt{\text{inertia}}$$

The speed in various substances is as follows (See Section 5.6.1):

| | | |
|---|---|---|
| wire or rod: | $v = \sqrt{Y/\varrho}$ | Y = Young's modulus |
| fluid (gas or liquid) | $v = \sqrt{B/\varrho}$ | B = bulk modulus |

The speed of sound also increases with temperature.

Forced vibrations occur when a series of waves impinge upon an object and cause it to vibrate. Natural frequencies are the intrinsic frequencies of vibration of a system. If the forced vibration causes the object to vibrate at one of its natural frequencies, the body will vibrate at maximal amplitude. This situation is called *resonance*. Note also that energy and power are proportional to the amplitude squared, so these two are also at a maximum.

Hearing is subjective but its characteristics are closely tied the physical characteristics of sound. These relations are:

SENSORY: loudness      PHYSICAL: intensity (I)
            pitch                        frequency (f)
            quality                      waveforms

The *quality* depends on the number and the relative intensity of the overtones of the waveforms. Frequency, and, therefore, *pitch*, are perceived by the ear from 20 to 20,000 Hz (Hertz = cycles/second). Frequencies below 20 Hz are called infrasonic. Frequencies above 20,000 Hz are called ultrasonic. *Sound intensity* (I) is the rate of energy (power) propagation through space:

$$I = \text{Power/area} \propto f^2 A^2$$
$$f = \text{frequency and } A = \text{amplitude}$$

## 5.11.1.1 THE HUMAN EAR

The human ear is divided into an *external ear* (pinna and auditory canal), the *middle ear* (the tympanic membrane and the three bones—malleus or hammer, incus or anvil, and stapes or stirrup), and the *internal ear* (the cochlea, the semicircular canals, and the origin of the vestibulocochlear nerve). The *tympanic membrane* (eardrum) is attached to the *malleus* which attaches to the *incus* which attaches to the *stapes* which attaches to the *oval window* of the cochlea. The outer and middle ear function to match the impedance of the air outside and the fluid of the cochlea inside. This mechanism results in more efficient transmission of sound. Sound waves are transmitted from the stapes via the oval window to the fluid in the *cochlea*. This fluid sets up vibrations in the *basilar membrane* which causes special hair cells to send impulses to the auditory part of the vestibulocochlear (VIII) nerve which transmits them to the auditory cortex in the temporal lobe of the cerebrum. The basilar membrane, tectoral membrane, and hair cells run the full length of the cochlea and together constitute the *organ of Corti*. The distance from the oval window that the vibration of the basilar membrane is a maximum determines the *frequency (pitch)* of the sound—highest frequencies are closest to the oval window. The *round window,* at the other end of the cochlea, serves as a release of pressure imparted to the cochlear fluid by the stapes.

The *vestibular system* is continuous anatomically but not functionally with the cochlea. The system is filled with fluid (endolymph) and contains the sacculus, the utricle and three perpendicular *semicircular* canals. Each *semicircular canal* has an *ampulla* region which contains hair cells sensitive to changes in angular acceleration. The *utricle* and *sacculus* contain a special sensory region called the *macula* which has crystals of calcium carbonate on it. These regions are sensitive to changes in gravity (position) and linear acceleration. Impulses travel from these special regions via the vestibular portions of the vestibulocochlear nerve (VIII) to the central nervous system. The vestibular system helps maintain posture, balance, spatial orientation, and stabilization of eye movements.

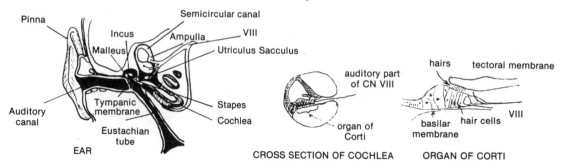

*Fig. 5.32 — The Human Ear*

The *loudness* varies with the amplitude. The ears are most sensitive (hear sounds of lowest intensity) at approximately 2,000 to 4,000 Hz. $I_0$, taken to be $10^{-12}$ watts/cm², is barely audible and is assigned a value of 0 (zero) dB (decibels).

Then the intensity level (I) of a sound wave in dB is,

$$dB = 10 \log (I/I_0)$$

$$I = \text{intensity at a given level}$$

$$I_0 = \text{threshold intensity.}$$

Examples of some values of dB's are: whisper (20), normal conversation (60), subway car (100), pain threshold (120) and jet engine (160). Continual exposure to sounds greater than 90 dB can lead to hearing impairment.

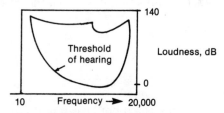

*Fig. 5.33—Audible Sound Intensities*

When sounds of different frequencies are heard together, they interfere (Section 5.10.1). Constructive interference results in *beats*. The number of beats per second is the absolute value of the difference of the frequencies ($|f_1 - f_2|$). Hence, the new frequencies heard include the original frequencies and the absolute differences between them.

The *Doppler Effect* is the effect upon the observed frequency caused by the relative motion of the observer (o) and the source (s). If the distance is decreasing between them, there is a shift to higher frequencies and shorter wavelengths, (to higher pitch for sound and toward the blue-violet for light). If the distance is increasing between them, there is a shift to longer wavelengths and lower frequencies (to lower pitch for sound and toward red for light). The summary equation of the above in terms of frequency (f) is:

$$fo/(V \pm v_0) = fs/(V \pm v_s)$$

$$fo = fs(V \pm v_0)/(V \pm v_s)$$

$$V = \text{speed of wave}$$

$$v = \text{speed of observer (o) or source (s).}$$

Choose the ($+$) or ($-$) such that the frequency varies as you would predict. If the o or s is moving toward the other the f should increase and vice versa. Predict the results and select the sign for the s and o independently of the motion of the other.

### 5.11.2     Questions to Review Sound

(1)    Sound waves:

    (a) are transverse waves
    (b) are produced by vibrating matter
    (c) may be transmitted in a vacuum
    (d) all of the above

(2)    The speed of sound is:

    (a) proportional to the square root of the elastic restoring force of the medium
    (b) inversely proportional to the square root of the inertia of the particles of the media
    (c) neither
    (d) both

(3)     The speed of sound is _____ by an increase of temperature.

(a) decreased
(b) increased
(c) does not change

(4)     When an object is forced to vibrate at one of its natural frequencies of vibration,

(a) resonance exists
(b) energy is a minimum
(c) work is a minimum
(d) the amplitude of vibration is a minimum

(5)     Which sensory (as interpreted by the brain) aspect of sound is incorrectly paired with its physical correlate of sound?

(a) loudness-intensity
(b) pitch-frequency
(c) quality-waveforms
(d) all are correctly paired

(6)     A human with normal hearing probably could not hear sound at:

(a) 100,000 Hz
(b) 20,000 Hz
(c) 5,000 Hz
(d) 20 Hz

(7)     The intensity (pressure per unit area) of a sound is

(a) inversely proportional to the square of the frequency
(b) directly proportional to the square of the frequency
(c) inversely proportional to the frequency
(d) directly proportional to the frequency

(8)     Decibels are used in describing:

(a) light
(b) sound
(c) electricity
(d) magnetism

(9)     The effect upon the frequency of sound observed when the source of the sound is moving relative to the observer is explained by the:

(a) Doppler Effect
(b) Compton Effect
(c) Theory of Relativity
(d) none of the above

(10)    If the density of a gas is quadrupled ($\times 4$), the speed (v) of sound through it is:

(a) decreased by a factor of ½
(b) increased by a factor of 2
(c) increased by a factor of 4
(d) not changed

(11)    If the elasticity (restoring force) of medium #1 is four times the elasticity of medium #2, then the sound will travel

(a) twice as fast in #1 as in #2
(b) twice as fast in #2 as in #1
(c) four times as fast in #1 as in #2
(d) four times as fast in #2 as in #1

(12) If the tension (F) in a string is increased by a factor of 4, the speed (v) of a wave in that string will be:

(a) quadrupled ($\times 4$)
(b) doubled
(c) reduced by $\frac{1}{2}$
(d) reduced to $\frac{1}{4}$ the original

(13) Three notes of 128, 256, and 512 are sounded; the frequencies heard are:

(a) 128, 256, 384, 512, 640, 768
(b) 512, 640, 768
(c) 128, 256, 384, 512
(d) 128, 256, 512

(14) A sound has an intensity 100 times that of the standard intensity. How many decibels is it?

(a) 10
(b) 20
(c) 50
(d) 100

(15) If a source which is emitting sound is moving toward an observer, the frequency of sound heard by the observer is _____ the frequency emitted by the source.

(a) the same as
(b) less than
(c) greater than

(16) If a source which is emitting light is moving away from an observer, the wavelength of light seen by the observer is _____ the wavelength emitted by the source.

(a) the same as
(b) shorter than
(c) longer than

(17) An observer is moving toward a source at 170 m/sec. The source is moving toward the observer at 130 m/sec and is emitting sound at a frequency of 10,000 hertz. The frequency of sound heard by the observer (assume speed of sound is 330 m/sec) is :

(a) 15,000 hertz
(b) 7,500 hertz
(c) 25,000 hertz
(d) 5,000 hertz

(18) The threshold of human hearing lies between:

(a) 20 Hz - 20,000 Hz
(b) 10 Hz - 10,000 Hz
(c) 18 Hz - 8,000 Hz
(d) 12 Hz - 1,200 Hz

(19) Given $I_0 = 10^{-12}$ watts/cm$^2$, find the intensity in watts/cm$^2$ of sound, given the intensity in dB = 100.

(a) 100 W/cm$^2$
(b) 1000 W/cm$^2$
(c) $10^{-10}$ W/cm$^2$
(d) $10^{-2}$ W/cm$^2$

(20) Find the magnitude of loudness in decibels at the threshold of human hearing:

(a) 0 dB
(b) 20 dB
(c) 200 dB
(d) 2,000 dB

(21) Given the intensity of sound of a subway car is 100 dB and the intensity of sound of a whisper is 20 dB. Compare their intensities in watts/cm².

(a) $I_1/I_O = (I_2/I_O)^5$
(b) $I_1 = \frac{1}{5}I_2$
(c) $I_1 = 5I_2$
(d) $I_2 = 5I_1$

(22) An ambulance, traveling 24m/sec, is moving toward an approaching car which is traveling at a speed of 14m/sec. The siren emits a frequency of 1,000 Hz, what is the frequency heard by the driver of the car? Speed of sound = 350m/sec.

(a) 1,000 Hz
(b) 1,116 Hz
(c) 1,350 Hz
(d) 1,038 Hz

(23) Frequency (pitch) is determined in the ear by the:

(a) oval window
(b) basilar membrane
(c) tympanic membrane
(d) medial geniculate body

(24) Which structure is not found in the middle ear of humans?

(a) cochlea
(b) tympanic membrane
(c) anvil
(d) incus

(25) Organ of Corti:

(a) brain
(b) eye
(c) ear
(d) bone

(26) Hearing is localized in which lobe of the cerebral cortex?

(a) frontal
(b) parietal
(c) temporal
(d) occipital

(27) All are components of the vestibular system except:

(a) semicircular canals
(b) sacculus
(c) organ of Corti
(d) utricle

(28) Semicircular canals are sensitive to:

(a) linear acceleration
(b) angular acceleration
(c) gravity
(d) all of the above

(29) The vestibular system is important for all except:

(a) balance
(b) posture
(c) spatial orientation
(d) voluntary movement

## 5.11.3    Answers to Questions in Section 5.11.2

( 1) b  ( 2) d  ( 3) b  ( 4) a  ( 5) d  ( 6) a  ( 7) b  ( 8) b  ( 9) a  (10) a  (11) a
(12) b  (13) c  (14) b  (15) c  (16) c  (17) c  (18) a  (19) d  (20) a  (21) a  (22) b
(23) b  (24) a  (25) c  (26) c  (27) c  (28) b  (29) d


## 5.11.4    Discussion of Answers to Questions in Section 5.11.2

*Questions #1 to #9* Adequately discussed in the Section.

*Question #10* (Answer: a)

$$v \propto 1/\sqrt{\varrho} \qquad \varrho = \text{density}$$

$$\frac{v_2}{v_1} = \frac{1/\sqrt{\varrho_2}}{1/\sqrt{\varrho_1}} = \frac{1}{\sqrt{\varrho_2}} \cdot \frac{\sqrt{\varrho_1}}{1} = \frac{\sqrt{\varrho_1}}{\sqrt{\varrho_2}} = \sqrt{\frac{\varrho_1}{\varrho_2}} = \sqrt{\frac{\varrho_1}{4\varrho_1}} = \sqrt{\tfrac{1}{4}} = \tfrac{1}{2}$$

$$\frac{v_2}{v_1} = \tfrac{1}{2}$$

$$v_2 = \tfrac{1}{2}v_1. \qquad\qquad \varrho_2 = 4\varrho_1$$

*Question #11* (Answer: a)

Speed of sound $(v) \propto \sqrt{\text{restoring force}} = F$

$$\frac{v_2}{v_1} = \frac{\sqrt{F_2}}{\sqrt{F_1}} = \sqrt{\frac{F_2}{F_1}} = \sqrt{\frac{F_2}{4F_2}} = \sqrt{\tfrac{1}{4}} = \tfrac{1}{2}$$

$$\frac{v_2}{v_1} = \tfrac{1}{2}$$

$$2v_2 = v_1 \qquad\qquad F_1 = 4F_2$$

*Question #12* (Answer: b)

$$v \propto \sqrt{F}$$
$$F_2 = 4F_1$$
$$v_2/v_1 = \sqrt{F_2}/\sqrt{F_1} = \sqrt{F_2/F_1} = \sqrt{4F_1/F_1} = \sqrt{4} = 2$$
$$v_2 = 2v_1$$

*Question #13* (Answer: c) The frequencies heard are the original frequencies plus all new frequencies resulting from the differences of the original frequencies:

$$512 - 128 = 384 \text{ (This is the only new frequency.)}$$

*Question #14* (Answer: b)
$$dB = 10 \log I/I_0 = 10 \log(100/1)$$
$$= 10 \log 100 = 10(2) = 20$$
$$(\log 100 = 2).$$

*Question #15* (Answer: c) As the observer and source move together the observed frequency increases.

*Question #16* (Answer: c) If the distance between observer and source is increasing, the wavelength observed increases as the frequency decreases.

*Question #17* (Answer: c) Use Doppler's relation as given in the Section:

$$f_O = f_S (V \pm v_O)/(V \pm v_S).$$

Since the source (s) is moving toward the observer (o), this tends to increase the $f_O$ over the $f_S$; for the $f_O > f_S$ must use $V - v_S$ because as the denominator decreases the fraction increases and this makes $f_O > f_S$

Since the o is moving toward the s, this tends to increase the $f_O$ over the $f_S$; for the $f_O > f_S$ need $V + v_O$ because as the numerator increases the fraction increases and this makes $f_O > f_S$.

Then:

$$f_O = f_S(V + v_O)/(V - v_S) \text{ for this problem}$$
$$f_O = (10{,}000)(330 + 170)/(330 - 130) = (10{,}000)(500/200) =$$
$$f_O = (10{,}000)(5/2) = 25{,}000 \text{ hertz.}$$

*Question #18* (Answer: a) Review the loudness-frequency graph, Fig. 5.33.

*Question #19* (Answer: d)

$$dB = 10 \log \frac{I}{I_O}$$

$$100 = 10 \log \frac{I}{10^{-12}}$$

$$10 = \log I + \log 10^{12} = \log I + 12$$
$$-2 = \log I \qquad I = 10^{-2} \text{ watts/cm}^2$$

*Question #20* (Answer: a) $I = I_O$ for threshold hearing

$$dB = 10 \log \frac{I}{I_O}$$

$$= 10 \log \frac{I_O}{I_O} = 0$$

*Question #21* (Answer: a)

$$100 \quad = 10 \log \frac{I_1}{I_O}$$

$$20 \quad = 10 \log \frac{I_2}{I_O}$$

Dividing, $5 = \log \dfrac{I_1}{I_O} / \log I_2/I_O$

$$5 \log \left(\frac{I_2}{I_O}\right) = \log \frac{I_1}{I_O}$$

(Review Vol. II: *Skills Development for the Medical College Admission Test*—logarithms)

$$\therefore I_1/I_O = (I_2/I_O)^5$$

*Question #22* (Answer: b) v = sound speed

$$f_O = f_S \left(\frac{v + v_O}{v - v_S}\right)$$
$$= 1000 \frac{(350 + 14)}{(350 - 24)}$$
$$= 1000 \frac{(364)}{(326)} = 1{,}116 \text{ Hz}$$

*Questions #23 to #29* Adequately discussed in Section.

## 5.11.5 Vocabulary, Concepts, etc. Checklist for Sound

_____ production of sound
_____ intensity
_____ speed of sound
_____ beats
_____ loudness
_____ middle ear
_____ outer ear
_____ tympanic membrane
_____ basilar membrane

_____ pitch
_____ decibel scale
_____ resonance
_____ Doppler Effect
_____ inner ear
_____ utricle
_____ stapes
_____ cochlea
_____ round window

## 5.12    OPTICS

### 5.12.1    Review of Optics

#### 5.12.1.1    THE HUMAN EYE

Anatomically, the eye is separated by the *lens* into an anterior region filled by the *aqueous humor* and a posterior region filled by the *vitreous humor*. There are three layers in the eye. The *sclera* (dense connective tissue) is the outermost. It is covered anteriorly by the conjunctiva (whites of the eyes). It is continuous with the clear portion called the *cornea* which is important in focusing light. Inside the sclera is the *choroid* which contains the blood vessels and black pigment to prevent light scattering. Continuous with the choroid in front are the *iris* (which gives the eye its color and opens and shuts to let light in through the *pupil*) and the *ciliary muscle* (which controls the shape of the lens and helps to focus or accommodate the eye to distance). The innermost layer is the retina which is the light sensitive layer containing rods and cones. *Rods* are located peripherally in the eye, are concerned with vision in dim light and peripheral vision, and contain *rhodopsin* (retinal from Vit A and a protein called opsin). Light converts retinal from a *cis* to a *trans* form which causes rhodopsin to fall apart and somehow sets up an impulse which is eventually transmitted to the optic nerve (Cranial Nerve II). Cones are located more centrally, are concerned with bright light and color vision, contain *iodopsin* (light sensitive substance) and are maximally concentrated at the *fovea* (or macula area) which has the highest visual acuity (ability to see clearly points that are close together).

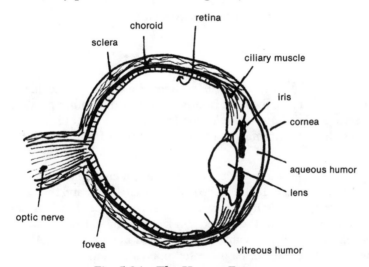

*Fig. 5.34—The Human Eye*

*Light passes* through the cornea where it is refracted (bent). It then passes through the aqueous humor and then through the pupil. The pupil size is regulated by the iris which is regulated by the parasympathetic (causes pupil to get smaller) and the sympathetic (causes pupil to get larger) systems. Next, the light passes through the lens where it is refracted further and focused upon the retina (after it passes through the vitreous). The lens is flat for objects far away (ciliary muscle relaxed), and it is rounded for objects nearby (ciliary muscle contracted—parasympathetic). Light then stimulates the cones and rods of the retina. From here nerve impulses are transmitted via the Ocular nerve (II) to the visual center in the occipital cortex of the cerebrum.

*Emmetropia* means that light is focused on the retina (by the cornea-lens system) when objects are near or far. *Myopia* (near-sightedness) means light is focused on the retina only when objects are near but not when objects are far away. A cause may be an eyeball that is too long and correction is by diverging (concave) glasses (i.e., lens). *Hypermetropia* (far-sightedness) means light is focused on the retina when objects are far away and not when they are near. A cause may be an eyeball that is too short and correction is by converging (convex) glasses. To *summarize* (Fig. 5.35) the problem in myopia is a cornea-lens system that refracts light relatively (for the eyeball length) too strong and focuses light in front of the retina when the object is far away. In hypermetropia, the problem is a cornea-lens system that refracts light relatively too weak and focuses light behind the retina when objects are near.

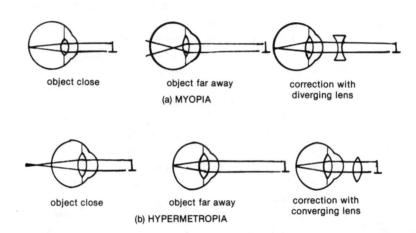

**Fig. 5.35—Myopia (a) and Hypermetropia (b)**

### 5.12.1.2    REFLECTION

Reflection is the process by which light rays (imaginary lines drawn perpendicular to advancing wave fronts) bounce back into a medium from a surface with another medium (versus being refracted or absorbed). The *Laws of Reflection* are: (1) The angle of incidence (I) equals the angle of reflection (R) at the normal (N, perpendicular to surface), and (2) the I, R, N all lie on the same plane.

Mirrors may have a plane surface a nonplane surface; only spherical nonplane mirrors will be discussed. For a plane mirror, all incident light is reflected in parallel off it and therefore all images seen are virtual, erect, left-right reversed and appear to be just as far (perpendicular distance) behind the mirror as the object is in front of the mirror. A *virtual image* has no light rays passing through it and cannot be projected upon a screen. A *real image* has light rays passing through it and can be projected upon a screen.

*Spherical mirrors* may have the reflecting surface convex (diverges light) or concave (converges light). Note the images formed by a converging mirror (concave) are like those for a converging lens (convex); and diverging mirrors (convex) and diverging lens (concave) also form similar images. The terminology for spherical mirrors (see Fig. 5.36) is:

    R = radius of curvature
    C = center of curvature
    F = focal point
    V = vertex (center of mirror itself)
 axis = line through C and V
    f = focal length (distance from F to V)
    i = image distance (distance from V to object along axis)
    o = object distance (distance from V to object along axis)
   AB = linear aperature (chord connecting ends of mirror, larger aperature
        means better resolution).

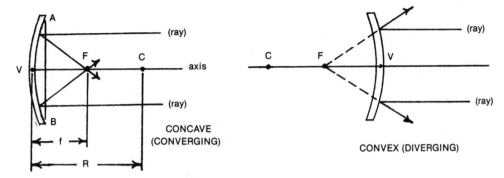

*Fig. 5.36—Reflection by Spherical Mirrors*

With *concave mirrors (spherical)* the incident light is converged (toward the axis). The path of light rays is as follows:

    (1) incident rays parallel to the axis reflect through F;
    (2) incident rays along a radius (of curvature) reflect back on themselves
        (rays through C);
    (3) incident rays through F reflect parallel to the axis.

The image formed by an object depends on the position of the image relative to the F and C (or f and R). General rules for image formation are:

    (1) if o < f, then image is virtual and erect;
        if o > f, then image is real and inverted;
    (2) if o = f, then no image is formed;
    (3) if o < R, then image is enlarged in size;
        if o > R, then image is reduced in size;
        if o = R, then image is same size.

These relations are similar to those for a converging lens (convex).

With *convex (spherical) mirrors*, the incident light is diverged (from the axis) after reflection. It is the backward extension (dotted lines above) that may pass through the F. The path of light rays are as follows:

    (1) incident rays parallel to the axis have backward extension of their
        reflections through F (see above);
    (2) incident rays along a radius (that would pass through C if extended)
        reflect back along themselves;
    (3) incident rays that pass through F (if extended) reflect parallel to the axis.

The image formed for a convex mirror is always virtual, erect and smaller than the object.

The *mirror equation* and derivations from it allow the above relations between object and image to be calculated instead of memorized. The equation is valid for convex and concave mirrors:

$$1/i + 1/o = 1/f$$
$$f = R/2$$
$$M = \text{magnification} = -i/o$$

    conventions: for i and o, positive values mean real, negative values mean
                    virtual,
        for R and f, positive means converging, negative is diverging,
        for M, positive means erect, negative is inverted.

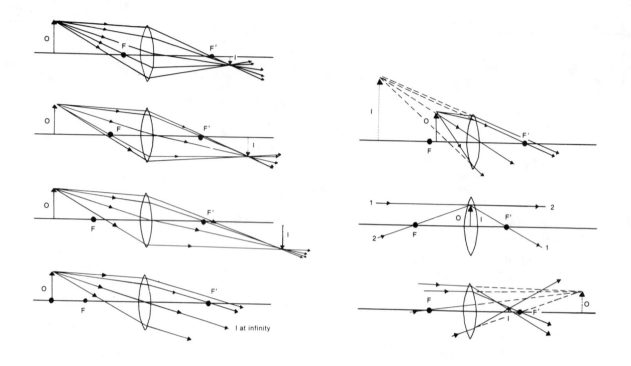

*Fig. 5.37(a)—Refraction through Convex Lens*

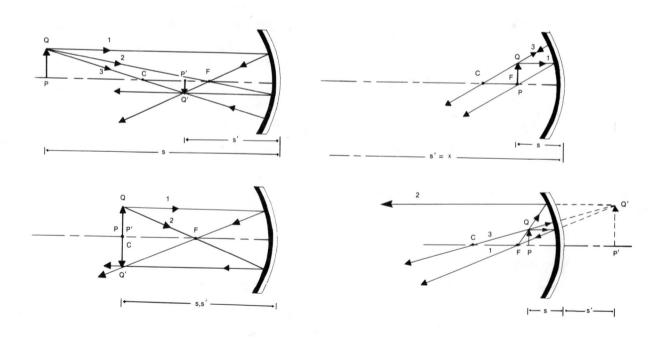

*Fig. 5.37(b)—Reflection from Concave Mirrors*

## 5.12.1.3   REFRACTION

*Refraction* is the bending of light as it passes from one transparent medium to another and is caused by the different speeds of light in the two media. If $\Theta_1$ is taken as the angle (to the normal) of the incident light and $\Theta_2$ is the angle (to the normal) of refracted light, where 1 and 2 represent the different media, the following relations hold (*Snell's Law*)(Fig. 5.38):

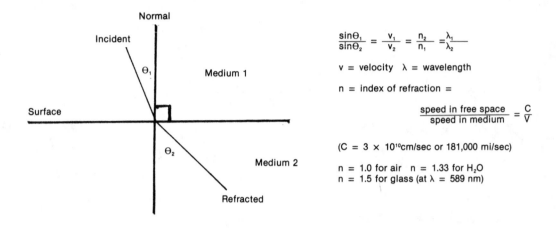

$$\frac{\sin\Theta_1}{\sin\Theta_2} = \frac{v_1}{v_2} = \frac{n_2}{n_1} = \frac{\lambda_1}{\lambda_2}$$

v = velocity   λ = wavelength

n = index of refraction =

$$\frac{\text{speed in free space}}{\text{speed in medium}} = \frac{C}{V}$$

(C = $3 \times 10^{10}$ cm/sec or 181,000 mi/sec)

n = 1.0 for air   n = 1.33 for $H_2O$
n = 1.5 for glass (at λ = 589 nm)

*Fig. 5.38—Refraction*

Note that the $\Theta$ is smaller (closer to the normal) in the more optically dense (higher n) medium. Also the smaller the wavelength of the incident light (i.e., toward the violet end), the closer is $\Theta_2$ to the normal (i.e., it is smaller than $\Theta_1$). This means longer wavelengths travel faster in a medium than shorter wavelengths. This leads to dispersion which is the separation of white light (all colors together) into the individual colors by this differential refraction. For example, a prism disperses white light. The *Laws of Refraction* are:

(1) The incident ray, the refracted ray and the normal ray all lie in the same plane.
(2) The path of the ray (incident and refracted parts) is reversible.

When light passes from a more optically dense (higher n) medium into a less optically dense medium, there exists an angle of incidence such that the angle of refraction ($\Theta_2$) is 90°. This special angle of incidence is called the critical angle ($\Theta_C$). This is because when the angle of incidence is less than $\Theta_C$, refraction occurs. If the angle of incidence is equal to $\Theta_C$, then neither refraction nor reflection occur. And if $\Theta_1 > \Theta_C$, then *internal reflection* (ray is reflected back into the more dense medium) occurs. The $\Theta_C$ is found from Snell's Law:

$n_1 \sin \Theta_C = n_2 \sin \Theta_2$
$n_1 \sin \Theta_C = n_2(1)$     (Since $\Theta_2 = 90°$ and sin 90° = 1)
$\sin \Theta_C = n_2/n_1$
    e.g., $\Theta_C = 42°$ for glass and air.

When looking at an object under water from above the surface, the object appears closer than it actually is. This is due to refraction. In general:

apparent depth/actual depth = $n_2/n_1$

$n_2$ = medium of observer
$n_1$ = medium of object.

A *lens* is a transparent material which refracts light. Converging lenses refract light toward the axis, and diverging lenses refract the light away from the axis. A converging lens is wider at the middle than at the ends, and a diverging lens is thinner at the middle than at the ends (Fig. 5.39).

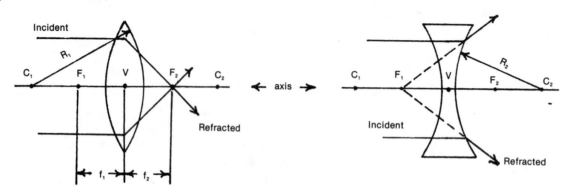

*Fig. 5.39—Lens*

R = radius of curvature

If the surface (note) is convex, the R is positive ($R_1$, e.g.). If the surface is concave the R is negative ($R_2$, e.g.). Subscript 1 refers to the incident side, subscript 2 refers to the refracted side.

C = center of curvature
F = focal point
V = optical center of the lens
axis = line through C and V

f = focal length is distance between V and F
i = image distance (from V to image)
o = object distance (from V to object)

The path of rays through a lens is:

(1) incident rays parallel to the axis refract through $F_2$ of a converging lens, and appear to come from $F_1$ of a diverging lens (backward extensions of the refracted ray, see dotted line on diverging diagram);

(2) an incident ray through $F_1$ of a converging lens or through $F_2$ of a diverging lens (if extended) are refracted parallel to the axis;

(3) incident rays through V are not deviated (refracted).

For a *converging lens* (biconvex, e.g.) the image formed depends on the object distance relative to the focal length (f). The relations (note similarity to a converging mirror) are:

(1) if $o < f_1$, the image is virtual and erect,
    if $o > f_1$, the image is real and inverted,

(2) if $o = f_1$, no image is formed,

(3) if $o < 2f_1(R)$, image is enlarged in size,
    if $o > 2f_1$, image is reduced in size,
    if $o = 2f_1$, image is the same size.

For a *diverging lens* (biconcave, e.g.), the image is always virtual, erect and reduced in size as for a diverging mirror.

The above relations can be calculated rather than memorized by the use of the *lens equation* (similar to the mirror equation) and derivations from it,

> (1) $1/o + 1/i = 1/f$ (lens equation, same as mirror equation)
> (2) *dioptres* (D) $= 1/f$ where f is in meters
>    Measures the refractive power of the lens, the larger the dioptres (D) the stronger the lens. It has a $+D$ for converging lens and a $-D$ for diverging lens. To get the refractive power (D) of lenses in series just add the dioptres which can then be converted into focal length:
>
> $$D_T = D_1 + D_2 = 1/f_T$$
>
> (3) Note that you cannot add focal lengths except as reciprocals:
>    $1/f_T = 1/f_1 + 1/f_2.$
> (4) $M = $ magnification $= -i/o$
>    $M = M_1 M_2$ for lens in series.

Conventions:

> (1) for i and o, positive values are real, negative values are virtual,
> (2) for R, see above,
> (3) for f, positive means converging, negative is diverging,
> (4) for M, positive means erect, negative is inverted.

The lens equation holds only for thin lenses—the thickness is small relative to other dimensions.

For a combination of lenses not in contact with each other, the image is found for the first lens (nearer the object) and then this image is used as the object of the second lens to find the image formed by it (see questions for examples).

## 5.12.2    Questions to Review Optics

(1)    Using the diagram below, select the *incorrect* statement of the Laws of Reflection of light from surfaces

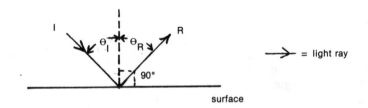

(a) $\Theta_I = \Theta_R$
(b) $\Theta_I + \Theta_R = 90°$
(c) I, N and R all lie in the same plane
(d) both (a) and (c)

(2)    All are true of images seen in plane (flat) mirrors *except:*

(a) they are always virtual
(b) they appear at a distance behind the mirror equal to the distance (perpendicular) of the object in front of the mirror
(c) they are right-left reversed
(d) they are inverted

(3)    A virtual image:

(a) cannot be projected onto a screen
(b) has light rays passing through it
(c) cannot be formed by plane (flat) mirrors
(d) all are correct

(4)    The reflected light rays from a smooth concave mirror:

(a) converge
(b) diverge
(c) are parallel
(d) are diffuse

(5)    The reflected rays from a convex mirror:

(a) diverge
(b) converge
(c) are parallel
(d) are diffuse

(6)    In terms of the reflected light and images, concave mirrors are most like:

(a) triangular prisms
(b) square prisms
(c) concave lens
(d) convex lens

(7)    In terms of reflected light and images, a convex mirror is most like a(n):

(a) convex lens
(b) concave lens
(c) triangular prism
(d) square prism

(8)    For the spherical convex mirror below:
($f_1 = f_2$; $R_1 = R_2$; f = focal length; R = radius of curvature)

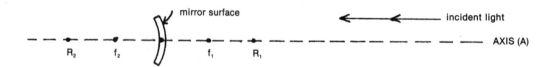

(a) incident rays parallel to A reflect through $f_1$
(b) incident rays passing through $R_1$ reflect through $R_2$
(c) the forward extensions of incident rays that reflect through $f_2$ pass through $f_1$
(d) the backward extensions of reflected rays that result from incident rays parallel to A pass through $f_2$

(9)    For the spherical concave mirror below:

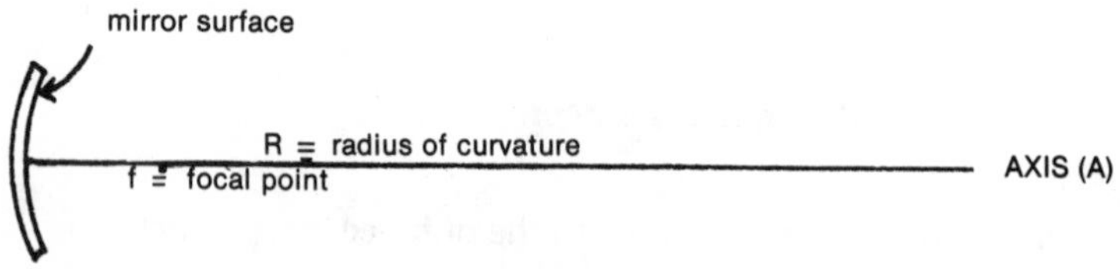

mirror surface

R = radius of curvature
f = focal point          AXIS (A)

(a) incident rays parallel to A reflect through f
(b) incident rays passing through R reflect parallel to A
(c) incident rays through f reflect through R
(d) all of the above are correct

(10)    For a convex mirror with f = focal length, R = radius of curvature, and o = object distance (along the axis) from the mirror, then

(a) images are always virtual, erect and reduced in size
(b) if o > f, the image is virtual and inverted
(c) if o = R, the image and object are the same size
(d) if o > R, the image is larger than the object

(11)    For a concave mirror with f = focal length, R = radius of curvature and o = distance (along the axis) of the object from the mirror, then

(a) if o < f, then the image is real and inverted
(b) if o = f, then no image if formed
(c) if o > f, then the image is virtual and erect
(d) if o > R, then the image is larger than the object

(12)    The mirror equation is:
(f = focal length, o = object distance, i = image distance)

(a) $f = o + i$
(b) $f = 1/o + 1/i$
(c) $1/f = o + i$
(d) $1/f = 1/o + 1/i$

(13)    If f = focal length, R = radius of curvature of a spherical mirror, then:

(a) $f = 2R$
(b) $f = R/2$
(c) $f = R^2$
(d) $f = \sqrt{R}$

(14)    If i = image distance and o = object distance from a mirror, then linear magnification (m) is:

(a) $m = -i/o$
(b) $m = (i)(o)$
(c) $m = -o/i$
(d) $m = 1/(i)(o)$

(15)    The phenomenon of refraction ("bending" of light rays) is attributable to

(a) the particle character of light
(b) the varying speeds of light in different media
(c) the longitudinal wave character of light
(d) none of the above

(16)    Given the diagram below for refraction of light, the correct relationship between the angles (Θ) shown and the velocities (v) of light in the media is:

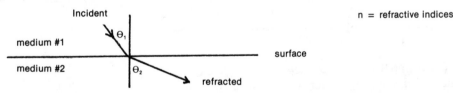

(a) $n_2\sin\Theta_1 = n_1\sin\Theta_2$
(b) $n_1 \Theta_1 = n_2\Theta_2$
(c) $\sin\Theta_1/\sin\Theta_2 = n_2/n_1$
(d) $\Theta_1/\Theta_2 = n_1/n_2$

(17)    The index of refraction of a medium is

(a) the speed of light in free space divided by the speed of light in that medium
(b) the density of the medium divided by the density of air
(c) the absorption of light in the medium divided by the absorption of light in water
(d) none of the above

(18) Dispersion of white light into its component colors (as in a prism) occurs by the process of:

(a) diffraction
(b) polarization
(c) refraction
(d) reflection

(19) A critical angle of incidence ($\Theta_c$)

(a) is reached when light passes from a lower optically dense medium into a higher optically dense medium
(b) means that the angle of refraction is 90°
(c) means that at all angles of incidence less than $\Theta_c$, light is reflected
(d) all of the above

(20) A converging lens should be

(a) of equal width at the middle and ends
(b) wider at the ends than at the middle
(c) wider at the middle than at the ends
(d) may be any of the above

(21) A concave lens:

(a) diverges light
(b) converges light
(c) both
(d) neither

(22) Select the correct statement concerning the lens below:
V = vertex; F = focal point; C = center of curvature

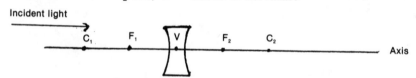

(a) If the incident rays are parallel to the axis, the backward extensions of the refracted rays pass through $C_1$
(b) If the forward extension of an incident ray would pass through $F_2$, then the backward extension of the refracted ray would pass through $F_1$
(c) Incident rays through V are not refracted
(d) All of the above are correct

(23) Select the correct statement concerning the lens below:
F = focal points; C = center of curvature; V = vertex

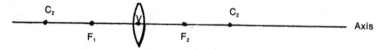

(a) Incident rays parallel to the axis refract through $C_2$
(b) Incident rays through $F_1$ refract parallel to the axis
(c) Incident rays through V refract along the axis
(d) All of the above are correct

(24) Concerning the image formed by a converging lens, select the *incorrect* statement:
(f = focal length, o = object distance from lens)

(a) If o < f, the image is virtual and erect
(b) If o = f, no image is formed
(c) If o > f, the image is real and inverted
(d) If o < 2f, the object is reduced in size

(25) Select the correct statement concerning the image formed by a diverging lens:
(f = focal length, o = object distance)

(a) If o > f, the image is virtual and inverted
(b) If o < 2f, the image is real and reduced
(c) All images are virtual, erect and reduced
(d) All images are real, inverted and enlarged

(26) Dioptres:

(a) the number of degrees of visual acuity
(b) a type of lens that corrects astigmatism
(c) the refractive power of a lens
(d) the reflective power of a mirror

(27) A concave mirror with a focal length (f) = 4 cms forms an image (i) of an object (o) placed 10 cms from it. The magnification (M) of this image is:

(a) ⅓ of the object
(b) ⅔ of the object
(c) ⅚ times the object
(d) 3 times the object

(28) An object (o) is placed 10 cms from a concave mirror with focal length (f) = 2 cms. The image is:

(a) real, inverted, reduced and 2.50 cms from the mirror
(b) virtual, erect, enlarged and 8 cms from the mirror

(29) An image formed by a concave mirror is 5 cms from the mirror, erect and virtual. If the focal length of the mirror is 2 cms, the object is how far from the mirro?

(a) ⅚ cms
(b) 2 cms
(c) ¹⁰⁄₇ cms
(d) ⅜ cms

(30) Optically dense media have high indices of refraction. From the diagram below, select the correct statement:

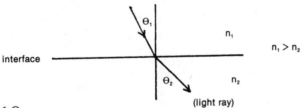

(a) $\Theta_1 < \Theta_2$
(b) $\Theta_1 = \Theta_2$
(c) $\Theta_1 > \Theta_1$
(d) need more information

(31) The index of refraction (n) for water is 1.5. The speed of light in water is:

(a) $4.5 \times 10^{10}$ cm/sec
(b) $2 \times 10^{10}$ cm/sec
(c) $3 \times 10^{10}$ cm/sec
(d) need the frequency of light in water to determine the speed

(32) If violet light and red light both have the same angle of incidence, which statement is correct concerning the angles of refraction?

(a) the angles of refraction are equal
(b) the angle of refraction of the violet light is larger
(c) the angle of refraction of the red light is larger
(d) need velocities in the media to evaluate

(33)   A ray of light passing from a type of glass into air has a critical angle ($\Theta_c$) of:
(n = index of refraction, n of air = 1.00 and n of glass = 2.00)

(a) 5°
(b) 15°
(c) 30°
(d) 45°

(34)   A fish is 8 meters from the surface in a tank of water. Looking from the air surface, the fish would appear to be how deep?
(n of air = 1.00, n of water = 1.33)

(a) 6 m
(b) 8 m
(c) 10.67 m
(d) need the angles of incidence and refraction

(35)   An object is 15 cms from a converging lens with a focal length of 5 cms. The image formed is:

(a) no image is formed
(b) virtual, erect, reduced
(c) real, erect, enlarged
(d) real, inverted, reduced

(36)   An object is placed 8 cms from a biconcave lens with a focal length of 10 cms. The image formed is:

(a) virtual, erect, reduced
(b) real, inverted, reduced
(c) real, erect, enlarged
(d) virtual, inverted, reduced

(37)   An object is placed 5 cms from a diverging lens with a focal length of 10 cms. The image formed is:

(a) virtual, inverted, enlarged
(b) virtual, erect, reduced
(c) real, inverted, enlarged
(d) real, erect, reduced

(38)   A 20 cm tall object is placed 5 cms from a convex lens with a focal length of 10 cms. The image is:

(a) real, erect, 2.5 cms from lens and 10 cms tall
(b) virtual, erect, 10 cms from lens and 40 cms tall
(c) real, inverted, 10 cms from lens and 40 cms tall
(d) virtual, inverted, 2.5 cms from lens and 10 cms tall

(39)   An object 10 cms tall is placed 20 cms from a concave lens with a focal length of 5 cms. The image is:

(a) virtual, inverted, 40 cms from lens and 20 cms tall
(b) virtual, erect, 4 cms from lens and 4 cms tall
(c) real, inverted, 40 cms from lens, 20 cms tall
(d) real, erect, 4 cms from lens and 4 cms tall

(40)   A lens with a focal length of 10 cms is how many dioptres?

(a) 0.10
(b) 1
(c) 10
(d) 100

(41) A lens of 2 dioptres has a focal length equal to:

(a) 50 cms
(b) 25 cms
(a) 4 cms
(d) 0.5 cms

(42) A diverging lens of focal length (f) 20 cms is placed in contact with a converging lens of focal length (f₂) 10 cms, the focal length (f) of the combination is:

(a) $^{10}/_3$ cms
(b) 10 cms
(c) 20 cms
(d) 30 cms

(43) Which of the following is not a converging lens?

(44) Which structure is anterior to the lens in the human eye?

(a) aqueous humor
(b) vitreous humor
(c) retina
(d) choroid

(45) From the outside in, the sequence of layers of the eye is:
(C = choroid, R = retina, S = sclera)

(a) S,C,R
(b) C,R,S
(c) R,S,C
(d) S,R,C

(46) Select the incorrect association of structure and function in the eye:

(a) cornea—scatters light
(b) choroid—prevents light scattering
(c) iris—regulates amount of light that enters eye
(d) ciliary muscle—controls shape of the lens

(47) Select the *incorrect* statement concerning rods and cones of the eye:

(a) rods are for vision in dim light
(b) rods are located peripherally in the eye
(c) cones are for color vision
(d) cones contain rhodopsin

(48) All are function or properties of cones of the eye except:

(a) provide for high visual acuity
(b) peripheral vision
(c) color vision
(d) vision in bright lights

(49) Select the correct path of light through the eye (anterior to posterior):

(a) cornea, aqueous humor, lens, vitreous humor, retina
(b) lens, aqueous humor, cornea, vitreous humor, retina
(c) cornea, vitreous humor, lens, aqueous humor, retina
(d) retina, cornea, aqueous humor, lens, vitreous humor

(50)   Select incorrect statement:

    (a) converging lenses will correct for myopic eyes
    (b) light is focused in front of the retina when objects are distant in myopic eyes
    (c) light is focused behind the retina when objects are near in hypermetropic eyes
    (d) convex lens will correct hypermetropic eyes

## 5.12.3     Answers to Questions in Section 5.12.2

( 1) b  ( 2) d  ( 3) a  ( 4) a  ( 5) a  ( 6) d  ( 7) b  ( 8) d  ( 9) a  (10) a  (11) b
(12) d  (13) b  (14) a  (15) b  (16) c  (17) a  (18) c  (19) b  (20) c  (21) a  (22) c
(23) b  (24) d  (25) c  (26) c  (27) b  (28) a  (29) c  (30) a  (31) b  (32) c  (33) c
(34) a  (35) d  (36) a  (37) b  (38) b  (39) b  (40) c  (41) a  (42) c  (43) d  (44) a
(45) a  (46) a  (47) d  (48) b  (49) a  (50) a

## 5.12.4     Discussion of Answers to Questions in Section 5.12.2

*Questions #1 to #26* Adequately discussed in the Section.

*Question #27* (Answer: b) Use the mirror equation:

$$1/f = 1/o + 1/i$$
$$f = +4 \text{ cm because of converging mirror}$$
$$\tfrac{1}{4} = \tfrac{1}{10} + 1/i$$
$$20i(\tfrac{1}{4}) = 20i(\tfrac{1}{10}) + 20i(1/i)$$
(note 20i is the least common denominator)
$$5i = 2i + 20$$
$$3i = 20$$
$$i = \tfrac{20}{3} \text{ cms from the mirror and is real}$$

$$m = -i/o = (-\tfrac{20}{3})/10 = (-\tfrac{20}{3})(\tfrac{1}{10}) = -\tfrac{2}{3} \text{ of the object}$$

    The image is inverted (because it is negative).

*Question #28* (Answer: a) Use the mirror equation:

$$1/f = 1/o + 1/i$$
$$f = +2m \text{ because of converging mirror}$$
$$\tfrac{1}{2} = \tfrac{1}{10} + 1/i$$
$$10i(\tfrac{1}{2}) = 10i(\tfrac{1}{10}) + 10i(1/i)$$
$$5i = i + 10$$
$$4i = 10$$
$$i = \tfrac{10}{4} = +\tfrac{5}{2} = 2.50 \text{ cms from the mirror}$$

Since, o (10 cms) > f (2cms), the image is real and inverted.
Since, o (10 cms) > R (4cms), the image is reduced
$$R = 2f = 2 \cdot 2 = 4.$$

*Question #29* (Answer: c) Use the mirror equation:

$$1/f = 1/o + 1/i$$
$$i = -5cm \text{ because it is virtual}$$
$$f = +2cm \text{ because the mirror is converging}$$
$$\tfrac{1}{2} = 1/o - \tfrac{1}{5}$$
$$10o(\tfrac{1}{2}) = 10o(1/o) - 10o(\tfrac{1}{5})$$
$$5o = 10 - 2o$$
$$7o = 10$$
$$o = \tfrac{10}{7} \text{ cms.}$$

*Question #30* (Answer: a) The angle to the normal is smaller in the more optically dense medium for refraction of light.

*Question #31* (Answer: b)

$$n = \text{speed in free space/speed in medium (s)}$$
$$1.5 = (3.0 \times 10^{10} \text{ cm/sec})/s$$
$$s = (3.0 \times 10^{10})/1.5 = (2)(10^{10} \text{ cm/sec}) = 2 \times 10^{10} \text{ cm/sec.}$$

*Question #32* (Answer: c) For light, the smaller the wavelength, the closer the refracted ray to the normal. Since violet light has a shorter wavelength than red, red light will be refracted through a larger angle.

*Question #33* (Answer: c)

$$\sin \Theta_c = n_2/n_1 = 1.00/2.00 = 0.5$$
$$n_2 = \text{less optically dense (air)}$$
$$n_1 = \text{more optically dense (glass)}$$
$$\Theta_c = 30°$$

You should remember that $\sin 30° = \frac{1}{2}$
or recall that in a 30°-60° right
triangle the following is true:

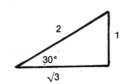

$$\sin 30° = \frac{1}{2}$$

*Question #34* (Answer: a) apparent depth $(D_a)$/actual depth $= n_2/n_1$

$$n_2 = \text{of observer} = 1.00$$
$$n_1 = \text{of object} = 1.33$$
$$D_a/8 = 1.00/1.33 = 1/(\frac{4}{3}) = \frac{3}{4}$$
$$D_a = (\frac{3}{4})(8) = 6 \text{ meters.}$$

*Question #35* (Answer: d) Since the object distance is greater than the focal length, the image is real and inverted. Since the object distance is more than twice the focal length, the image is reduced in size.

*Question #36* (Answer: a) A biconcave lens is a diverging lens. The image is always virtual, erect and reduced in size.

*Question #37* (Answer: b) All images formed by diverging lenses are virtual, erect and reduced.

*Question #38* (Answer: b) Use the lens equation:

$$1/f = 1/o + 1/i$$
$$f = +10 \text{cm because of converging lens}$$
$$\frac{1}{10} = \frac{1}{5} + 1/i$$
$$10i(\frac{1}{10}) = 10i(\frac{1}{5}) + 10i(1/i)$$
$$i = 2i + 10$$
$$-i = 10$$
$$i = -10 \text{ cm}$$
this means the object is virtual (negative sign) and 10 cms from the mirror
$$M = \text{magnification} = -i/o = -(-10)/5 = +2$$
∴ the image is erect (positive sign) and is $2(20) = 40$ cms tall.

*Question #39* (Answer: b) A concave lens is a diverging lens. Use the lens equation:

$$1/f = 1/o + 1/i$$
$$f = -5 \text{cms because of diverging lens}$$
$$\tfrac{1}{-5} = \tfrac{1}{20} + 1/i$$
$$20i(\tfrac{1}{-5}) = 20i(\tfrac{1}{20}) + 20i(1/i)$$
$$-4i = i + 20$$
$$-5i = 20$$
$$i = -4 \text{cms (negative means virtual)}$$
$$m = \text{magnification} = -i/o = -(-4)/10 = \tfrac{4}{10} = \tfrac{2}{5}$$

positive M means the object is erect; the image is $(\tfrac{2}{5})(10) = 4$ cms tall.

*Question #40* (Answer: c)

$$\text{dioptres} = 1/\text{focal length in meters} = 1/(\tfrac{1}{10}) = (1)(\tfrac{10}{1}) = 10$$
$$10 \text{ cms} = \tfrac{1}{10} \text{ meter}$$

*Question #41* (Answer: a)

$$\text{dioptres (d)} = 1/\text{focal length in meters (f)}$$
$$d = 1/f$$
$$f = 1/d = \tfrac{1}{2}m$$
$$\tfrac{1}{2}m = (\tfrac{1}{2}m)(100 \text{ cms}/1m) = 50 \text{ cms.}$$

*Question #42* (Answer: c) The focal length of lenses in contact is found by:

dioptres: lens #1: $20 \text{ cm} = \tfrac{1}{5}m$
$$D_1 = -5 \text{ (because diverging)}$$
lens #2: $10 \text{ cm} = \tfrac{1}{10}m$
$$D_2 = 10$$

Total dioptres: $D_T = D_1 + D_2 = -5 + 10 = +5$
Then $f_T = f = 1/D_T = \tfrac{1}{5}m$ or 20 cm

*Question #43* (Answer: d) A converging lens is smaller at the edges than the middle—this holds for (a), (b) and (c). The lens in (d) is larger at the ends than in the middle.

*Questions #44 to #50:* Adequately discussed in the Section.


## 5.12.5    Vocabulary, Concepts, etc. Checklist for Optics

_____ reflection
_____ virtual image
_____ real image
_____ combination of lenses
_____ spherical mirror
_____ Snell's Law
_____ total internal reflection
_____ center of curvature
_____ aqueous humor
_____ sclera
_____ choroid
_____ pupil
_____ ciliary muscle
_____ rods
_____ retinal
_____ cones
_____ fovea
_____ hypermetropia

_____ diverging lens
_____ dioptres
_____ plane mirror
_____ lens equation
_____ mirror equation
_____ focal length
_____ converging lens
_____ vitreous humor
_____ cornea
_____ iris
_____ lens
_____ retina
_____ rhodopsin
_____ opsin
_____ iodopsin
_____ emmetropia
_____ myopia

## 5.13 NUCLEAR STRUCTURE, AND ATOMIC AND QUANTUM PHYSICS

### 5.13.1 Review of Nuclear Structure, and Atomic and Quantum Physics

#### 5.13.1.1 REVIEW OF NUCLEAR STRUCTURE

An atom is made of a *nucleus* containing protons (mass = 1 a.m.u., charge +1) and neutrons (mass = 1 a.m.u., charge = O ). The *atomic number (AN)* is the number of protons in the nucleus of an atom. An *element* is a group of atoms with the same AN; i.e., it is the number of protons that make elements different from each other. The *mass number* (MN) is the sum of protons and neutrons in a given atom (not element!). *Isotopes* are atoms of the same element with different MNs, i.e., they have the same number of protons but different numbers of neutrons. The *atomic weight* (AW) is the weighted average of all naturally occurring isotopes of an element. Note that it is the number of protons that distinguishes one element from another, and it is the electron configuration (Section 3.1.1) of a given element that determines its chemical reactivity.

Coulomb repulsive force (between protons) in the nuclei are overcome by *nuclear forces.* The nuclear force is a nonelectrical type of force that binds nuclei together and is equal for protons and neutrons. The *nuclear binding energy* ($E_b$) is a result of the Coulomb and nuclear binding forces. Einstein derived the relation between energy and mass changes associated with nuclear reactions,

$$\Delta E = \Delta mc^2 = \text{ergs if m = grams and c = cm/sec}$$
$$\Delta E = \text{energy released or absorbed}$$
$$\Delta m = \text{mass lost (\textit{mass deficit}) or gained, respectively}$$
$$c = \text{speed of light} = 3.0 \times 10^{10} \text{ cm/sec}$$

conversions:

$$1 \text{ gram} = 9 \times 10^{20} \text{ ergs}$$
$$1 \text{ amu (atomic mass unit)} = 931.4 \text{ MeV}$$
$$1 \text{ amu} = \tfrac{1}{12} \text{ the mass of } 6C^{12}$$

The above is a statement of the *Law of Conservation of Mass and Energy.* The value of $E_b$ depends upon the mass number (MN) as follows,

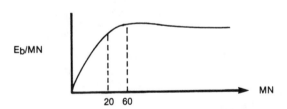

$E_b$/MN = binding energy per nucleon; this is the energy released by the formation of a given nucleus.

*Fig. 5.40—Binding Energy Diagram*

Note that the peak $E_b$/MN is at MN = 60. Also, the $E_b$/MN is relatively constant after MN = 20. *Fission* is when a nucleus splits into smaller nuclei. *Fusion* is when small nuclei combine to form a larger nucleus. Energy is released from a nuclear reaction (see diagram above) when nuclei with mass number ≫ 60 undergo fission or nuclei ≪ 60 undergo fusion.

Not all combinations of protons are equally likely or stable. An even number of protons or an even number of neutrons, in general, means the nuclei are more stable. The *most stable* nuclei are those with an even number of protons and an even number of neutrons. The *least stable* nuclei are those with an odd number of protons and an odd number of neutrons. Also, as the atomic number (AN) increases, there are more neutrons (N) needed for the nuclei to be stable (Fig. 5.41).

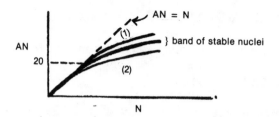

*Fig. 5.41—Stability of Atoms*

Up to AN = 20 (Calcium) the protons equal the neutrons, aftre this there are more neutrons. If an atom is in region #1 above, it has too many protons or too few neutrons and must decrease its protons or increase its neutrons to become stable. The reverse is true for region #2. Also all nuclei after AN = 84 (Polonium) are unstable.

Unstable nuclei can become stable nuclei by fission (splitting) to smaller nuclei or by absorbing or emitting small particles. Spontaneous fission is rare. *Spontaneous radioactivity* (emitting particles) is common. The common particles are (1) *alpha (α) particle* $_2He^4$ (helium nucleus); (2) *beta (β) particle* $-1e^0$ (an electron); (3) a *positron* $+1e^0$; (4) gamma (γ) ray—no mass, just energy; and (5) *orbital electron capture*—nucleus takes electrons from K shell and converts a proton to a neutron. If there is a flux of particles such as neutrons ($_0n^1$), the nucleus can absorb these also.

*Nuclear reactions* are reactions in which changes in nuclear composition occur. An example of nuclear reactions and the terminology is:

$$_{92}U^{238} + 1H^2 \rightarrow _{93}Np^{238} + 2_0n^1$$

Note:

$U^{238} \leftarrow \text{mass number} \rightarrow ^{238}U$
$^{92} \leftarrow \text{atomic number} \rightarrow ^{92}$

the sum of the lower (higher) numbers on one side of the equation equals the sum of the lower (higher) numbers on the other side.

Another way of writing the above reaction is:

$$_{92}U^{238}(_1H^2, 2_0n^1)_{93}Np^{238}$$

Spontaneous radioactive decay is a *first order process*. This means that the rate of decay is directly proportional to the amount of material present:

$$\Delta m/\Delta t \propto m$$

$\Delta m$ = change in mass
$\Delta t$ = change in time
$m$ = mass present at a given time
$\Delta m/\Delta t$ = rate of decay.

This relation is equalized by adding a proportionality constant called the *decay constant* (k),

$$\Delta m/\Delta t = -km \text{ (equation #1)}$$

The minus sign indicates that mass is disappearing. The meaning of k is:

$k = -(\Delta m/m)/\Delta t$ = fraction of the mass that decays with time.
(equation #2)

Note that k = 1/time. If time is seconds, then k = 1/secs. This means that if k = 0.1/sec, then $\frac{1}{10}$ of the substance (that is present at that time) will disappear in the next second.

The *half-life* ($T\frac{1}{2}$) of a radioactive atom is the time required for one-half of it to disintegrate. The $T\frac{1}{2}$ is related to k as follows,

$$T\frac{1}{2} = 0.693/k.$$

This is derived from equation #1 by calculus. Although not exactly correct, the amount left after n half-lives is:

amount left = $(\frac{1}{2})^n$ m

m = mass began with

n = number of half-lives = elapsed time/$T\frac{1}{2}$

Or, the amount that has disappeared can be calculated using k from equation #2 and is:

amount decayed = $\Delta m$ = (k)($\Delta t$)(m)

k = decay constant

$\Delta t$ = elapsed time

m = mass began with.

## 5.13.1.2   REVIEW OF ATOMIC AND QUANTUM PHYSICS

The energy that an electron contains is not continuous over the whole range of possible energies. Rather, electrons in an atom may contain only discrete energies and occupy certain orbits. Electrons of each atom are restricted to these discrete energy levels. These levels have an energy below zero. This means energy is released when an electron moves from infinity into these energy levels. A representative set of energy levels of an electron in an atom may be:

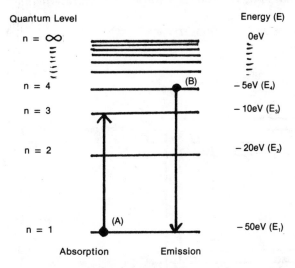

Fig. 5.42—*Absorption and Emission Spectra*

If there is one electron in the atom above, its *ground state* will be in the n = 1, or lowest energy level available. Any other energy level, n = 2 or n = 3, e.g., is considered an *excited state* for that electron. The difference in energies (E) between the levels gives the energy and, hence, frequency (f) of light necessary to cause the excitation (absorption, electron A):

$E_3 - E_1$ = hf

$E_1$ = energy level one

$E_3$ = energy level three

h = Planck's Constant

f = frequency of light absorbed.

So, if light is passed through a substance (gas, e.g.), certain wavelengths (since $\lambda$ = c/f, c = speed of light, $\lambda$ = wavelength) will be absorbed, which corresponds to the energy needed for the electron transitions. An *absorption spectrum* will result that has dark lines against a light background. Multiple lines result because there are possible transitions from all quantum levels occupied by electrons to any unoccupied levels (e.g., n = 1 to n = 2, n = 3, etc., n = 2 to n = 3, n = 4, etc.).

An *emission spectrum* results when an electron is excited to a higher level by another particle or by an electric discharge, for example. Then, as the electron falls from the excited state to lower states, light is emitted that has wavelength (frequency) corresponding to the energy difference between the levels. As an example (emission, electron B):

$$E_1 - E_4 = hf$$

The resulting spectrum will have light lines against a dark background.

The absorption and emission spectrums should have the same number of lines but often will not. This is because in the absorption spectrum, there is rapid radiation of the absorbed light in all directions, and transitions are generally from the ground state initially. These factors result in fewer lines in the absorption than in the emission spectrum.

*Flourescence* is an emission process that occurs after light absorption excites electrons to higher electronic and vibrational levels. The electrons spontaneously lose excited vibrational energy to the electronic level and then emit light as they fall to the ground vibrational and electronic states. There are certain molecular types that possess this property, e.g., some amino acids (tryptophan).

The *fluorescence* process is depicted as follows:

Step 1 — absorption light
Step 2 — spontaneous deactivation of vibrational levels to zero vibrational level for electronic state
Step 3 — fluorescence with light emission (longer wavelength than absorption).

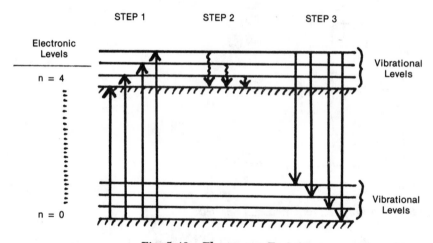

*Fig. 5.43—Fluorescent Emission*

### 5.13.2    Questions to Review Nuclear Structure, and Atomic and Quantum Physics

(1)    A proton is _____ charged and has a mass of _____ amu(s).

(a) positively, one
(b) negatively, $\frac{1}{1845}$
(c) neutral, one
(d) none of the above

(2)    The sum of protons and neutrons in a nucleus is called the:

(a) electron number
(b) atomic number
(c) atomic weight
(d) mass number

(3)    Isotopes have the _____ atomic numbers and _____ mass numbers.

    (a) same, same
    (b) same, different
    (c) different, same
    (d) different, different

(4)    The particles that distinguish one element from another are the:

    (a) neutrons
    (b) protons
    (c) electrons
    (d) mesons

(5)    The particle of the nucleus that has mass and is neutral is called the:

    (a) neutron
    (b) proton
    (c) neutrino
    (d) meson

(6)    Which particle has no mass?

    (a) neutron
    (b) meson
    (c) neutrino
    (d) electron

(7)    The nuclear binding energy of nuclei depends on:

    (a) coulomb forces
    (b) nuclear forces
    (c) both
    (d) neither

(8)    If $\Delta E$ = the energy change, $\Delta m$ = mass change and c = the speed of light, the correct relation between these for describing the conversion of mass and energy is

    (a) $\Delta E = \Delta m/c$
    (b) $\Delta E = c^2/\Delta m$
    (c) $\Delta E = \Delta mc$
    (d) $\Delta E = \Delta mc^2$

(9)    Which of the following statements is correct concerning binding energy $(E_b)$?

    (a) binding energy depends on protons only
    (b) binding is relatively constant at all mass numbers
    (c) the peak in binding energy per nucleon is at mass number = 60
    (d) none of the above

(10)    Which of the following particles is emitted by nuclei in spontaneous radioactivity?

    (a) $\alpha$-particle
    (b) $\beta$-particle
    (c) $\gamma$-ray
    (d) all of the above

(11)    The particle composed of two protons and two neutrons is the:

    (a) $\gamma$-ray
    (b) $\alpha$-particle
    (c) neutrino
    (d) positron

(12)    The rate of radioactive decay

   (a) is independent of the amount of material present
   (b) is inversely proportional to the amount of material present
   (c) varies unpredictably but does depend on the amount of material present
   (d) is directly proportional to the amount of material present

(13)    The radioactive decay constant

   (a) is the fraction of mass that decays in a given amount of time
   (b) is the amount of mass that decays in one half-life
   (c) is not related to the half-life
   (d) none of the above

(14)    The atomic number is the number of _____ contained in the nucleus.

   (a) neutrons
   (b) electrons
   (c) protons
   (d) positrons

(15)    The atomic weight of an element is

   (a) the weighted average of naturally occurring isotopes
   (b) the sum of protons and neutrons
   (c) twice the number of protons
   (d) none of the above

(16)    Carbon has an atomic number (AN) of 6. One of its isotopes has a mass number (MN) of 13. The number of neutrons in this isotope is:

   (a) 6
   (b) 7
   (c) 13
   (d) 19

(17)    An isotope of boron has 5 protons and 6 neutrons. The atomic number (AN) of boron is:

   (a) 11
   (b) 10
   (c) 6
   (d) 5

(18)    Suppose the natural abundance of the isotopes of berylium (atomic number = 4) is 90% of mass number = 8; 10% of mass number = 9. The atomic weight (AW) is:

   (a) 9.00
   (b) 8.50
   (c) 8.10
   (d) 8.00

(19)    An atom has an atomic number (AN) = 18 and a mass number (MN) = 38. Letting P = # of protons and N = # neutrons, which atom below is an isotope of this atom?

   (a) P = 18, N = 19
   (b) P = 20, N = 18
   (c) P = 19, N = 18
   (d) none of the above

(20)    A nuclear reaction proceeds with a mass deficit (mass loss) of $5 \times 10^{-5}$ gms. The amount of energy released is:

   (a) $1.5 \times 10^{6}$ ergs
   (b) $4.5 \times 10^{16}$ ergs
   (c) $9.0 \times 10^{20}$ ergs
   (d) none of the above

(21) The radioactive decay of a substance has a half-life ($T_{1/2}$) of 10 secs, the decay constant (k) is:

(a) 1.4 secs$^{-1}$
(b) 0.069 secs$^{-1}$
(c) 6.9 secs$^{-1}$
(d) none of the above

(22) After 20 days, how much of a substance with a half-life of 5 days is left if there were 10 gms initially?

(a) 2.50 gms
(b) 2 gms
(c) $5/8$ gm
(d) none of the above

(23) How much of 5 gms of radioactive substance with a half-life of 10 secs has decayed in 2 seconds?

(a) 1.38 gms
(b) 1.0 gms
(c) 0.69 gms
(d) none of the above

(24) What is the missing particle in the following reaction?   $_{27}Co^{59} + ? \rightarrow _{27}Co^{60}$

(a) proton
(b) electron
(c) neutron
(d) none of the above

(25) What is the missing particle in the following reaction?   $_{92}U^{238} + ? \rightarrow _{94}Pu^{239} + 3\,n$

(a) $\beta$-particle
(b) proton
(c) $\gamma$-ray
(d) none of the above

(26) Determine the amount of phosphorus left after 4 weeks if we start with 100 gms of $_{15}^{32}P$ (half-life = 14 days).

(a) 50 gms
(b) 37.5 gms
(c) 25 gms
(d) 12.5 gms

(27) The half-life of a substance called JUNKIUM is 11.5 hrs. How much time will it take to lose 25% of its original starting mass?

(a) 2.88 hrs
(b) 46 hrs
(c) 5.75 hrs
(d) 4.77 hrs

## 5.13.3    Answers to Questions in Section 5.13.2

( 1) a  ( 2) d  ( 3) b  ( 4) b  ( 5) a  ( 6) c  ( 7) c  ( 8) d  ( 9) c  (10) d  (11) b
(12) d  (13) a  (14) c  (15) a  (16) b  (17) d  (18) c  (19) a  (20) b  (21) b  (22) c
(23) c  (24) c  (25) d  (26) c  (27) d

## 5.13.4    Discussion of Answers to Questions in Section 5.13.2

*Questions #1 to #15* Adequately discussed in the Section.

*Question #16* (Answer: b)

$$MN = \text{protons (P)} + \text{neutrons (N)}$$
$$13 = 6 + N \ (AN = P)$$
$$7 = N.$$

*Question #17* (Answer: d) The AN is the number of protons.

*Question #18* (Answer: c) The AW is the weighted average of the naturally occurring isotopes. This is simply found by multiplying the percent abundance (as a decimal) of each isotope times the mass number of that isotope and adding all of these together:

$$AW = (0.90)(8) + (0.10)(9) = 7.2 + 0.9 = 8.1$$

*Question #19* (Answer: a) The AN = the number of protons and this must be the same because isotopes are of the same element. Therefore, the answer is (a).

*Question #20* (Answer: b)

$$\Delta E = \Delta mc^2 = (5 \times 10^{-5} \text{ gms})(3.0 \times 10^{10} \text{cm/sec})^2$$
$$= (5 \times 10^{-5})(9 \times 10^{20}) = 45 \times 10^{15} = 4.5 \times 10^{16} \text{ ergs.}$$

*Question #21* (Answer: b)

$$k = 0.693/T\tfrac{1}{2} = 0.693/10 \text{ secs} = 0.0693 \text{ secs}^{-1}$$

*Question #22* (Answer: c)

$$\text{amount left} = (\tfrac{1}{2})^n m = (\tfrac{1}{2})^{20/5}(10) = (\tfrac{1}{2})^4(10)$$
$$= (\tfrac{1}{16})(10) = {}^{10}\!/_{16}$$
$$= \tfrac{5}{8} \text{ gms}$$

*Question #23* (Answer: c) One may use $T\tfrac{1}{2}$ or k to find the amount left. In this case it is easier to use k:

$$k = 0.693/T\tfrac{1}{2} = 0.693/10 \text{ secs} = 0.069 \text{ secs}^{-1}$$
$$\text{amount left} = (k)(\Delta t)(m)$$
$$= (0.069)(2)(5) = (0.069)(10) = 0.69 \text{ gms}$$

*Question #24* (Answer: c) Adding the top numbers (the sum of protons and neutrons):

$$59 + x = 60$$
$$x = 1$$

Adding the bottom numbers (the number of protons):

$$27 + y = 27$$
$$y = 0.$$

The particle is then: $0^{?1}$
which fits the neutron; $0n^1$.

*Question #25* (Answer: d) See question #30 for steps:

top numbers
$$238 + x = 239 + 3(1) = 242$$
$$x = 242 - 238 = 4$$
bottom numbers
$$92 + y = 94 + 3(0) = 94$$
$$y = 94 - 92 = 2.$$

The particle is: $2^{?4}$
which fits the $\alpha$-particle (or helium nucleus): $2\,He^4$.

*Question #26* (Answer: c)

$$\frac{m}{m_O} = (\tfrac{1}{2})^{t/t_o}$$

$$m_O = 100 \text{ gms}$$
$$t_O = 14 \text{ days}$$
$$t = 4 \text{ weeks} = 28 \text{ days}$$
$$m = \text{mass left} = m_O(\tfrac{1}{2})^{t/t_o}$$
$$= 100(\tfrac{1}{2})^{28/14}$$
$$= 100(\tfrac{1}{2})^2 = 25 \text{ gms.}$$

*Question #27* (Answer: d)

$$t_O = 11.5 \text{ hrs.}$$
$$m_O = \text{starting mass}$$
$$\text{mass lost} = 0.25 \, m_O$$
$$\text{mass left} = m = m_O - 0.25 \, m_O = 0.75 \, m_O$$

$$\frac{m}{m_O} = (\tfrac{1}{2})^{t/t_o}$$

$$\frac{0.75 m_O}{m_O} = (\tfrac{1}{2})^{t/11.5}$$

$$0.75 = (\tfrac{1}{2})^{t/11.5}$$

$$\log 0.75 = \left(\frac{t}{11.5}\right) \log(\tfrac{1}{2})$$

$$\log 3 - \log 4 = \left(\frac{t}{11.5}\right) (\log 1 - \log 2)$$

(See Vol. II: *Skills Development for the Medical College Admission Test*—remember logs of common numbers)

$$4771 - 0.6021 = \frac{t}{11.5} (0 - 0.3010)$$

$$-0.1249 = \left(\frac{t}{11.5}\right) (-.3010)$$

$$t = 4.77 \text{ hrs.}$$

## 5.13.5    Vocabulary, Concepts, etc. Checklist for Nuclear Structure

_____ atomic number
_____ atomic weight
_____ binding energy (nuclear)
_____ neutrons
_____ protons
_____ half-life
_____ decay constant
_____ mass deficit

_____ $\Delta E = \Delta mc^2$
_____ mass number
_____ isotopes
_____ electrons
_____ $\beta$-particle
_____ nuclear reactions
_____ $\alpha$-particle

## 5.14    REFERENCES FOR REVIEW OF PHYSICS

Beiser, Arthur. *Basic Concepts of Physics*. 2nd or latest ed. (Addison-Wesley Publishing Company, Inc.)

Halliday, D., and R. Resnick. *Fundamentals of Physics*, 2nd or latest ed. (John Wiley and Sons, Inc.)

Harris, N. C. and E. M. Hemmerling. *Introductory Applied Physics*. 4th or latest ed. (McGraw-Hill Book Company)

Tippins, P. E. *Applied Physics*. 3rd or latest ed. (McGraw-Hill Book Company)

tz
blishing
mpany, Inc.

01-340-0030
00-634-4365

## like to order:

end the attached postcard
r write:
**Customer Service**
**etz Publishing Company**
. O. Box 34631
ethesda MD 20817

## ve to a friend:

give one of the attached postcards to a friend or fill in the name and address and send it direct to us:
**Customer Service**
**Betz Publishing Company**
P. O. Box 34631
Bethesda MD 20817

## ut us on mailing list

fill in and return the attached postcard to be placed on our mailing listor write:
**Information Services**
**Betz Publishing Company**
P. O. Box 34631
Bethesda MD 20817

# Help me to place an order.

( ) Please send me an order form and booklist.
( ) Please send us ______ poster(s) with 25 order forms and group discount information.

name:____________________

street address:____________________

city:____________________ state:__________ zip:________

telephone:____________________ today's date:__________

**please let us know your area of interest:**____________________

college:____________________ group or organization:____________________

# Please send ordering information to:

name:____________________

street address:____________________

city:____________________ state:__________ zip:________

college:____________________

telephone:____________________ today's date:__________

**Area of interest:**____________________

____________________

____________________

____________________

# Please add us to your mailing list:

name:____________________

college:____________________ title:____________________

street address:____________________

city:____________________ state:__________ zip:________

telephone:____________________ today's date:__________

**Area of interest:**____________________ **Size of group:**__________

Betz Publishing Company accepts institutional purchase orders and prepaid orders.
( ) Our Institutional Purchase order is in the mail.
( ) Please send individual order information.
( ) Please send group order and discount information.

# Betz
# Publishing
# Company, Inc.

**P O Box 34631**
**Bethesda MD 20817**

**301-340-0030**
**800-634-4365**

---

## BUSINESS REPLY MAIL
First Class      Permit No. **310**      Bethesda, MD

Postage will be paid by addressee:

**Betz Publishing Company, Inc.**
P. O. Box 34631
Bethesda, MD 20817

---

*"Preparation for graduate*
*education in the*
*health professions:*

- *MCAT study guides*
- *pre-MCAT exam*
- *admissions manuals*
- *test prep materials*
- *premedical information*
- *preveterinary resources*
- *also podiatry/osteopathic*
- *self-directed study mater*
- *group discounts*

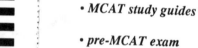

## BUSINESS REPLY MAIL
First Class      Permit No. **310**      Bethesda, MD

Postage will be paid by addressee:

**Betz Publishing Company, Inc.**
P. O. Box 34631
Bethesda, MD 20817

---

*"Materials for students*
*and advisors in*
*preprofessional health*
*education."*

- *See our booklist*
- *Order by mail or phone*
- *Visa and Mastercard*

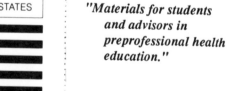

## BUSINESS REPLY MAIL
First Class      Permit No. **310**      Bethesda, MD

Postage will be paid by addressee:

**Betz Publishing Company, Inc.**
P. O. Box 34631
Bethesda, MD 20817